T0201105

Looking through the Speculum

Looking through the Speculum

Examining the Women's Health Movement

JUDITH A. HOUCK

The University of Chicago Press
Chicago and London

The University of Chicago Press, Chicago 60637
The University of Chicago Press, Ltd., London
© 2024 by The University of Chicago
Published 2024
Printed in the United States of America

33 32 31 30 29 28 27 26 25 24   1 2 3 4 5

ISBN-13: 978-0-226-83084-1 (cloth)
ISBN-13: 978-0-226-83086-5 (paper)
ISBN-13: 978-0-226-83085-8 (e-book)
DOI: https://doi.org/10.7208/chicago/9780226830858.001.0001

Library of Congress Cataloging-in-Publication Data

Names: Houck, Judith A. (Judith Anne), author.
Title: Looking through the speculum : examining the women's health movement /
    Judith A. Houck.
Description: Chicago : The University of Chicago Press, 2024. | Includes
    bibliographical references and index.
Identifiers: LCCN 2023020236 | ISBN 9780226830841 (cloth) | ISBN 9780226830865
    (paperback) | ISBN 9780226830858 (ebook)
Subjects: LCSH: Reproductive health services—United States. | Women's health
    services—United States. | Feminism—United States.
Classification: LCC RA564.85 .H677 2024 | DDC 613/.0424—dc23/eng/20230527
LC record available at https://lccn.loc.gov/2023020236

♾ This paper meets the requirements of ANSI/NISO Z39.48-1992
(Permanence of Paper).

For Judy, Mariamne, and Nancy: activists, teachers, scholars

Contents

From the Speculum to the Clinic:
A History of Feminist Health Praxis

A gynecologist's office. Naked except for a scratchy paper gown, open in the front. The indignity of the position—feet in stirrups, legs apart. A paper sheet covering the ignominious area and the doctor's mysterious manipulations. The shock of the cold steel, the feel of sweat trickling between breasts and in clenched fists, the tense knot in the stomach. And the doctor says "Relaaaax!"[1]

In the 1970s and beyond, women across the country compared their experiences of the pelvic exam. *Humiliating. Traumatic. Infantilizing. Enraging.* They complained about the literal intrusion into their bodies that was always uncomfortable and sometimes painful. Women noted physicians' carelessness and ineptitude that made a fraught procedure worse; they railed against the physicians who seemed intentionally rough—"He really jams that speculum up there." They shared the intrusive questions about their sex lives and the off-color jokes that sometimes accompanied the exam. They protested the vulnerability the exam created: women on their backs, nearly naked, their feet in stirrups, their legs splayed, their vision of the procedure obstructed by a sheet. And women described their physicians' attitudes toward them: callous, bored, patronizing, distracted, unwilling to share details of the procedure and cagey about what they found. For many women, the pelvic exam symbolized women's relationship with medicine in general: passive and vulnerable female patients examined by male physicians who guarded and controlled information about women's bodies.[2]

Women understood what was at stake. In dorm rooms and in bookstores, in apartments and in libraries, women connected their relationship with medicine to their larger role in society. Physicians controlled information, devices, medications, and procedures that shaped women's lives. Without the ability to control their bodies—especially their reproduction—women could not control their lives.

The women's health movement, beginning in 1969 and taking hold in the 1970s, was a broad-based movement seeking to increase women's bodily knowledge, reproductive control, and well-being. It was a political movement which insisted that bodily autonomy, acquired through bodily knowledge and sisterly connection, provided the key to women's liberation. It was also an institution-building movement that sought to transform women's relationship with medicine, dedicated to increasing women's access to affordable health care without the barriers of homophobia, racism, and sexism. But not only did the movement focus on women's bodies, it also encouraged activists to reimagine their relationships with each other, to develop their relationships in the name of personal and political change, and, eventually, to discover and confront the limitations of the bonds of womanhood.

Women and the Medical Landscape

Before we delve into the history of the women's health movement, joining the feminist activists who demanded change and transformed health care, it is useful to look at a few snapshots of medicine and reproductive health care at the dawn of the movement.

- Medicaid, created in 1965, provided health coverage for poor people, but physicians were under no obligation to accept patients covered by Medicaid.[3]
- In the 1960s, Black women in the South were sterilized so frequently—often against their will and without their knowledge—that the procedure was known as the "Mississippi appendectomy."[4]
- The birth control pill, on the market for contraception since 1960, had revolutionized the sexual lives of women, especially married women, by separating sex and contraception and by affording reliable fertility control. Single women used the pill too, but some physicians resisted prescribing contraception for the unmarried, believing it condoned premarital sexual behavior. In some states, physicians lacked the authority to prescribe oral contraceptives for unmarried women. In 1969, a female journalist published an exposé suggesting that the pill had endangered the health of countless women.[5]
- Legal abortion was unavailable to most women. Women with the wherewithal might secure a so-called "therapeutic" abortion if they could convince three physicians and maybe a psychiatrist that their mental or physical health required terminating their pregnancy. In

1965, two hundred women, mostly women of color, died from illegal abortions.[6]

- Pregnant women could be forced to take unpaid leave from their jobs. Sometimes they were fired outright.[7]

- In 1970, only 7 percent of American physicians were women. On a practical level, the paucity of women physicians meant that most patients would never see a female doctor. Patients eager to be seen by a female provider would be unlikely to find one. On a theoretical level, medicine was a bastion of male authority and privilege. Male physicians guarded medical knowledge, distinguished between health and illness, developed and deployed medical treatments, and limited access to contraception and abortion.[8]

- In 1970, few people could name a famous woman with breast cancer. Many women received a diagnosis and endured treatment without ever divulging the nature of their illness. No one raced for the cure.[9]

- Lesbians in 1970 could be legally denied housing or employment, their discrimination buttressed by the psychiatric profession's claim that they were sick. (Psychoanalysts might demur, claiming instead that lesbians merely suffered from immature or arrested development.) When they sought medical care, lesbians frequently hid their sexual identity in order to prevent an "upsetting confrontation" with their physicians; lesbians who could not or would not "pass" frequently avoided medical care altogether.[10]

- Trans people seeking gender-affirmation surgeries were routinely denied treatment at the very few medical centers that performed the procedures. Instead, trans people frequently acquired transition hormones on the street, and, if they had significant money, they could access surgery in Casablanca. Trans people seeking general medical care—a Pap smear, treatment for the flu, pain relief during a sickle cell crisis—were frequently denied medical care outright if their trans identity was discovered.[11]

These details help us understand the health care landscape at the beginning of the 1970s. Inspired and nurtured by the larger feminist movements simultaneously underway, women across the country demanded better. They created a social movement determined to educate women about their bodies, challenge the authority of the male medical profession, and increase women's control over their own bodies and lives.

Feminists were not the only activists eager to change the medical system. Indeed, critics from within medicine and from without had launched a series of attacks on the United States health care industry, excoriating its economic and geographic inaccessibility, its racist and classist foundations, its role as an agent of social control, and its narrow focus on the treatment of disease rather than support for health. America's health care system, then, was widely understood as broken. As one 1972 publication put it, "The United States has failed to provide adequate health services to the vast majority of its citizens."[12] Consequently, the moment was ripe for creative responses to mainstream medicine. Health activists and reformers created new provider categories, developed innovative models of health care delivery, and directly challenged medical institutions and prerogatives.[13] Women's health activism was an important element of a larger critique of medicine.

In this book, I focus on the politics, institutions, and relationships created by and within the women's health movement—primarily from the perspective of the activists who shaped its priorities, fought its battles, and struggled with its shortcomings. I ask four central questions: Who did the women's health movement serve? What did the women's health movement hope to achieve? How were the movement's politics reflected in its institutions? How did the women's health movement change over time? These questions guide this project.

All Women or Every Woman?

Who did the women's health movement serve? Although early feminist health activists believed they were working on behalf of all women, they were quickly accused of creating a movement that primarily benefited white, middle-class, heterosexual women. What did a plastic speculum offer women who couldn't afford medical care? Which women felt a "sisterly" connection with other women as they gathered in a church basement to see their cervices? Where did feminists locate their health centers? How did the movement address lesbians' reproductive health needs? These questions suggest how the movement to liberate women's bodies from patriarchy and medical domination struggled to look beyond the needs of "all women" to consider the circumstances and needs of each woman and, alternatively, mapped the needs and desires of one type of woman onto the banner of "all women."

The women's health movement has frequently been understood as a predominantly white movement, but the reality was more complex. Clearly, some high-profile organizations were staffed exclusively by white women, at least in the beginning. The Boston Women's Health Book Collective stands as one obvious example. Feminist health clinics, especially in some locations, had few women of color in leadership; likely some had none. But women of color contributed to the women's health movement from the beginning. They promoted self-exams, founded and staffed health clinics, and organized self-help groups. Any claim that the women's health movement appealed only to white, middle-class women erases the considerable efforts of some of the women you will meet here—women like Byllye Avery, Carol Ervin, Mary Lisbon, Loretta Mears, and Rita Shimmin. It also ignores the work of those whose stories are left for others to tell.

To highlight the women of color involved in the movement does not deny that some, perhaps most, white women in the movement struggled to understand their obligation to confront and address how structural racism shaped the experience of health, illness, and self-care among women of color. Certainly, women's health activists overwhelmingly denounced racism and espoused their solidarity with "Third World women." Some health feminists explicitly highlighted the importance of a race- and class-inflected theory for the movement. Barbara Ehrenreich and Deirdre English, for example, insisted in their pathbreaking 1973 pamphlet *Complaints and Disorders* that "a movement that recognizes our biological similarity but denies the diversity of our priorities cannot be a women's health movement, it can only be *some women's* health movement."[14] On the ground, however, white health activists frequently concentrated on issues most salient to women like themselves rather than focusing on the health needs of the most underserved and vulnerable women.

For at least the first decade of the movement, feminist health activists typically sought to explicate women's shared oppression rather than experiences of difference. Reflecting the larger feminist movement at the time, health feminists in the 1970s believed in a "sisterhood" that could bond women together to fight their shared oppression. In her important study of the women's health movement, *Bodies of Knowledge* (2010), the historian Wendy Kline argued that activists' "attempts at creating a universalist notion of shared oppression . . . ultimately stymied" the movement.[15] Although Kline identified an important dynamic of the movement, she ended her study just as this particular trend shifted. The historian and former feminist health activist Susan Reverby noted, "As in other places in the second wave of the women's movement, the essentialism of a gender-only argument proved to be unstable ground as an earthquake of demands hit us broadside."[16] In the early 1980s, women of color, in tandem with white allies, shook the movement up, demanding more inclusion and diversity. They urged their white colleagues to take difference among women seriously, to diversify the staffs of their clinics, and to reach out to groups who had been underserved in the movement's first decade. In a process rife with conflict, clinic spaces diversified and became more responsive to the varied needs in their communities.

But for some women of color, working in coalition with white women was not the end point of their activism. Black women—some of whom cut their

activist teeth within the women's health movement—created their own organizations to meet the specific needs of their communities. They developed
bonds of sisterhood among themselves, shaped in part by their shared experiences of oppression. I tell some of their stories here.

Although other scholars have discussed conflicts over race within women's
health and reproductive rights movements,[17] no historian has given sustained
attention to the place of lesbians in the movement. Did the women's health
movement serve lesbians, or did it focus on the reproductive health needs
of straight women, as some have accused? Lesbians participated widely in
the women's health movement from the beginning. Many of them believed
that self-help, reproductive control, and bodily knowledge would benefit all
women, lesbian and straight alike. But they also worked within their own collectives and organizations to identify and accommodate lesbians' particular
health needs. For some, this was enough. Others turned their attention to
forging and enacting a lesbian health agenda that put lesbian issues at the
center of their work. This eventually led lesbian health activists to confront
their own version of the movement's animating question: Which lesbians—
and, eventually, which people—did their efforts serve?

A Means to Varied Ends

By 1974, "tens of thousands" of women considered themselves part of the
women's health movement.[18] As a mass movement, health feminism supported a variety of projects and politics. When women joined the feminist
health movement, they brought with them inchoate hopes and dreams.
Different priorities brought them in: to help women secure safe and affordable abortions; to be part of something larger than themselves; to improve
their medical school applications; to meet other feminist women; to improve
women's health care; to liberate women; and to liberate themselves. College-
age women looked for an entrée into feminism; women with children wanted
to change the world for their daughters; nurses saw a pathbreaking way to use
their skills.

Surely, some goals loomed large: increased reproductive autonomy, enhanced bodily knowledge, an end to medical paternalism. But this book captures some of the diversity of ideas and politics of the movement. It demonstrates that while some activists and organizations saw their work in the
service of a larger feminist revolution, other activists and organizations had
less expansive goals in mind. Some of these women wanted to bring a feminist
sensibility into medicine, offer women more health care options, and transform medicine from within.

The Feminist Politics of Health Institutions

Cervical self-exam provided a "traveling technology" for women's liberation.[19] Self-help advocates packed speculums in their suitcases and crisscrossed the country on Greyhound buses and in VW vans. Self-help proponents flew across oceans, introducing audiences in Europe, New Zealand, and the Middle East to the power of self-exam. But many health activists sought to give self-help and feminist health care a stable home. In the 1970s, feminist health activists built health centers to centralize health organizing and clinics to provide health services, frequently guided by self-help politics. Throughout the decade, women on the coasts and in the heartland founded more than fifty health centers and clinics.

Bringing feminist health politics into clinical spaces—spaces that required licensing, bookkeeping, outside funding, and medical support—proved challenging on many levels. This book highlights those challenges and analyzes the difficulties of maintaining feminist health praxis in an increasingly conservative regulatory landscape. The clinics showcased here are a handful of clinics in Northern California that were founded to enact a variety of health politics; they hoped to meet women's need for health care, channel feminist political hunger for social change, fund additional political projects, and demonstrate a woman-centered approach to health care. Over time, these clinics became less like showcases for the possibility and promise of feminist health care and more like other community health clinics and reproductive health centers. And yet, each of these clinics continued to meet local health care needs into the twenty-first century.

In 1995, the feminist sociologists Myra Marx Ferree and Patricia Yancey Martin famously asserted that feminist organizations provided "tangible evidence" of the women's movement "in the social and political life of the nation." They claimed that "the women's movement exists because feminists founded and staffed these organizations to do the movement's work. . . . All these organizations sustain women and are sustained by them."[20] This book's focus on women's health centers and clinics demonstrates both that much of the "movement's work" occurred in institutional spaces, and that some of those institutions continued, in one form or another, well beyond the moment that created them.

Struggle and Change

While historians of feminist health activism generally agree that the women's health movement began in the late 1960s or early '70s, they are less clear on when it came to a close. Many of the vital interventions of the movement occurred in the '70s: the birth of gynecological self-exam and menstrual extraction; the emergence of women's health clinics; the publication of *Our Bodies, Ourselves*; the creation of the National Women's Health Network; the efforts to protect vulnerable populations from unwanted and coerced sterilization; and the protests against the Dalkon Shield. But if we keep looking, the movement turns a corner in the 1980s with the creation of the Black women's health movement; the development of a lesbian health agenda; the emergence of HIV/AIDS; and the rise of an increasingly violent antiabortion activism. In the 1990s, as more people who rejected the gender assigned to them at birth became politically active, they insisted that they, too, deserved compassionate health care, free from hostility and discrimination. Health activists joined this movement at different moments for different reasons, and they stayed for varied lengths of time. As a result, the movement continually grappled internally with new practical concerns and political commitments. These "generational" differences caused significant but often productive tensions, forcing the movement to respond to newly urgent health needs.

This book follows the movement and its institutions as they changed over time in response to internal struggles and outside pressures. The institutions in this story are long-term artifacts of the movement. As of this writing, the major clinics described in here survive, in one form or another. (Some of the smaller players do not.) The survival of these clinics is atypical. The vast majority of the feminist clinics founded in the 1970s failed to make it out of the twentieth century.[21] Nevertheless, by privileging the survivors, we can explore how health activists responded to women's continued demand for reproductive control and general health care. By following these clinics into the twenty-first century, we can see how they changed their goals and their policies as the political landscape changed around them. In some cases, this story of change reads like a prolonged battle to protect ever-eroding feminist principles. In other cases, we see how change created more capacious institutions that met the needs of a more diverse set of stakeholders.

Because the major clinics here survive, the endpoint for this book is jagged. I have documented and explained each clinic's moments of major change and crisis. While some clinics weathered the most significant of their challenges in the twentieth century, at least one clinic was struggling to survive as I prepared this book for press in 2022.

Embodied Feminism

Women's health activism was inspired by and part of second-wave feminism, a movement beginning in the 1960s and focused on increasing women's rights and securing women's liberation.[22] The term *second-wave feminism*, widely contested, describes a mass movement of women organizing for a variety of goals with a diverse set of tactics. Second-wave feminists also espoused a variety of beliefs about women and their difference from and similarity to men. As with earlier women's movements,[23] many second-wave feminists came to feminism through their bodies, challenging women's inability to control their reproduction,[24] protesting their vulnerability to sexual assault and domestic violence,[25] and objecting to the constraints of the sexual double standard. Many activists joined the health movement with feminist credentials from participating in other areas of the women's movement, and they saw clinic building or self-help promotion as a fulfilling channel for their feminist energies. Others came to feminism through the self-help movement itself, inspired by the light shining on a glistening cervix or grateful for the ride across the Santa Cruz Mountains to secure an abortion. One health worker, with a broken-down car and unclear prospects, stumbled into a feminist clinic and found a life's work. In each case, health feminism, anchored in women's embodied needs, provided clear evidence of the need for and value of feminism.

For the most part, health activists understood the category of woman as a self-evident category associated with a particular anatomical configuration that centered on the vagina, the uterus, and, to a lesser extent, the breasts. While health activists understood that not all women have uteri—in the context of medical removal through hysterectomy—they did not, in general, consider the health needs of trans women. Only the lesbian health clinics explicitly considered the category of woman, at least as it influenced who might be understood as a lesbian.[26]

The women described in this history explored and developed their political commitments to an improved world in a variety of ways. In the early 1970s, most of the activists described in this book donated their labor to their cause—staffing abortion referral hotlines, developing self-help protocols, writing lesbian health pamphlets, launching feminist health clinics. Over time, some of them found ways to earn a living—some barely and some more comfortably—doing the work they once did for free. Others joined the women's health movement under conditions of employment, as AmeriCorps VISTA workers, social workers, health care providers, and receptionists. Still others wrote grants to cover salaries, and some continued to donate their labor for free. These women made professional and social decisions to work toward their political commitment to women's self-determination and empowerment, feminist health care, and social change.[27]

Documenting the Movement

This book contributes to an already rich and vibrant history of the women's health movement and other struggles for women's bodily autonomy and reproductive rights.[28] It begins with the speculum, wrested from medical hands and deployed by women to give them literal and symbolic control over their bodies. It follows the women as they peer into their own bodies and those of their movement "sisters" to ascertain just what they saw that moved them so. It examines the internal decision-making of health activists as they created health centers, and it shares their struggles as they tried to keep the centers afloat even when they could no longer recognize their politics in the clinical work. It illuminates conflict within the lesbian community over just who belonged at a lesbian clinic and whether lesbians were at risk for HIV/AIDS. It explores how Black women created their own feminist health organizations. It documents how white activists confronted charges of racism and how they stumbled repeatedly as they created more diverse organizations.

I relied on a variety of sources for this history. Oral interviews provide an important thread. Over a long decade, I talked with more than seventy-five health activists who shared with me their stories of the women's health movement and their role within it. These activists shared their passion, pride, struggles, and disappointments. Their accounts identified themes, filled gaps, revealed connections, and captured moments. This project would have been impossible without them. The overwhelming majority of people I asked to interview, BIPOC and white activists alike, agreed. Nevertheless, most women who declined were women of color. As a result, certain stories are told without the perspectives of activists who could provide a more complete account of events.

The women who shared their stories occasionally also shared their files. "Perhaps these might help," they said as they handed me meeting minutes, planning notebooks, self-help pamphlets, handwritten correspondence, interview transcripts, and much more. These documents from attics and basements, squirreled away because they couldn't just be tossed, were a historian's dream. Many of the accounts in this book came to light only because women thought that maybe their histories were worth preserving, and they were willing to share that history with a stranger.[29] The executive directors of two clinics, Lyon-Martin Health Services and Women's Health Specialists, provided access to their historical files.[30] Although none of us knew what I was looking for or what I might find, they gestured to their file cabinets and let me dig. More formal archives also provided administrative clinic records and other health movement ephemera.

Published sources round out the evidence base for this history. The feminist and gay press in particular documented the changing goals and central conflicts of the movement. Newsletters from feminist clinics and other health-focused organizations highlighted their specific preoccupations, politics, and projects. Newspapers provided a perspective that didn't privilege the activists.

These sources illuminate some aspects of the feminist health movement more fully than others. Clearly, they privilege activists rather than the women and men who sought services at health clinics. They also privilege the perspectives of the founders of collectives and clinics who left behind foundational documents and whose work has been memorialized in retrospective accounts of the organizations. They fail to capture the perspectives of short-term participants whose efforts did not leave a paper trail.

Organization

This book is organized into eight paired chapters. The first chapter in each dyad takes on a feminist health project that engaged the women's health movement. The second chapter of each pair examines the same issue as it was taken up by feminist health clinics. This approach provides both a national and a local perspective. Women across the country promoted self-help, defined a feminist abortion politics, built a lesbian health agenda, discovered the promise of sisterhood, and demanded increased diversity. They also built clinics in particular cities and neighborhoods. The book focuses on four women's health clinics in California. One was located in San Francisco, while the others were founded in college towns in the far northern part of the state. Each of these clinics illustrate some of the distinctive approaches to women's health nurtured by the movement. They provided different services for different communities with different politics. Considered together, they highlight both the diversity of the movement and the similarities of their struggles. Despite their differences and their geographic separation, these clinics were linked informally in a larger feminist health network. They often shared information, inspiration, training, and clients. These connections then demonstrate the contours of a social movement as opposed to individual health-based projects.

Chapters 1 and 2 feature the creation and deployment of cervical self-exam and the self-help gynecology movement it anchored. From its origins in a feminist bookstore in 1971, self-help spread quickly across the country, allowing women to see and understand their bodies in new ways. Women in different regions all were inspired and emboldened by the promise of self-help, and many of them eagerly sought to make self-exam the basis of a feminist health care praxis. Others promoted self-help as the revolutionary key to women's liberation. Chapter 1 tries to understand why self-exam was so popular with and inspirational to so many women. What did women get from peering into their bodies? What kind of work did self-exam do? Why did its advocates see it as revolutionary?

Many health advocates understood, however, the limits of self-help as it took place in homes, gymnasiums, and conference rooms. They wondered aloud whether self-help gynecology could translate into health care services. In towns and cities across the country, health feminists tested the practical limits of the speculum and the self-exam as epistemological and political tools by founding feminist health clinics. Chapter 2 explores the creation of two feminist health clinics in Northern California to understand how the movement's political commitment to women's health in women's hands played out within institutions designed to provide health care services. Their significant differences highlight the personal and professional investments of the women involved, the geographic proximity to and isolation from health movement networks, and the particular contexts of their origins. They also highlight the breadth of the political commitments within the women's health movement. They separately enacted a feminist health politics that reflected the needs of their communities and the activists themselves.

The second chapter dyad explores the place of abortion in the women's health movement. The movement began as efforts to reform and repeal abortion laws picked up steam. Before and after *Roe*, feminist health activists generally regarded access to safe, legal, and affordable abortion as a precondition to women's self-determination. Without the ability to control her reproduction, a woman could not control her life. Nevertheless, these feminists understood that abortion was not inherently good for women. Abortions could be and often were sites for the exploitation, co-optation, coercion, humiliation, and colonization of women. At least some feminists understood that context mattered: who performed the abortion, on whom, with what tools, and for what ends created the social and personal meaning of abortion. Chapter 3 examines the abortion politics of the Federation of Feminist Women's Health Centers, a group of loosely affiliated health clinics united by their commitment to self-help gynecology, as imagined and shaped by the health activist

Carol Downer. It argues that the Feminist Women's Health Centers (FWHCs) simultaneously highlighted the need for abortion services, fought for a particular model of woman-centered abortion provision, and condemned efforts to use abortion as a tool of exploitation and control.

Although most women's health clinics that emerged out of the women's health movement did not provide abortions, chapter 4 focuses on one that did. The Chico Feminist Women's Health Center opened and began providing abortions in 1976; the clinic remains an important abortion provider in Northern California. This chapter traces the clinic's steadfast efforts to provide abortions in a feminist space while confronting a variety of opponents, ranging from local physicians and medical societies to state party politics and national religious mobilization. It argues that the continual threats to abortion changed the clinic's focus from a broad-based effort to empower women in all aspects of health care to a narrower but crucial focus on access to abortion.

Although the women's health movement has long been associated with (and castigated for) its focus on reproductive issues and the needs of heterosexual women, chapters 5 and 6 highlight the movement's role in creating and providing lesbian health. Many of the women active in the women's health movement identified as lesbians. Lesbians counseled women about abortion, wrote prescriptions for contraceptives, provided information about sexually transmitted diseases, and taught women about their bodies. Nevertheless, some lesbians in the movement and some who felt excluded by it complained that it prioritized the reproductive issues of heterosexual women while ignoring the health care and reproductive needs of lesbians. Chapter 5 explores the place of lesbians within the women's health movement and the creation of a movement focused on lesbian health. It highlights how sexual identity politics informed and shaped the lesbian health movement. Chapter 6 examines what happened when lesbian health activists moved their projects into clinic spaces. It focuses on Lyon-Martin Women's Health Services, a San Francisco clinic founded in 1979 by three white lesbians to provide sensitive and competent health care to the lesbian community. The founders believed that the clinic was necessary to combat the heterosexism and homophobia pervasive in society and medicine at the time. This chapter traces the history of this health clinic from its founding, exploring the sexual, racial, and gender politics at the center of its history.

The last pair of chapters explores the explicit expansion of the feminist health movement to involve and serve more women of color. Women involved in the movement often promoted an antiracist, anti-imperialist, and anti-capitalist agenda. They understood that women experienced gendered oppression in different ways. Still, health activists in the 1970s frequently believed that their efforts for women's liberation would benefit all women without explicitly addressing the specific health needs of different groups of women, especially women of color. They envisioned (sometimes literally) an embodied sisterhood, and they articulated a politics of commonality. Black women in the movement, however, increasingly understood the health consequences of racist oppression, and they created organizations to acknowledge and heal their wounds together. Chapter 7 examines the efforts of Black feminists, some with experience in the larger health movement, to create approaches to self-help that created pathways to personal well-being and community health.

Through the 1970s, feminist health clinics were staffed overwhelmingly by white women and generally served white women. Over time—frequently in response to prodding by women of color—these organizations worked to understand the racialized consequences of the movement's commitment to a common sisterhood; they vowed to diversify their clinics at all levels. Chapter 8 examines the strategies and confrontations around these efforts, focusing in depth on one clinic that successfully diversified its staff and clientele, but not without significant change to its politics and mission.

Each chapter pair illuminates the struggles and successes of bringing feminist dreams into clinical spaces. In every chapter, this book is also about women who turned their rage, wonder, and determination into a movement. The women profiled in this book all sought to shape their communities and the place of women in them. They exposed their privates—their bodies, their shame, their trauma—believing that in the act of exposure, by revealing their vulnerability, they laid the foundation for trust and political action. In ways big and small, through efforts lasting and ephemeral, they intervened in the world, hoping to improve their lives and the lives of other women.

With a Flashlight and a Speculum: Envisioning a Feminist Revolution

In the summer of 1973, "city sisters" from Portland and Eugene traveled to Mountain Grove, an intentional feminist community in southern Oregon. They brought with them flashlights, mirrors, plastic specula, and a new feminist practice—cervical self-exam. Against a backdrop of songs and snacks, the city women demonstrated how they could use a speculum to gain a new perspective on their bodies. Jean of Mountain Grove described the power of this "revolutionary afternoon": "We lay on our backs . . . feet to the big sun-filled window. Our awareness of nudity and modesty faded in the presence of women like ourselves—all eager, barefoot, laughing, thoughtful, encouraging, curious." Jean's cervix was initially elusive, but she and her self-help partner persevered. "'No, not yet. Try the left; push down a little. There!' What a sense of accomplishment!" After Jean's success, she helped another woman in her community with her search. "I went back to help hold the mirror, to offer my knees to a struggling woman as she tried to catch that first glimpse of the inner, hidden gateway to her uterus, at that moment to join the thousands of sisters who are facing their fears, their feelings of shame and uncleanliness, their ignorance, and asking for knowledge to control their bodies and their lives."[1]

These cervix-seeking women shared their curiosity and their vulnerability, and they collectively lost their modesty. But significantly, they were not only connected to the women around them—those who provided a backrest or those who held a mirror. They were also connected to a larger movement of women who rejected shame and ignorance and demanded power and knowledge. A view of a cervix, framed as a glimpse of the forbidden, simultaneously made women aware of their common oppression and gave them a tool to fight it.

In the 1970s, across the country and around the globe, women gathered
to peer into the inner recesses of their bodies, to see parts of themselves that
had long been controlled and surveilled by men—especially their husbands
and their physicians. They perhaps struggled to maneuver the plastic speculums, and they fidgeted a bit against the pillows as they figured out where to
shine the flashlight and how to get the angle of the mirror just right. They
often felt self-conscious about their exposed bodies, at least at first, surrepti-
tiously glancing at the woman next to them, wondering if they, too, had hair
on their thighs, wishing fervently to stop sweating. Perhaps they wondered if
something on their body was too big or too small, too wrinkly or not there
at all. But through their shame and their fear, spurred by their curiosity and
their excitement, women—college students, clerical workers, faculty wives,
high school students, feminist activists—looked; they looked at each other,
and they looked at themselves.

What women saw when they peered between their legs varied tremen-
dously. Some found a short-lived political project, while others found a road
map to the rest of their lives. Some saw eternity, others the passageway of life.
Still others merely saw their cervix. This collective view of women's previously
unseen interiors played a critical role in the emerging women's health movement. With a plastic speculum, a mirror, and a flashlight, cervical self-exam
allowed women to see into the previously hidden recesses of their bodies,
share their bodies with other women, and, in theory, wrest control of their
healthy bodies from the domination of the medical profession.

From its 1971 debut, the cervical self-exam—also called gynecological
and vaginal self-exam, symbolized by the plastic speculum in an upraised
female fist—spread quickly across the nation (and less quickly and less completely around the globe). Despite its widespread appeal, gynecological self-
exam and the self-help health movement it encouraged have been criticized
from many angles, both by its contemporaries and in retrospect. At the time,
feminists and nonfeminists alike dismissed self-exam as trivial, distasteful,
individualistic, apolitical, and downright dangerous. More recently, several
feminist critics of cervical self-exam have focused on its appropriation of the
medical gaze for feminist ends. For example, in her admittedly caricatured
portrayal, Donna Haraway simultaneously described and dismissed the self-
exam: "Land ho! We have discovered ourselves and claim the new territory
for women."[2] Haraway and other scholars have located both the irony and
the inadequacy of substituting one set of conquering eyes for another and of
insisting that seeing transformed easily into either knowledge or power.

This chapter examines why self-exam was so popular with and inspirational to so many women. What did women get from looking at their bodies?

What kind of work did self-exam do? If self-exam was an important tool of the feminist movement, what were its uses? To answer these questions, this chapter argues that self-exam was not one thing, frozen symbolically in a particular political or epistemic frame. Instead, I show that as a feminist practice, gynecological self-exam was always carried out in particular contexts, and that those contexts created and sustained a variety of meanings, goals, and outcomes. To demonstrate the varied work of self-exam, this chapter looks at several instantiations of the self-help method. Examined and analyzed together, these examples demonstrate the epistemic flexibility of the gynecological self-exam, able in different contexts to elicit or provoke revelation, inspiration, connection, and confrontation. Indeed, it is likely that the multivalent nature of self-exam explains why so many women felt compelled to go public with their privates.

This chapter provides a social history of gynecological self-exam.[3] It analyzes self-exam within particular contexts to better understand its power, influence, and significance. Only by following the speculum-wielding women into bookstores, conference rooms, church basements, and clinics can we understand how this tool transformed women into feminists, patients into providers, and shame into wonder.

Cultural Critiques of Medicine and Alternative Approaches to Care

Cervical self-exam and the self-help gynecology movement it anchored emerged amid several other cultural developments and social movements, including a widespread critique of medicine. Although some Americans grumbled about organized medicine as early as the 1920s, the voices of discontent grew louder and more powerful in the late 1960s and into the '70s.[4] Demands for change took many forms. Left-leaning activists in New York City, for example, concerned about the increasing power of the "medical industrial complex" and the widespread medical neglect of the most economically and socially vulnerable, formed the Health Policy Advisory Center (Health/PAC) in 1968. Although especially focused on urban health care issues, Health/PAC provided a forum for a political examination of the economic and social effects and failures of medicine.[5] Reflecting a quite different constituency, in 1969, Lester Breslow, then former director of the California State Department of Health Services, convened a Citizens Board of Inquiry into Health Services for Americans staffed with a variety of "community stakeholders"—business executives, public health workers, patients. In 1972, the board published *Heal Your Self*, which indicted the US health care system for its many shortcomings and documented widespread patient dissatisfaction. It concluded: "The

United States has failed to provide adequate health services to the vast majority of its citizens."[6] On yet another front, intellectuals like Irving Zola and Ivan Illich argued that medicine was both a powerful vector of social control and, ironically, a barrier to well-being. In 1974, Illich, for example, published *Medical Nemesis*, a scathing examination of the damage caused by medicine and medicalization, opening with a provocation: "The medical establishment has become a major threat to health."[7]

Many physicians were themselves frustrated by the medical status quo, and some doctors and medical students led the charge for a more accessible and responsive medical system, working sometimes for revolution, more often for reform.[8] One group of physicians aimed to change medical delivery by changing the patient. Advocating variously for the "smart patient," the "activated patient," and the "health consumer," these physicians hoped to challenge or at least adjust the power imbalance at the heart of the medical encounter.[9]

The passive patient was a frequent target of these efforts to "reform" patients. For example, the physicians Arthur and Stuart Frank insisted that the "medical care business thrives on the passivity of the patient and reinforces the mysticism of medicine."[10] Indeed, much of this literature sought to banish medical mystique from medical practice.[11] In one particularly vivid (and perhaps alarming) exhortation to patients, a physician insisted, "You've got to get off your knees."[12] Assuming that the imagined passive patient was male, the context of this demand was likely religious, or at least supplicant; regardless, it was designed to shock.

The encouragement of the active patient overlapped with a larger cultural acceptance of a variety of self-help projects. Rooted in traditions of nineteenth-century mutual aid on the one hand and ideals of self-reliance and individualism on the other, self-help initiatives and groups proliferated in the 1970s.[13] These projects varied in purpose and style, but many focused on self-care and self-help as a way to improve health.

One version of these efforts centered on patient education. Physicians and health care institutions frequently spearheaded patient education programs as a useful complement to medical care. The physician Keith W. Sehnert, for example, pioneered a patient education course in 1970 to give people tools to make better decisions about their health and health care. Sehnert named it the Course for Activated Patients, describing activated patients as those who "become active participants in their own health care rather than assume the passive role traditionally assigned to them."[14] While these efforts championed engaged patients, they also generally provided information that conformed to dominant medical perspectives. In contrast, *Women and Their*

Bodies, the 1970 precursor to the broadly influential milestone *Our Bodies, Ourselves*, provided a feminist version of patient education that highlighted and validated women's perspectives. Indeed, *Women and Their Bodies* offered an explicitly demedicalized view of health-and-wellness education. Despite their significant differences, both of these projects encouraged people to learn about their bodies and their health.[15]

Self-help gynecology, then, reflected both the critique of mainstream medicine and the proliferation of lay initiatives in health care. It adopted tools of education and reform and transformed them into tools of revolution and liberation.

Origin Story

The story of Carol Downer, the bookstore, and the speculum has been described by many authors as a foundational moment in the women's health movement.[16] Though Downer often referred to herself as a housewife with six children, any image of a life devoted to domesticity, leaving the political world to others, gives the wrong impression. In the mid-1960s, Downer, a white, working-class woman, engaged with various political causes, including urban renewal and protesting the Vietnam War. Influenced perhaps by her Chicano husband, Downer worked to increase the political representation of Chicanos in California through the Mexican American Political Association, and she participated in the National Chicano Moratorium Committee's march in Laguna Park. Gradually, however, she grew disillusioned with volunteer efforts and electoral politics. She hoped that the emerging feminist movement might provide a fruitful outlet for her passion and her energies.

In 1969, Downer attended a National Organization for Women (NOW) meeting in Los Angeles, but she felt little connection to most of the career women at the meeting because they had not shared Downer's "radicalizing experiences." Still, when asked to contribute, she joined the Abortion Committee, chaired by Lana Clarke Phelan. Phelan, also a white, working-class woman, was already a veteran of abortion politics as one of the famous Army of Three, a California group that, beginning in 1965, demanded the repeal of all abortion laws.[17] Phelan's knowledge of abortion and her passion for change inspired Downer, who threw herself into abortion politics. She, Phelan, and another abortion activist, Mary Petrinovich, worked on a variety of levels, speaking to civic groups, organizing demonstrations, writing policy papers, and transporting women to abortion providers. During this work, Petrinovich invited Downer to meet Harvey Karman, an abortionist with dubious credentials but a long work history. She visited his Santa Monica Boulevard clinic and watched as Karman inserted an intrauterine device (IUD) into a patient. As she recounted the story:

> I found myself looking into the woman's vagina, which was held open by a plastic speculum, and I saw her beautiful pink cervix. . . . I was transfixed, looking at her rosy, knob-like cervix with a tiny opening. I thought of Lana's brilliant political analysis and I felt the frustration of our century-long suffering from these unjust laws. I had six children at this time, and I had never looked carefully at my genitals. . . . I marveled at how close the cervix is; how simple it is and how accessible it is with the use of an inexpensive, plastic speculum.[18]

Here Downer connected her ignorance of her own body—an ignorance supported by the cultural insistence that women's bodies required cover and the medical assumption of authority over bodies—to the political control of women. Ignorance created and reinforced bodily alienation. Alienation encouraged women to inhabit their bodies passively, turning them over to men for surveillance and control. This moment in Karman's office provided both a literal and a figurative revelation; Downer saw in this woman's body the possibility for women's liberation.[19]

In April 1971, Downer invited thirty or so women to Everywoman's Bookstore in Los Angeles to consider how women could take control of their reproduction. More specifically, they planned to discuss the feasibility of launching their own illegal abortion clinic.[20] Quite unexpectedly—at least, to some of the women in attendance—Downer hiked up her long flowy skirt, pulled down her underpants, inserted a plastic speculum into her vagina, and showed the assembled women her cervix. And self-help gynecology was born, taking much of the women's liberation movement by storm.[21]

Downer and another self-help pioneer, Lorraine Rothman, repeated this story or some version of it countless times over the next four decades. They described it in press releases and publications. It provided the starting point for self-help demonstrations and clinics. It supposedly marked the beginning of a revolution. As an origin story, this account serves many purposes. Perhaps most clearly, it credits an individual with the invention of an allegedly revolutionary tool for women's liberation. It highlights Downer as a feminist celebrity and provided justification for her authority over the direction of gynecological self-help.[22] Second, it insists on a political rather than domestic birth of the movement. Downer was not fiddling around on a couch when she first saw her cervix; instead, she brought her cervix into view at a feminist meeting about reproductive rights. Further, self-exam debuted in a space that straddled the public-private divide. While the bookstore was not open for business at the time and thus not completely public, Downer revealed herself beyond a circle of friends and family. Her actions rejected the need for modesty.[23] Finally, this story suggests the necessary role of supportive women. Downer hitched up her skirt to reveal her body to create shared knowledge and to build community. Self-exam depended on and created trust among women. In sum, self-help gynecology was born political among women who instantly validated the revolutionary potential of the gesture.

Demonstrations

Perhaps awestruck by the potential of her own invention, Downer looked for outlets to share it widely. She chose a National Organization for Women convention in Los Angeles in the summer of 1971 for self-help's next public showing. This venue allowed word of self-help to spread to feminist audiences across the nation. As a result, NOW chapters and other women's groups inundated Downer with requests to share her technique and her message.[24] Responding to the enthusiasm, she and Rothman elaborated and standardized a cervical self-exam demonstration and set out on the road, stopping in church basements, living rooms, school cafeterias, and hotel rooms, at music festivals, and on college campuses. In these settings, to largely supportive if not always enthusiastic audiences, a facilitator began by showing slides.[25] The slides showed and identified what the audience would eventually see in person—the vaginal walls, the hymen tags, the cervix, and the os. The presentation highlighted how women's bodies change over the course of their menstrual cycle and over the course of their lives. To this end, the demonstration included slides of cervices during ovulation, pregnancy, and menstruation.[26] Perhaps most significantly, the slides tried to capture the range of female variation, implicitly reconceiving as normal many conditions medically considered pathological. Indeed, by including photos of tipped uteri and cervices exhibiting yeast imbalances, these slides challenged how medicine had created and deployed the very categories of normal and abnormal. After the slideshow, the facilitator would demonstrate how to use a speculum and give each woman the opportunity to view a willing volunteer's perineum. If the settings were small and private enough, the women in the audience might be invited to view their own interiors.[27]

The goals of these demonstrations were modest but strategically important to the women's health movement. They were meant to provide a basic map of women's bodies, to encourage and validate curiosity about those

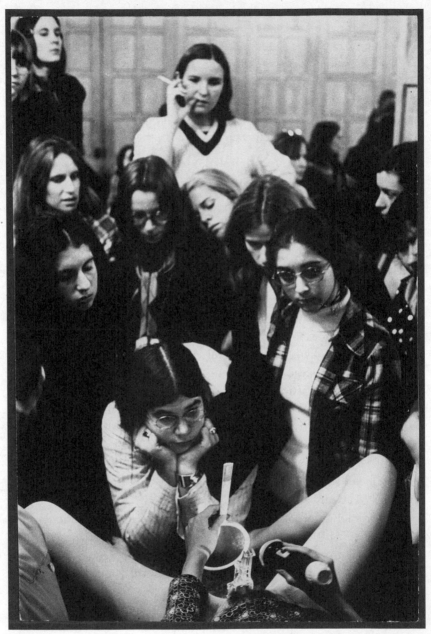

FIGURE 1.1. A 1972 self-help demonstration in Los Angeles. Image by Bettye Lane. Courtesy of Schlesinger Library, Harvard Radcliffe Institute.

bodies, to chip away at women's bodily shame, and to inspire discussion and trust among women. Most ambitiously, they attempted to recruit women into a self-help movement that could wrest control of women's bodies from the medical profession and thereby further the cause of women's liberation.

Did it work? Did women come away from slideshows feeling less alienated by their bodies or, in extreme cases, ready to devote their lives (or at least an evening or so a week) to the cause of women's liberation? Clearly, most of the women who saw the slideshow, who peered into a stranger's vagina, left no record of their impressions. Still, the evidence suggests, not surprisingly, that women reacted in a variety of ways to the spectacle of vaginas on stage and screen. Some women apparently could not bring themselves to watch the demonstrations even though their presence testified to their curiosity.[28] Others, however, found in self-exam something worthwhile and perhaps sustaining. A woman in Omaha, Nebraska, for example, noted in the aftermath of a cervical demonstration, "I think I'm in a state of shock. I've found my freedom and I am looking for women to share it with."[29] An Indiana woman learned from a demonstration some basic anatomy and some self-care. She looked at her vagina, felt her uterus and her ovaries, then looked at and felt the vaginas and uteri of the other women in her group. Despite all the knowledge she gained, what she valued most was that "we gave each other permission to do these things, to talk to other women about our bodies and to call each other up for help when we need it."[30] Yet another woman described her first experience with self-exam: "The first cervix I ever saw belonged to my mother. Everyone said, Look! That's where you came out! . . . That tiny little os, no bigger than the point of a pencil, was the gateway through which I made my debut on earth. . . . And from that first moment, my life was changed. We opened ourselves up to each other in a final triumph of sisterhood. . . . We talked and talked and haven't stopped since that fateful October day."[31] Finally, Eileen Schnitger didn't even know what a cervix was when she saw posters announcing their display in 1974. After her college roommate dragged her to the demonstration, Schnitger became a convert, believing immediately that gynecological self-exam and self-help could liberate women by allowing them to seize control of their bodies. She devoted forty years of her life to the feminist women's health centers and the women's health movement. Taken together, these examples highlight both how these demonstrations could elicit varied responses from their audiences and how women extracted different meanings from their exposure to self-exam. An illuminated cervix, in the context of a wider movement, offered, at least for the moment, a chance for knowledge, freedom, connection, and liberation.

As news of self-exam spread, both in the feminist press and by word of mouth, proponents sometimes brought it to unlikely audiences. For example, the women of the Salt Lake City Feminist Women's Health Center (SLC FWHC) brought self-exam and the message of self-help to the Utah State Fair in 1974. Sandwiched between a booth selling electric organs (Lady of Spain to any tempo) and a man selling portable toilets, the women of the SLC FWHC handed out literature about the self-help movement and showed a movie that culminated in cervical self-exam. Most women hurried by the booth, their eyes averted, but others entered the booth, their curiosity piqued. Although some viewers walked out of the film before it was finished, many others seemed at least receptive; a few were reportedly "really excited."[32] By insisting on bringing self-exam to audiences beyond the feminist choir, these women introduced feminism and the tools of the women's health movement to audiences who would never have attended a NOW meeting, let alone a consciousness-raising (CR) group. In the hands of these health activists, the speculum and the flashlight were tools of exposure. Activists could not force the fairgoers to look, but they made visible the radical and perhaps revolutionary idea that women *could* look, and allowed some women to do so.

Although the Salt Lake City women faced some occasional harassment from passersby, other health activists used gynecological self-exam explicitly as a tool of defiance and confrontation. On several occasions, women from one of the Feminist Women's Health Centers loaded up their speculums and headed into hostile territory. For example, in December 1973, Laura Brown of the Oakland FWHC headed to Hawaii to demonstrate self-exam at a menstrual regulation conference sponsored jointly by the International Planned Parenthood Federation and the United States Agency for International Development.[33] Her actions defied the anti-natalist positions of the population-control establishment. Self-exam and the self-help movement it symbolized insisted that women—not doctors, not patriarchal governments—should oversee their own reproduction. Amid hostile audiences like these, the self-exam was not primarily intended to win converts. Instead, these women wielded the speculum as an act of defiance and confrontation. They were insisting that women were on the verge of reclaiming their bodies from the medical institutions that had so long oppressed them.

Self-help advocates used self-exam to achieve various goals. Its meanings and its power depended on both the intentions of the demonstrators and the perspectives of the viewers. It lasted only a moment, maybe an evening; but its engagement with the forbidden, its rejection of bodily shame, and its promise of access to hidden knowledge inspired tens of thousands of women to investigate further the wonder and power of their own bodies.

Self-Help Clinic

Typically, or so it seems, a handful of women who were exposed to self-exam at each demonstration yearned to know more about themselves and about the self-help gynecology movement. By the summer of 1971, Downer, Rothman, and a few other women had designed and publicized their vision for the next step: the self-help clinic. Although *clinic* may conjure up images of a health care facility, the self-help clinic referred to a group of women gathered together for a course of instruction.[34] Over several weeks, the women explored a curriculum that included information on female anatomy, the menstrual cycle, contraception and fertility, and breast exams. They learned to recognize common conditions, and they experimented with "natural" treatments. By recognizing vaginal yeast imbalances and applying a dab or two of yogurt for relief, women extended the terrain of their self-care practice. Advanced self-help clinics elaborated on the basic information acquired in an initial clinic by using women's own bodies to create further knowledge about their health. Many of these advanced groups focused on one issue, exploring topics such as menopause, nutrition, natural birth control, physical fitness, and artificial insemination in depth.[35] While most self-help clinics were short-term projects, some women met with their self-help clinic cohort for years, occasionally decades.

The original articulation of the self-help clinic described the efforts of a group of women who gathered to "rap" about the "care of their reproductive and sexual organs." They commiserated over how little they knew about their bodies and how often knowledge about an itch, twinge, or discharge was guarded by the medical profession. To gain access to information about their own bodies, women had to schedule an appointment and pay for a medical exam, an opinion, and treatment. The cervical self-exam figured prominently in the self-help clinic, allowing women to assess the nature of their secretions, plot their fertility, and identify their reproductive anatomy. With a speculum and a group of curious and resourceful "sisters," women could learn about their bodies and decrease their dependence on medicine, at least for routine care.[36] Sometimes, then, the benefits of self-help clinics were framed in practical terms: they communicated and generated knowledge that encouraged women to make informed decisions about their bodies and their health.[37]

In addition to the practical appeal, activists promoted self-help clinics to "demystify" women's bodies and medical control of them. In many accounts, demystification justified the entire self-help movement and formed the centerpiece of its challenge to medicine. Ina Clausen and Jack Radey, for example, claimed in 1974 that the main function of self-help groups was "to demystify the status of doctors and not let them make us feel intimidated."[38] Another self-helper valued self-help clinics because they demystified women's bodies in addition to medical practice.[39] Because self-help clinics provided access to information once shrouded in mystery and guarded by physicians, self-help advocates believed the clinics enabled women to regard medical professionals as resources rather than authority figures and encouraged women to claim responsibility for their own bodies.[40] Ideally, by allowing women to gain knowledge and discard bodily shame, self-help clinics shifted the balance of power in a variety of contexts, including the medical encounter.[41]

These references to demystification were consistent with the larger efforts to reform medical practice at the time.[42] Feminist self-help advocates, however, also explicitly framed self-help as a challenge to medical misogyny. Participants in the feminist health movement believed that individual women suffered from sexism and racism on the examining table and that women as a group suffered because of medicine's ideological validation of "power inequalities based on race, sex and class."[43] They argued that medicine surveilled and controlled much of women's lives—childbirth, contraception, mental health, menopausal care, and the treatment of disease—and that medicine was infused with the sexism that pervaded American society and beyond. Consequently, women's bodies and, in turn, much of their lives were governed by the sexist and male-dominated medical profession. By demystifying women's bodies, by empowering women to look at and learn about themselves, self-help challenged the medical control of women. "Only by knowing our bodies and having within the community of women the skills and technology to control our own reproduction," self-helpers believed, could women challenge their oppression. Ultimately for Downer and other advocates, feminist self-help provided the practical knowledge and the psychological power to reject "an image of ourselves as powerless, isolated victims of the male, medical establishment."[44]

But promoters of self-help also claimed that it posed a broader challenge to patriarchy in general by insisting that women's bodies did not belong to men—fathers, doctors, lovers, husbands. As one advocate put it, "The first time a woman looks into her own vagina, she knows that what she has between her legs is no longer HIS secret—not her doctor's, not her lover's, and not Norman Mailer's."[45] Another self-help clinic participant noted that before she became involved in self-help, "I really thought that [my vagina] belonged to my doctor or was only a vessel for a penis."[46] These comments suggest that self-help clinic provided a political as well as a practical education. Ultimately, self-help feminists believed that it could convince women that they had the "right to control their own bodies."[47]

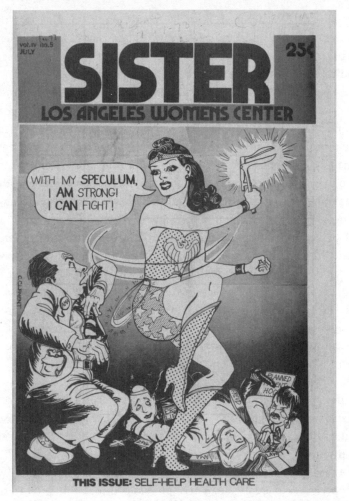

FIGURE 1.2. This 1972 illustration captured self-help as an empowering tool. Women armed with specula were able to vanquish the sources of women's oppression, including Freud, the American Medical Association, Planned Parenthood, the church, Zero Population Growth, and the law. Image by Carol Clement. Courtesy of Schlesinger Library, Harvard Radcliffe Institute.

For many feminist health activists, the ultimate value of self-exam and self-help came from its use by a group. For its proponents, "the power of self-help depended on collective knowledge, collective experiences, [and] collective training."[48] As a result, most self-exam advocates insisted that a woman alone with a speculum was not performing self-help. In part, the group was important because it allowed women to know their own specific bodies within a context of varied female embodiment more generally. By showing their bodies to each other, women discovered that there was no representative vagina, no typical uterus. This led to the understanding that the very categories of normal and abnormal, healthy and diseased, were medical constructs, designed in some degree to convince women to subject their bodies to medical surveillance and control.

But the collective experience provided more than bodily information. It also worked powerfully—perhaps most powerfully—to build community and connection among women. As Downer described the dynamics of the self-help clinic: "It wasn't just my cervix . . . that made it an experience, but it was me talking about that with you; with you, with other women. . . . We're building ties to each other, and we're being responsible for each other and we're taking care of each other and I think in that sense we're building—we're building something that's bigger than any one of us."[49] Other proponents of self-help likewise stressed the importance of the group. Spokeswomen for the Portland Women's Health Center, for example, insisted that self-help was not about self-care for the individual: "Only in a group can we emerge from our self-doubts and isolation."[50] Clearly, for proponents, the power of self-exam and self-help extended beyond the development of alternative knowledge, whether they be based on physical examinations or the shared revelations of consciousness-raising. Trust, nurturance, and interdependence among women were fundamental elements of self-help.

The power of the group encounter in the self-help clinic recalls a variety of other group encounters that were part of contemporary efforts to effect social and personal transformation. Most obviously, the self-help clinic resembled in goal and form the consciousness-raising groups that had provided much of the inspiration, theory, and organization for women's liberation.[51] Begun in the late 1960s, CR groups brought women together to discuss their lives and their experiences to identify axes of oppression. Through these conversations, women linked their personal struggles to the systemic oppression of women. Based on this analysis, the slogan "The personal is political" became a rallying cry for many radical feminists of the era.

The self-help clinic caught on quickly.[52] Descriptions and justifications of self-help demonstrations and clinics featured prominently in the burgeoning feminist press.[53] The mother-daughter team Lolly and Jeanne Hirsch created the *Monthly Extract: An Irregular Periodical* to be the "community network of the global self-help movement."[54] Feminist health centers—many of them inspired by the power of self-help—often sponsored self-help clinics and demonstrations as a central aspect of their programming. Stoking the enthusiasm created by Rothman and Downer's tours, a group of women called the West Coast Sisters (also known as Self-Help Clinic One) distributed a pamphlet describing the goals of self-help clinics with tips on how to start one.[55]

Although women on the West Coast seemed particularly receptive to the self-help message, women created self-help clinics in every region of the country.[56] In Colorado Springs, for example, a group of women decided to throw their energy into the women's health movement. They visited health centers in Los Angeles and San Francisco to learn more, and they attended the first self-help conference in Iowa City, organized by Downer, Rothman, and other Los Angeles–based self-help advocates in October 1972. Their focus on feminist self-help, they explained, enabled more women to reclaim "control of [their] bodies from the medical industry, Madison Avenue, and big business."[57] A clinic in New Hampshire adopted self-help as its "underlying philosophy" and the means to achieve its goals. By practicing and promoting self-help, they provided a "model for woman controlled health care" and a road map for "women to act as . . . agents of social change."[58]

The self-help clinic even spread overseas. Women in Berlin, for example, inspired by the power of self-help demonstrations and clinics, founded their own Feministisches Frauengesundheitszentrum.[59] On separate trips in 1972 and 1973, the self-help advocates Debra Law and Carol Downer traveled to Rome to demonstrate the power of self-help.[60] Health activists also established self-help clinics in New Zealand. When Rothman visited in 1973, New Zealand already boasted more than twenty-five.[61]

Self-help advocates often strove to create self-help clinics that were heterogeneous, bringing together women of different ages, races, ethnicities, and sexualities. When created, sometimes these groups worked productively, if not easily. But more frequently, women wished to share their bodies and experiences of embodiment with women who were, at least along some axis, like them. As a result, groups that focused on commonality frequently emerged. Self-help clinics that focused on the needs of lesbians or menopausal women were common.[62] Other groups were designed for women who had undergone mastectomies and hysterectomies. Yet others focused on the needs of girls; feminists in Southern California planned a self-help group for Girl Scouts.[63]

Feminists promoted self-help clinics as a meaningful step toward female empowerment, self-knowledge, medical demystification, and bodily autonomy. They insisted that even if women employed the knowledge gained through self-help primarily for their own personal use, it was still "political" because it marked the "very first steps in freeing ourselves from helpless dependency on the medical profession," and because it would lead women to "remove additional shackles." But advocates understood that the "physical liberation" of women required further effort. They utilized the community-building aspect of the self-help clinic to organize further feminist health actions. Self-help clinics urged their participants to use the clinic as a start-ing point to promote a host of health care causes, including self-abortion techniques, complete and accessible sex education, responsive health care, and paramedic training. The clinics also publicized self-help and its power by teaching self-help methods to others.[64]

Self-Help for Whom?

Women active in the self-help gynecology movement were largely white and, to a lesser degree, middle class.[65] Despite the general racial and class homo-geneity, proponents of self-help argued that the goals they championed— claiming control over and knowledge of women's bodies in the service of women's liberation—benefited all women. Indeed, one of the goals of self-help was to demonstrate commonalities across race, class, and sexuality and to identify common mechanisms of oppression. These women did not deny the role of racism and poverty in women's lives, but they urgently believed in "sisterhood," and they believed that self-help clinics offered an opportunity to identify and nurture it.[66] As a result, some predominantly white groups sought to include women of color in their self-help clinics or to inspire women of color to create their own.[67] Their results were mixed. In Concord, New Hampshire, for example, the women's clinic unsuccessfully attempted to organize self-help clinics in Spanish-speaking and Black neighborhoods. Efforts to bring self-help to Asian American and Latinx communities also failed. Some self-help adherents blamed these failures on the cultures of the nonwhite women, citing "cultural values and morals strongly prohibiting them from publicly exposing or touching their bodies in the presence of other women."[68] As Michelle Murphy described it, because their "unraced woman-focused politics . . . imagined itself as welcoming all women," they failed to incorporate the insights and analysis of women of color into their body poli-tics.[69] Self-help enthusiasts believed in the potential of their technique; when it failed to inspire and liberate as expected, they blamed "culture" rather than examining the limits of self-help.

Some women of color did reject gynecological self-help, but not on cul-tural grounds. Some Black women dismissed self-help as "trivial," especially when compared to the "serious health problems black women faced."[70] As communities of color struggled against poverty and racism, with high rates of illness and little access to medicine, self-exam seemed to some like a privi-leged luxury of white, middle-class women; cervix viewing was dismissed as feminist navel-gazing.

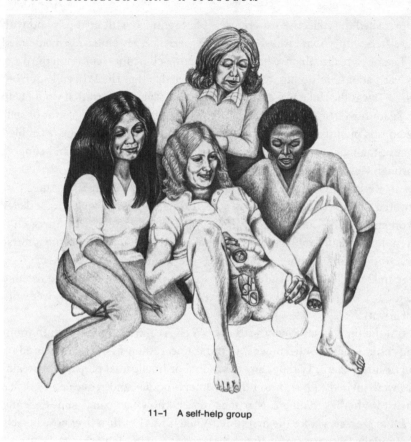

11–1   A self-help group

FIGURE 1.3. A self-help group as imagined by the Federation of Feminist Women's Health Centers. Note the diversity of the group. Self-help encouraged women to look beyond their differences and bond around their commonality. From the Federation of Feminist Health Centers, *A New View of a Woman's Body: A Fully Illustrated Guide* (Simon and Schuster, 1981), 152. Permission given by Suzann Gage.

Nevertheless, women of color did participate in self-help clinics, and some embraced the technique as a tool of liberation. In Oakland and Detroit—cities with large African American communities—Black women more frequently joined self-help efforts, sometimes providing leadership.[71] The radical alternative press also presented the value of self-help to women of color. In an April 1972 article in *Gidra*, the unofficial voice of the Asian American movement, Julia Aihara described her powerful experience with self-exam: "I was handed a mirror and met my own cervix for the first time. . . . I was discovering my body and thought it was beautiful. Then the other women looked at my cervix and I could feel my excitement regenerated in their eyes." Writing as "A Sister," Aihara appreciated the self-knowledge generated by self-exam, but she most appreciated the collective experience: "I felt reunited with my body and with my sisters with whom I was sharing this experience. My embarrassment faded as I came to realize that we had all come to the clinic for a common purpose: to learn about our bodies, to seek the knowledge that [had] been kept from us. . . . It was the collective effort toward knowledge and trust that would help us again turn insights into our femaleness."[72] Although this account of self-exam was published in an Asian American journal, the language resembled that of the many white women who found beauty, knowledge, and support through viewing their cervices.

In Berkeley, California, the Latina feminist Luz Alvarez Martinez discovered the power of self-exam in 1978 through her work with the Berkeley Women's Health Collective (BWHC). Martinez, a mother with three children, had recently returned to college at age thirty-four to become a nurse practitioner. She became involved with the women's center at Merritt College in Oakland and recruited guests for its speaker series. As she listened to the women from the BWHC, she realized she needed to be involved with their work.[73]

At the time, involvement with the BWHC required a seven-month training commitment. Unbeknownst to the trainees, their first lesson focused on cervical self-exam. Without any emotional or intellectual preparation, trainees were invited to peer into other women's bodies and requested to reveal their own bodies to others. Martinez recalled how "amazing" and "exciting" it felt to see a cervix for the first time. When it was her turn to expose herself, she initially felt nervous. As they began sharing with each other, she "just got into it." She remembered thinking, "What a wonderful thing . . . that we can look at each other and learn this way, and be so intimate with each other. . . . I got into it right away."[74]

Martinez stayed with the BWHC for about five years. She and other women of color encouraged the collective to diversify its staff and clientele; eventually, she helped establish its clinic for women of color. Her work with the BWHC introduced her to a network of other health activists, including Byllye Avery and other participants in what became the Black women's health movement, which helped her imagine an organization committed to Latina health. In 1986, Martinez and three other women founded the National Latina Health Organization.[75]

Because some women of color like Aihara and Martinez embraced self-help, white women in the movement often failed to grasp why women without white, middle-class, heterosexual identities might not want to share their bodies in group settings. For example, women from Salt Lake City described their experiences with a Chicana woman, Renee, who was active in a self-help group but who was certain that it would not appeal in general to Chicana women. She insisted that "we have too much body shame" to ever want to participate in self-exam. The white women in her group protested that they, too, had shame and claimed that self-exam was just as hard for them. Renee remained skeptical and asked whether the white women had ever "done a clinic with non-white women." When they assured her that they had, Renee asked, "Was it any different?" When the white women said no, Renee probed further, "Are we any different?" The white woman who narrated this story then stepped back to explain her interpretation of Renee's questions: "That was the real gut level thing. 'Are we different?' And I think that's where we all start: 'I must be different from everybody else. I must not be quite okay. I must not be normal.'"[76]

For this white woman and probably many others, this was the crux of the problem, the explanation why many women of color might be resistant to self-exam. In her analysis, women of color were afraid that they were not like white women. Nevertheless, this woman reasoned, self-exam could put that very fear to rest; therefore, women of color had even more reason to reveal their bodies to themselves and others. That the cultural baggage of bodies, the political and personal uses of bodily propriety, and the level of tolerance for physical vulnerability might differ among groups of women seemed lost on many white self-exam advocates. Self-exam's potential to reveal bodily similarities ironically blinded these women to the apparent experiential and political differences of embodiment. In other words, white women's limited understanding of the embodied experiences at the intersection of racism and sexism sometimes led them to double down on their insistence that gynecological self-exam had the potential to unify all women, which often had the effect of further marginalizing women of color.

Some women of color found value in self-help and self-exam,[77] but they sometimes preferred to organize groups without white women. One such group was the Black Women's Self-Help Collective (BWSHC) of Washington, DC, founded in 1981.[78] The BWSHC viewed self-exam as an especially valuable tool for Black women because slavery and its legacy had denied Black women authority over their own bodies. Self-help, they believed, would embolden women to seize control. An explicitly Black feminist organization, the BWSHC sought to educate, empower, and liberate Black women through self-exam and self-help. For these women, then, self-exam was not an indulgence, not a distraction from their struggle for survival. Indeed, it was an important tool within that struggle. While they understood that self-exam was only one step toward the empowerment of black women, they considered it a necessary step.

Self-Help within Feminist Health Centers

Many, perhaps most, women who peeked at their cervices, who marveled at the sight of menstrual blood glistening on a barely open os, who charted their own menstrual periods and examined their cervical mucus, did not go on to become feminist health activists. Indeed, some of them never identified as feminists.[79] But for countless others, self-exam and self-help clinics launched activist careers. Inspired by the perceived potential of self-help, women across the country created educational materials, sponsored talks, founded collectives, offered pregnancy tests, counseled abortion seekers, and opened women's health centers.

Feminist health centers and *feminist health clinics* were terms that designated a wide variety of institutions. At one end of a spectrum, they provided a basic setting for self-help clinics and a collection and distribution point for health-related material. At the other end, some health centers provided health care services, including health screenings, contraceptive devices, and abortions. Some emerged as "women's nights" at a free clinic; others were freestanding facilities. Some relied on all-volunteer staffs. Others paid some or all of the workers. Within these divergent settings, self-exam—or, at least, the belief that women had the right to look at and learn about their bodies—provided much of the ideological foundation.

The health institutions most conspicuously devoted to the potential of self-exam were a loosely associated network of centers known as the Feminist Women's Health Centers. In the summer of 1972, Lorraine Rothman and Carol Downer founded the first Feminist Women's Health Center, a Los Angeles institution dedicated to achieving women's liberation by promoting gynecological self-help.[80] In the beginning, the Los Angeles FWHC served as a distribution center for publicity about self-help, a location for self-help clinics, and an abortion referral service. The center also advertised a "Women's Free Clinic." Whether this was a "clinic" in the sense of a course of study or a health services facility may have been intentionally ambiguous.[81] The Women's Free Clinic likely provided pregnancy testing, contraceptives, and some health screenings and treatments. The absence of credentialed care workers at the clinic affirmed its commitment to a woman-centered self-help approach to basic reproductive and sexual health care. (As we will see below, "treatment" in a clinic without medical oversight pushed the limits of lay feminist health practice.) In the wake of the Supreme Court's January 1973 decision in *Roe v. Wade*, the women of the Los Angeles FWHC expanded their health clinic, providing abortions and reproductive health care. Downer claims that this was the first "woman-owned, woman-controlled" abortion clinic in the United States.[82] In time, other self-help advocates began their own centers and clinics under the banner of the Feminist Women's Health Centers. Although five of these clinics were in California, activists founded them in cities across the country, including Tallahassee, Salt Lake City, Detroit, Atlanta, and Ames, Iowa. (After 1975, some of these centers joined a Federation of Feminist Health Centers. Over time, surviving FWHCs varied in their formal and informal connections to the Federation and to each other.) The hallmark of these centers was their belief in the power of self-help and their commitment to restoring women's health to women's hands.

Participatory Clinic

But how does a feminist health center offer health care services to women for money while preserving its dedication to self-help? Many feminist health clinics depended on laywoman health workers to provide much of the care at these facilities.[83] At some centers, abortion was the only procedure that required a physician. At the Jane Collective in Chicago, laywomen even performed the abortions themselves.[84] This commitment to lay health workers clearly challenged the patriarchal medical monopoly on women's health care. But was it enough to substitute laywomen for professional medical providers? Did it truly further the goals of women's empowerment? Responding perhaps to the frequent and often quite vituperative charge that women's health clinics betrayed the revolutionary mission and zeal of the gynecological self-help movement, some women attempted to bring the politics of self-help gynecology into the health center through the development of a new concept: the participatory clinic.[85]

In a participatory clinic, pioneered by the FWHCs but employed widely, women who needed routine services or exams—such as Pap smears, venereal disease and pregnancy testing, breast exams, and contraceptive options— would meet in a group with two lay health workers for roughly two hours. Women in this setting would learn how to perform cervical and breast self-exams, how to fit a diaphragm or a cervical cap, and how to do Pap smears. They would also talk to each other, describing their experiences with birth control, with their physicians, with their own bodies. Promoted as an antidote to the medical model wherein physicians reserved for themselves the authority to define and diagnose abnormality, the group setting of the participatory clinic "insure[d] [sic] a more egalitarian process." Women, in consultation with other women, would learn to value their own subjective experiences of their bodies along with objective measurements in order to "make educated decisions about their own health care." In many significant ways, self-exam in participatory clinic and in self-help clinics shared similar goals: to educate, demystify, and challenge medical authority over women's bodies. Nevertheless, in participatory clinic, the techniques of self-exam performed one further task: they transformed women from patients into health care providers who looked after their own bodily needs and the needs of other women in the group.[86]

The participatory clinic was a radical alternative to medical care as usual in a number of ways. It challenged, for example, traditional notions of expertise by validating the experiential knowledge of other women. Within a participatory clinic, women's advice about tender breasts and dry vaginas was transformed from ignorant "wives' tales" into useful information. It encouraged feminized collaborative knowledge production. Participatory clinic also insisted that women could and should assume responsibility for knowing about their bodies. It made a passive relationship to health care impossible, at least in the participatory clinic setting. Further, it dissolved the vulnerabilities created by the difference in social position between the generally male physicians and the female patient. By receiving care from peers instead of hierarchically positioned authorities, women may have felt more comfortable asking about the niggling things, the small embarrassments. Finally, the participatory clinic was perhaps most radical in its reframing of the distinctions between private and public bodies. The traditional medical consultation fetishized patient privacy; the draping of the body and the orchestrated props of medical professionalism contributed to the belief that female bodies should be covered and shared only with a medical professional. The participatory clinic, by insisting that bodies need not be relegated to private spaces, encouraged women to accept their own bodies—with their bulges, wrinkles, smells, and secretions— and to see other women's bodies as sources of information and wonder.

Cause Célèbre: The Great Yogurt Conspiracy

Although widespread in feminist and other alternative health facilities, the employment of lay health workers within clinic settings tested the boundaries of the law.[87] Was it "practicing medicine" to look at another woman's cervix or to teach women about the signs of pregnancy? Did it matter if a cervical exam ended with the identification of an overgrowth of yeast? What about if it included a diaphragm fitting? These questions went largely unanswered in the early 1970s even as new categories of health care professionals (e.g., nurse practitioners, physicians' assistants) and lay health workers proliferated. But in 1972, self-help gynecology and cervical self-exam performed within the Los Angeles FWHC—presumably the Women's Free Clinic—provided a test case.[88]

On September 20, 1972, ten policemen entered the Los Angeles FWHC to execute search warrants to support the accusation that the women of the center were practicing medicine illegally. The police officers confiscated specula, books, records, pregnancy test kits, IUDs, curettes, and menstrual extraction kits.[89] The search warrant also gave them permission to seize "yogurt used in the treatment of yeast infections."[90] (According to an article in the feminist periodical *Off Our Backs*, the police confiscated a carton of strawberry yogurt, at which point a woman protested, "You can't have that. . . . That's my lunch."[91]) The police officers also left arrest warrants for Carol Downer and Colleen Wilson, both original West Coast Sisters, alleging that the women were practicing medicine without a license. Downer and Wilson were not at the center at the time, but they turned themselves in the next day.[92]

The seeds of this event were planted in the spring, when John Urso, an investigator for California's Department of Consumer Affairs (DCA), received a complaint from a parent of a child at a local junior high school. The DCA sought to "protect" the state's consumers by setting industry standards, issuing licenses, and enforcing regulations on service-oriented professionals, including fumigators, accountants, real estate appraisers, and physicians. Allegedly, the complainant's daughter heard about the self-help clinic from a teacher at the school, and the woman was concerned that her daughter might learn about birth control and abortion if her daughter attended the clinic. The mother apparently took her concerns to the school board. From there, the complaint made its way to the DCA.[93] In response, the DCA launched an investigation, sending in undercover witnesses and a school guidance counselor to collect information about the Los Angeles FWHC's activities.[94]

The investigators witnessed a variety of allegedly illegal practices. They saw Downer and Wilson performing vaginal exams involving the use of a speculum, "diagnosing" yeast infections, and "treating" those infections with yogurt. In addition, Wilson allegedly fit several women with diaphragms, performed Pap smears, tested women for pregnancy, "dispensed" birth control pills, and "performed" a "menses extraction." She also advised a woman who feared she might be pregnant to pull on the string of her IUD to possibly cause an abortion.[95]

Although the application of yogurt to treat a yeast infection seemed the most benign of the practices seen by the investigator, it represented the crux of the case for Deputy City Attorney David Schacter. In his statement to the press, Schacter highlighted the issue: "They've been making a diagnosis and then prescribing a treatment. Who are they to diagnose a yeast infection and prescribe yogurt for it?"[96] Who, indeed? In this defense of physician prerogatives, Schatcher demonstrated that the offense was not the improper use of dairy; it was the nerve of improperly behaving women.

Based on these allegations, the state charged Wilson with eleven misdemeanor counts of practicing medicine without a license, including "performing a menstrual extraction, giving pelvic examinations, and testing for pregnancy."[97] These charges were clearly serious and potentially difficult to defend. In October 1972, the Office of the California Attorney General explicitly ruled that pelvic examinations fell within the practice of medicine. (The ruling did not, however, define a "pelvic examination," although it did describe in detail the procedure for a Pap smear.)[98] If found guilty, Wilson faced up to eleven years in jail.[99] Perhaps because of the odds against her acquittal and the potential consequences of a conviction, she pled guilty to one count of fitting a diaphragm. She received a twenty-five-day suspended sentence, paid a $250 fine, and served two years on probation.[100]

Downer was charged with one count of practicing medicine without a license, for "diagnosing a woman's illness as a yeast infection and treating it with yogurt."[101] She decided to fight the charges, seeing the trial as an opportunity to test the interpretive limits of "diagnosing and treating" disease and to publicize and garner support for self-help and the larger women's health movement.[102]

After the raid and the arrest, Downer and the FWHC moved quickly to mobilize feminist outrage and support. In language designed to shock, they publicized their account of the "raid" as "Feminist Rape," thereby stressing the inherent violation involved in the intrusion of the police and the state into women's bodily care practices. By referring to it as rape, they also argued that the state and police were trying to exert their power over women's bodies in response to women's efforts to claim their bodies as their own.[103]

The defense team solicited notarized messages of support for self-help. Many women and organizations responded. A dental hygienist from Honolulu, for example, described how she felt ethically bound to instruct her patients to examine their own mouths for signs of disease and how to keep their mouths clean. She argued that the same principle should hold true for reproductive organs, and she concluded that "any attempt by the state of California to stop or punish the actions of . . . Carol Downer is in opposition to the true ethics of the health professions."[104] Similarly, the Feminist Coordinating Council of Seattle compared self-help clinics to hygiene and nutrition instruction. They concluded by insisting, "We will practice self-help. We will fight harassment with all the resources available. . . . We will control our own bodies."[105] High-profile feminists, including Bella Abzug and Robin Morgan, also offered their support.[106]

Not all support was wholly enthusiastic, however. NOW's response, for example, was markedly tepid. Wilma Scott Heide, president of the national organization, acknowledged that medicine and law "consciously or unconsciously . . . have had a misogynist strain damaging to women" and that she supported "in principle" efforts to demystify women's bodies. Perhaps Heide's response was colored by her training as a nurse.[107] Consequently, NOW indicated its "special interest in this case" and hoped that women's right to understand their bodies was protected.[108]

Downer and her female lawyers, Diane Wayne and Jeanette Christy, launched a defense based on showing that the notion of practicing medicine without a license, especially the idea of "diagnosing and treating disease," was overly vague and capriciously enforced. In the press and presumably in the courtroom, Downer and her supporters repeatedly compared her case with mothers' efforts to care for their own children, using experiential knowledge and home remedies. Self-exam was akin to "applying eye drops to an eye infection or a Band-Aid to a bruised knee."[109] Downer and her defense also used Wilson's probation as evidence that the law was unclear. As part of her probation, Wilson had been directed to refrain from practices "that would require a license." When she asked what that might include, the judge, according to Downer, had replied, "Well, we're not sure." For Downer and her defense, a law with such fuzzy boundaries and unpredictable enforcement should not be used to prevent women from taking care of themselves and each other.[110] Downer also denied that the women of the Los Angeles FWHC offered services to "anyone who walk[ed] in." Instead, she described self-exam and menstrual extraction as performed within a closed self-help group.[111]

This claim warrants examination. Some accounts of this story suggest that Zsuzsanna Budapest, a "friend" or alternatively a "sister" who was at the center for a "class," had asked Downer to apply the yogurt. Clearly this could have occurred within the context of a self-help clinic. But the charges against Wilson—that she was accused of dispensing oral contraceptives and fitting diaphragms—do not closely follow the self-help clinic model. That the center's stationary also advertised a "Women's Free Clinic" in addition to the self-help clinic further suggests that perhaps the Los Angeles FWHC offered services in addition to instruction.[112]

The raid at the Los Angeles FWHC and the subsequent trial received widespread coverage in the feminist press and some coverage in the mainstream press.[113] Although most of the mainstream coverage took the trial seriously, some reporting described the raid in language that mocked Downer and the self-help movement. A *Time* magazine article, for example, began: "One extreme symptom of Women's Liberation has been the refusal of some feminists to submit to examination by male gynecologists." Although the medical context provided cover to the author for referring to self-help as a "symptom," it nevertheless presented women's liberation as a pathological condition, and its adherents as off kilter; it also misrepresented the position of the women who promoted self-help. The attitude continued as the author described the raid on "one of the self-help movement's temples," thus framing self-help adherents as swayed by faith in feminist politics rather than science. This depiction trivialized the event and the women involved. Tempering his scorn, perhaps, the author eventually admitted that the trial would likely focus on "women's right to know their own bodies" and conceded that the clinic remained open, and thus "continu[ed] to challenge the state by doing business as usual."[114]

On December 5, 1972, at the end of the eight-day trial, the jury of eight men and four women pronounced Downer not guilty of practicing medicine without a license.[115] In the aftermath, the foreman of the jury, Paul Barnum, gave Downer a note of appreciation: "Carol—You're not a downer—you're a real upper! . . . Good Luck."[116] At a press conference after the verdict, Downer insisted that the acquittal was not for her alone but was a "victory for all women," as it allowed women to explore their bodies and share information about those bodies without fear of legal reprisal.[117] In its press release, the Los Angeles FWHC claimed that the Great Yogurt Conspiracy was the "first Feminist trial in recent history where a woman has been challenged by the legal system for her beliefs and execution of those beliefs." They deemed it as a "landmark for the Women's Liberation Movement."[118]

In many ways, the Great Yogurt Conspiracy bolstered the FWHC. It gave Downer and her supporters a forum to publicize self-help as a way for women to take control of their lives. Perhaps more important, by the women challenging state and medical overreach and winning, the trial provided a compelling example of self-help's legitimacy and value.[119] Clearly, the state did not believe that women could be trusted with a speculum, yogurt, or woman-shared knowledge. The mainstream press, however, ridiculed women's liberation even as it publicized feminist issues. By portraying the trial with a tone of "Can you believe what these gals are doing now?" and misrepresenting self-help's relationship to medicine more generally, the coverage of the trial in the mainstream press likely reinforced health feminism and the women's movement as misguided, ridiculous, and perhaps dangerous.

Self-Help as Intellectual Property

Self-help gynecology was a widespread social movement. It was also an intellectual argument and a political strategy originally proposed and regularly elaborated by Downer, Rothman, and women associated with the Feminist Women's Health Centers. As the originators' visions clashed with new arguments for self-exam, as health feminists created their own protocols for self-help clinics, as activists failed to provide sufficient attribution to feminist foremothers, self-help became a battleground over credit and mission.

One area of conflict was the authenticity and pedigree of self-help depictions in the feminist press. The original self-help clinic document attributed to West Coast Sisters (Downer and Rothman, among others) was first published in July 1971 in *Everywoman*, a Venice, California, publication.[120] It was widely reprinted in whole or in part in a variety of feminist periodicals.[121] Second-generation discussions of self-examinations were themselves excerpted and reprinted. "Vaginal Politics" by Peggy Grau, likely a self-help feminist not affiliated with the West Coast Sisters or the Los Angeles FWHC, was published in *Everywoman* in August 1971.[122] In this article, illustrated by photographs and line drawings, Grau described how to perform a self-exam and argued for its political and practical utility. This and other self-help articles by Grau were reproduced widely.[123]

Perhaps because of a history of conflict over abortion politics, the articles written by Grau incensed Downer and Rothman. Now writing as the Feminist Women's Health Center, Downer and Rothman distanced themselves from Grau's articles and the information in them, claiming that "all articles written by Peggy Grau, although containing some of our self-examination techniques and findings, are not concerned with us in any way."[124] In turn, Grau publicly denied that she was connected to the Self-Help Clinic of the FWHCs. She alleged, however, that her article "Vaginal Politics" had been reprinted by the Self-Help Clinic without proper attribution.[125]

Similar arguments over the true self-help models emerged at the first national self-help conference in Iowa City in October 1972. Although self-help groups from across the nation anticipated this conference with enthusiasm, its appeal diminished in some quarters as the California founders of the movement used the conference to establish self-help orthodoxy. Participants at this conference, for example, decided that all future conferences should begin with the traditional anatomy slideshow "because we discovered that many women attending this conference who had not seen the presentation had not fully grasped the impact of SELF HELP."[126] For some leaders of the movement, self-help needed to include certain foundational steps and adhere to particular commitments. Agreement appears to have emerged around the need for women leading self-help clinics and promoting the movement to be paid for their work (or at least be reimbursed for their own outlays) and to remain independent of other women's health projects not dedicated to self-help, including "free clinics, Planned Parenthood, [and] reformist organizations aimed toward legislative or professional changes."[127]

Dissension also emerged within the Feminist Women's Health Centers. Twelve women who left (or were fired from) the Orange County FWHC, for example, complained that the FWHC acted as if it owned self-help. One ex-staffer noted in exasperation, "The idea of 'Self Help' has become a company and professionalized. It is FWHC *property*. No one near an FWHC would dare to hold a neighborhood 'Self Help' group without the FWHC present."[128] Perhaps she overstated the case, but FWHC women did believe that there was a right and a wrong way to offer self-help. As Laura Brown of the Oakland Feminist Women's Health Center described the misguided practices of the San Francisco Health Center, she complained that "from the very beginning [they proceeded] to distort and destroy the ideas of the self-help clinic. They never did, have not to this day, grasped what self-examination is about."[129]

Much of the appeal of self-exam was likely its political and material simplicity and accessibility. Feminists could easily offer a self-help clinic in a home, a community center, or a grange hall. But the debates over self-help orthodoxy suggest that the tool and its politics could not be controlled by the original intent of the founders. Although Downer, Rothman, and other feminists involved with the FWHCs attempted to imbue self-help with a particular meaning, the allegedly self-evident political potential of self-exam, along with its flexibility, gave self-exam its power to inspire versions of health activism different from the visions of its creators.

Self-Help Critiques

For feminist self-helpers, the cervical self-exam in its various incarnations provided a flexible tool for demystifying bodies, producing knowledge, nurturing community, and publicizing feminist health efforts. But self-help earned many detractors. These opponents, or at least skeptics, also publicized a variety of dangers and limits of self-exam. Doctors and other health care workers were among those who believed that self-exam was misguided and perhaps dangerous. The physician Arthur Levin, for example, promoted patient involvement and discernment in medical settings, and he applauded breast self-exam as an appropriate complement to professional health care; vaginal self-exam, however, clearly went too far. Levin regarded the use of vaginal self-exam to diagnose cervical cancer and the use of yogurt to treat vaginal infections as examples of suboptimal medicine. According to Levin, it would have been better for women to use their justifiable anger and frustration to demand better medical care. By doing so, they would benefit themselves as well as "their husbands and other men."[130] With this statement, Levin revealed his ignorance of the politics behind the feminist self-help movement and simultaneously validated its efforts.

Self-helpers frequently described their interactions with medical professionals who clearly disapproved of self-exam. In 1974, for example, Margaret Rossoff feared that she had injured herself during a self-exam, and so she went to the local ER for an examination. There she encountered a nurse who had never heard of self-examination, and who seemed shocked and "disgusted" by the procedure and perhaps by Rossoff herself for using it. Rossoff interpreted this nurse's reaction as an example of medicine's "resentment of nonprofessionals acquiring control of their bodies." "Conventional medicine," she argued, "is recognizing self help as a threat to their monopoly rip-off."[131] Another self-helper, Barbara Monty, reported a similarly shocked medical professional who suggested that she had "no business" examining her own cervix. "He . . . looked at me as if I were a rare species of caterpillar."[132] In these examples, health care professionals reacted to self-exam with a shock that only underscored the rationale behind it: women's bodies were the purview of physicians, who saw women's desires to see and know their own bodies as both jarring and inexplicable. Health professionals in these accounts regarded self-exam as evidence of feminist recklessness, and they defended the value of medical surveillance. Self-helpers, by contrast, used the health care professionals' reaction to self-exam in these accounts to highlight a lack of respect for female autonomy.

Some feminists feared self-exam might be unsafe. One woman who attended a presentation on self-exam in Princeton, New Jersey, found it full of misinformation and "man-hating." In her letter to the NOW chapter that sponsored the event, she warned readers, "Let us not play dangerous games." Instead, she insisted, health feminists should be fighting for more professional training for women and increased access to first-rate medical care.[133] Although NOW had been an important forum for the dissemination of self-help and self-exam, this letter writer suggests why the organization was generally associated with the liberal stream of feminism, dedicated to increasing women's rights and opportunities, rather than the radical stream, which advocated the overthrow of patriarchy and the rise of women's liberation.[134]

Some feminists—even feminists within the women's health movement— challenged the ultimate political utility of self-exam.[135] Susan Reverby, a feminist activist with the Health Policy Advisory Center (Health/PAC) in New York City, challenged the value of self-help in her 1973 review of *Our Bodies, Ourselves*. Reverby acknowledged the attraction of woman-centered knowledge production and self-care practices, but she also highlighted its limitations. In addition to her concern that self-help could lead to misdiagnosis and mistreatment (it had in her case), Reverby primarily challenged its political worth. She insisted that "we cannot equate control over some bodily processes with power over the body politic and the forces that control our lives. . . . Bodily knowledge is in no way a substitute for political challenge."[136] "Lorrien" was also dismissive after seeing her first self-help presentation at the June 1973 Women's Sexuality Conference in New York City, but perhaps for different reasons. She wrote that "these women have made a religion out of self-help. The speculum is their holy chalice. Feminists create a form of worship, . . . adoration of the physical body to the total exclusion of the mind and the universal spirit."[137] In her review of Ellen Frankfort's *Vaginal Politics*, published in 1972, the feminist essayist and eventual screenwriter Nora Ephron suggested that the self-help movement had become self-absorbed and, in the process, had come to ignore the need for broad political change. According to Ephron, self-exam demonstrated how "self-knowledge dissolves into high-grade narcissism."[138]

Frankfort herself, while more sympathetic to the power of self-exam, also worried that a focus on self-help risked ignoring the urgent need for broader institutional change.[139] As she famously quipped, "The speculum is a weapon, but giving women specula rather than helping them change the medical care system is like giving people guns in lieu of a battle plan."[140] A similar complaint came from the Far Left. In a 1974 *People's World* article, Stephanie Allan depicted self-examination as an inadequate response to the real unmet health needs of women. She wondered both whether or not the women examining themselves were truly competent judges of normal and abnormal bodies, and how self-help addressed the supposed health needs of "millions of women who never even receive bad medical care." She dismissed self-exam as "an individual solution that a few women can adopt to relieve their own personal anger and frustration at a system that literally kills and sterilizes thousands and thousands of women, many of them not white." She urged feminists to use their considerable skills and energies to change the institutions that had "for too long relegated medical care for women (and children, also) to the lowest priority."[141] For Allan, self-help gynecology highlighted and reinforced white, middle-class privilege and distracted from systemic change. Self-exam enthusiasts could afford to assume the care and surveillance of their well bodies, confident that if they found something wrong, they could secure professional health care. Because not all women could rely on medical backup, self-help represented to its left-leaning skeptics little more than cervix-gazing disguised as body politics.

Certainly not all women who viewed their cervix saw it as the gateway to their liberation or a meaningful challenge to medicine as usual. Many, perhaps most, considered the moment exciting, but its value and significance faded as they returned to their lives as students, workers, mothers, and activists. Surely some women found the self-help movement preposterous, heavy on exhibitionism and light on analysis. Others found it trivial, framed too narrowly around the perspectives of well women—often white and middle class—while neglecting the needs of medically underserved women.

And yet, gazing upon previously inaccessible parts of their bodies, in the presence of other women, allowed some to imagine a system where women could gain more control over their bodies and their lives. Inspired by the potential of the speculum and women's collective power, some women devoted their energy to the personal and political practice of feminist self-help, anchored by self-exam and self-help clinics. Sometimes their excitement and commitment lasted for a summer; for others, self-help and feminist health activism became their life's work. For these women, self-help challenged the medical control of women's bodies, exposed the needlessness of bodily shame, diminished personal ignorance, and charted a path to women's liberation. It promised to restore women's health to women's hands.

Feminist Health Services:
Moving beyond the Speculum

In the fall of 1973, a group of women gathered in Santa Cruz, California, and wondered what came next. Linked by their work in self-help groups and abortion counseling, many had grown frustrated by the limits of their current projects. They wanted to do more to meet women's health care needs, and they wanted to give women more options to avoid childbearing and -rearing. At some point, one of the women wondered aloud, "Why don't we start a clinic?" Incredulous at the audacity of the suggestion, many in the room insisted they were too young and inexperienced to successfully launch a clinic. And yet, after swallowing their fear and skepticism, buoyed by determination, some of the women vowed to make it happen. "We'll just do it," they agreed. In 1974, the Santa Cruz Women's Health Collective opened WomanKind, a health clinic offering abortion services and gynecological care. The founders imagined the center and its clinic as an outgrowth of their self-help politics and their commitment to empower and liberate women and meet their reproductive health needs.[1]

Women's health centers were institutional attempts to bring the women's health movement to knowledge-seeking and health-seeking female publics. Activists created women's health centers to provide a physical hub for their projects. At these centers, feminists offered a range of services, including self-help clinics and demonstrations, pregnancy screening, abortion counseling and referrals, and educational materials promoting the power of self-knowledge. For many feminist health activists, these services fulfilled their desire to meet women's most immediate (reproductive) health needs and publicize the potential power of self-help.

Activists at some health centers, however, strove to provide more than a critique of medicine or, in the case of pregnancy testing, an end run around medical gatekeeping. These health activists founded feminist health clinics to both meet individual women's needs and provide a woman-centered model of care dedicated to health education and political change. On the coasts and in the heartland, in cities big and small, feminists created with determination, idealism, rage, and naivete a loosely connected network of clinics striving to empower women and help them control their lives. Some of these clinics were short-lived ventures. Others, including those described here, survived in one form or another into the twenty-first century.[2]

This chapter examines the history of two feminist women's health collectives and their efforts to provide feminist health care. It demonstrates how political commitments and local idiosyncrasies created quite different models of feminist health care and body politics. Both the Santa Cruz Women's Health Collective and the Women's Health Collective of Humboldt Open Door Clinic (and later Northcountry Clinic) were part of a radical health movement that reimagined access to medical care and medical knowledge; they were also part of a feminist movement that deemed bodily control necessary for women's empowerment and liberation. They both offered affordable, woman-centered health services. But significant aspirational differences distinguished these organizations' politics and clinics. The women of the Santa Cruz Women's Health Collective (SCWHC) were simultaneously devoted to self-help and to feminist revolution, and they considered the SCWHC and the health center it eventually created vehicles for both. Their political commitments and goals influenced how they lived (and with whom), how they managed the SCWHC and its health center, and how they envisioned the provision of health care. Over time, however, the collective members struggled to keep their center and its clinical services aligned with their politics. Ironically, as their clinic expanded, their original feminist body politics receded from view. In contrast, the aspirations of the Women's Health Collective of Humboldt Open Door Clinic were less complex. They aimed to provide woman-centered health care free from sexist oversight. They transformed the self-help impulse to democratize medical knowledge into a new model for feminist care and a new pathway for health care provision. While they offered no explicit critique of medicine, they enacted their beliefs that women working together could deliver feminist health care.

New Models of Clinical Care

Feminist health clinics emerged in the 1970s from a larger social movement to revolutionize the delivery of health care. Health radicals and reformers decried the "medical industrial complex," medicine's focus on treatment rather than prevention, and its embrace of profit at the expense of health.[3] Activists in the 1960s and '70s sought to change the nature of medicine and make health care more accessible. Neighborhood health centers (NHCs) and free clinics offered new models of understanding and addressing the root causes of illness and widened access to health care.[4]

Neighborhood health centers, funded first by the newly created federal Office of Economic Opportunity (OEO) and later by the OEO and the Department of Health, Education, and Welfare (HEW), were developed in the mid-1960s as comprehensive health centers to treat illness and to address its socioeconomic roots. According to Dr. H. Jack Geiger, one of the major visionaries of the NHC concept, neighborhood health centers did not merely aim to prevent and treat disease; they sought to empower and transform communities. Community involvement and collaboration were key to their mission. As Geiger put it, community members must be given "an assured role in the design and control of their own health services."[5] These centers would create jobs, offer education, feed families, treat illness, and prevent disease.

While still a medical student, Geiger first saw the connection between medical care and community transformation while visiting the Pholela Health Center in Pholela, South Africa. Clinic founders Sydney and Emily Kark believed that social issues—including sanitation, access to employment, inadequate housing, and poor nutrition—influenced illness and health. As a result, the Karks focused on improving the environment, broadly understood, as a vital component of improving the community's health. Geiger recalled this experience in 1964, when he served as the Mississippi field coordinator for the Medical Committee for Human Rights (MCHR) during Freedom Summer. While most MCHR activists aimed only to provide care to civil rights activists, Geiger and others stayed in the South through the fall to establish health care facilities for poor African Americans in the region.[6]

United by their commitment to medical civil rights, Geiger collaborated with Count Gibson and John Hatch, both from the Preventive Medicine Department of Tufts Medical School, to propose the first NHC demonstration projects: one in Mound Bayou, Mississippi, one of the poorest counties in the nation, and another in a Columbia Point housing project in Boston. These projects sought to show how health centers with a social mission could strengthen communities as well as individuals. The OEO funded these and four other NHC projects in 1965.[7]

The NHC program grew quickly over the next six years. By 1971, a nationwide network of more than 150 centers served nearly one million people. More than 75 percent of these centers were in cities. Three hallmarks linked these clinics: significant federal funding, first from the OEO and then from

HEW; partnerships with elite institutions, including hospitals and universities; and mandatory community involvement through advisory boards and other mechanisms. At their best, these clinics demonstrated the potential for communities to identify their own health care needs and their ability to design institutional solutions to address them.

At roughly the same time, health activists from a loosely defined "radical health movement" promoted a different model. The free clinic movement began as a response to a brewing health crisis in California. In the summer of 1967, thousands of countercultural young people festooned with flowers planned to descend upon San Francisco to experience lives of peace and love, unfettered by the bourgeois constraints of their parents. (Many of these people likewise hoped to experience the drugs that were also headed to San Francisco.) This posed a multilevel crisis for city leaders. How would they cope with the housing, sanitation, and health care needs of the visitors? Robert Conrich, a former private investigator and LSD-inspired "dropout," envisioned a health center that would treat the drug-induced problems that were surely on their way. Imagining a free clinic staffed by volunteers, he floated the idea by his friend, David Smith, a toxicologist and chief of the Alcohol and Drug Abuse Screening Unit at San Francisco General Hospital. Smith eagerly signed on to become medical director for a clinic in the Haight-Ashbury district, the anticipated center for the Summer of Love.[8]

Conrich and Smith found great support for their idea from both the community and health professionals. Financial support (including a large gift from rock producer Phil Graham), in-kind gifts, and enthusiastic volunteers allowed the clinic to open in June 1967. The Haight Ashbury Free Clinic was immediately inundated with clients, seeking testing and treatments for infections, first aid for injuries, and rescue from bad trips and drug overdoses. Although most of the young people who flocked to San Francisco that summer left in the fall, the health problems, especially the drug problems, continued.[9] The Haight Ashbury Free Clinic also remained, surviving into the twenty-first century.

The model of the Haight Ashbury Free Clinic inspired communities across the country to launch their own community-funded, mostly volunteer-run free clinics to meet local needs. By 1971, there were roughly two hundred free clinics operating nationwide.[10] Some of them were short-lived experiments in alternative health care delivery. Others continue to offer health care to socially and economically marginalized communities.[11]

While many early free clinics were inspired by the Haight Ashbury Free Clinic, they were launched by individuals and groups with diverse medical and political agendas. Medical students, faith communities, recovered addicts, gay activists, recent immigrants, Young Patriots, countercultural radicals, and individuals from a variety of other constituencies founded clinics to meet local needs. Some of these clinics focused on drug-related health problems, while "VD" clinics provided testing and treatment for sexually transmitted infections. Some clinics concentrated on caring for the elderly; others catered to meeting the psychological and physical needs of street youth.[12]

Many of the high-profile free clinics were organized to meet the health needs of racial and ethnic minorities as part of a larger project of community empowerment and liberation. In the late 1960s, for example, the Black Panther Party began creating health clinics—People's Free Medical Clinics (PFMC)—as part of their larger effort to serve the people. By April 1970, Bobby Seale, building on these local initiatives, directed all party chapters to open health clinics in their communities. By 1972, thirteen cities boasted PFMCs. Like many other free clinics, the PFMCs relied on collaboration with medical experts and donated supplies and labor. As the sociologist Alondra Nelson wrote in her pathbreaking monograph on the history of the party's health projects, the clinics "embodied the Party's critique of medical authority, professionalization, and the medical–industrial complex."[13] Medical professionals were valued in these projects, both for the care they offered and for the skills they shared. Like many other radical health projects, the PFMCs encouraged the transfer of knowledge and skills from medical professionals to community members. The Brown Berets, a leading Chicano civil rights organization, also founded health clinics in low-income, Spanish-speaking neighborhoods of Los Angeles (El Barrio Free Clinic) and Chicago (Benito Juarez Health Clinic).

These clinics varied in size, duration, and services. Some struggled to open at all, barely managing to provide sickle cell anemia and blood pressure screenings. Others supplied a wide range of health screenings, first aid for injuries, treatments for minor complaints, and immunizations. They also often provided referrals for the treatment of more serious conditions and illness. But these clinics were never meant only to deliver health care; they offered legal aid, housing resources, and political education as well.[14]

Although some of the free clinics focused nearly exclusively on health care (e.g., VD clinics), others viewed themselves as centers for community organizing. In these clinics, "the mimeograph machine [was] as important as the stethoscope."[15] Clinic organizers offered a critique of medicine as usual, demanding "health care for people, not for profit," the demystification of medical knowledge, and the deprofessionalization of medicine.[16] Some of these clinics served as powerful symbols of community self-determination.

Over time, striking the right balance between creating social change and offering social services concerned many radical health activists. They feared that some free clinics had enabled the medical establishment to maintain its practices of oppression and exclusion by providing a Band-Aid rather than challenging the system. Indeed, they feared that within a few years, "the energy of the free clinic movement will . . . be at the service of the health power structure."[17] Some activists on the Left offered a stronger critique, claiming that free clinics were "counter-revolutionary" because they allowed mainstream medicine to continue as usual while providing inadequate care to the "socially stigmatized individuals or poor, inner city dwellers."[18]

Although men often founded these free clinics and provided most of the "medical" care, women often led their day-to-day operations. For example, at the Robert Taylor Clinic, organized in a housing project in Chicago, women filled all the "tenant" seats on the policy-making board. Women organized schedules, tested urine samples, raised funds, and saw patients as lay workers, nurses, and occasionally physicians.[19] In the case of the PFMCs, Alondra Nelson noted that the "Party health cadre was mostly composed of Black women."[20] Gloria Arellanes was the director of the El Barrio Free Clinic in Los Angeles. Indeed, sexism within some free clinics occasionally encouraged women to establish their own women's clinics.[21]

Free clinics and neighborhood health centers shared many characteristics and goals. Both frequently offered free or low-cost care and demonstrated the value of community involvement. But these two types of clinics differed significantly in their relationship with the federal government and with institutions of medicine. NHCs relied on federal money, subjecting them to federal regulation and oversight. Free clinics, although they sometimes employed AmeriCorps VISTA workers and depended on Medicaid or Medi-Cal (California's Medicaid program) for reimbursement, generally rejected federal funding as an option, believing that it would "co-opt Free Clinics" and "decrease their effectiveness as social change agents." Consequently, they were freer to experiment with health care delivery and to offer alternatives to mainstream, allopathic medicine.[22] Partnerships with medical institutions that were crucial to NHCs also limited their ability to offer a critique of medicine. Because free clinics lacked these partnerships and the resources that came with them, they rarely offered care beyond routine outpatient services. As a result, Geiger dismissed much of the free clinic movement as "playing house, not responding to the real need."[23]

The Rise of Feminist Clinics

Feminist health clinics emerged in the early 1970s alongside and sometimes within these other experiments in health care delivery and health politics.

Health feminists were inspired by the proliferation of alternative health institutions, women's need for abortion access, and the rise of women's health projects, including the Boston Women's Health Course Collective (later known as the Boston Women's Health Book Collective) and the self-help movement. Clinics provided a mechanism to meet material health needs— especially reproductive health needs—while simultaneously demonstrating in practice women's ability to control their bodies and their lives. As the anthropologist Sandra Morgen put it, feminist health clinics became "vanguard organizations" for the women's health movement.[24] Clinics provided a vehicle for activists to enact an alternative vision of health care, one that could empower as well as heal.

"Women's Night" at the Berkeley Free Clinic (BFC) may have been the first feminist clinic.[25] In November 1970, a group of about thirty white, middle-class women formed the Berkeley Women's Health Collective. They believed health care was a "right of all people," and they wanted to provide access to health care without regard to ability to pay. Consistent with other health movements of the time, the collective aimed to demystify medicine, deprofessionalize health care, and promote preventative health. They also wanted to "reclaim" their bodies from medical experts and gain the know-how to "care for ourselves."[26]

The collective approached the BFC and asked for access one day a week to provide a women's clinic. After the BFC agreed, the collective recruited medical personnel—physicians, nurses, pharmacy workers, and medics—to provide some of the health care. The Women's Clinic at the Berkeley Free Clinic opened in February 1971, claiming to be the "first women's clinic in the country."[27] The clinic, promoting "prevention not cure," offered health screenings and basic treatment to a clientele of mostly young, white women described as "transients, street people and students."[28] It also provided abortion and birth control counseling. If a woman chose abortion, the clinic volunteers provided a referral and a companion to accompany the client through the process.[29]

Other groups of women followed Berkeley's example. In the spring of 1971, women in Seattle and Baltimore established their own free clinics, and others quickly made similar plans.[30] Two January 1973 Supreme Court rulings—*Roe v. Wade*, legalizing early abortion in every state, and *Doe v. Bolton*, authorizing abortions outside of hospitals—encouraged the further expansion of the feminist health care marketplace. Some feminist clinics added abortion provision to their services, and women working independently and within feminist organizations founded new clinics to provide abortions in a woman-centered, feminist environment.[31] In Iowa City, for example, women involved in the Women's Resource and Action Center, an abortion referral service that also organized self-help groups, began planning their abortion clinic within hours of the *Roe* decision. In September 1973, they opened the Emma Goldman Clinic, providing the only outpatient abortions in Iowa.[32] In Oakland, the Feminist Women's Health Center, which had opened in 1972, began offering abortions in May 1973.[33] At least thirty-five feminist health centers operated by the end of 1973. By 1976, roughly fifty feminist health centers provided a range of health services.[34]

Feminist clinics varied widely in their approach health care, especially regarding their relationship with mainstream medicine. The Emma Goldman Women's Health Center, founded January 1974 by group of Chicago feminists, occupied one edge of a wide spectrum. (This clinic should not be confused with the Iowa City clinic of the same name.) Extending the self-help praxis many of the founders had deployed in their work with the underground abortion clinic known as Jane, the Chicago Emma Goldman center offered preventative services performed exclusively by lay health workers or, in their terms, "feminist paramedics." As the historian Wendy Kline has explained, these women argued that their approach was "revolutionary" because they dared to learn and perform "skills previously monopolized by the professional medical establishment."[35]

The Somerville Women's Health Project occupied a position on the other side of the spectrum. Developed by middle-class and working-class women to be a "political women's health project in a working-class community," the project did not adhere to the self-help model embraced by many other feminist clinics. Instead, the Somerville clinic hired doctors, nurses, and lab techs to provide basic outpatient services for men, women, and children. Although the clinic provided basic health services, it concentrated on the issues common to women's clinics: reproductive health and gynecological screening. The project founders envisioned the clinic as a "base for pressuring the health system, for organizing women in the community, and a model of decent, democratically controlled women-run health care." Its relationship to the larger women's movement may have been vexed. Conversations about whether the project should encourage the development of women's liberation groups in the community apparently "sometimes led to splits and people leaving the Project."[36]

Emma Goldman (Chicago)'s rejection of medicine and the Somerville Project's embrace of it likely reflected their different class constituencies. The Somerville Project responded to the community's vast unmet health care needs, describing Boston as a health care oasis while neighboring Somerville was a "desert."[37] The community prioritized securing access to basic medicine rather than challenging its excesses. By contrast, Emma Goldman's clients could receive preventative care at the feminist clinic while presumably seeking care at other facilities for illness.

Feminist health clinics focused primarily on women's gynecological and reproductive care for many reasons. First, reproductive control was key to women's social and bodily autonomy. Without the ability to make reproductive choices, women's life choices were similarly constrained. Second, the gynecological exam, featuring a nearly naked woman with her feet in stirrups examined by a male doctor, demonstrated some of the most gross inequities in women's health care: men examining and judging parts of women's bodies that were literally and metaphorically inaccessible to them. Third, reproductive health issues marked a border between men's and women's health care. While other free clinics might treat bronchitis in men and women equally well, women benefited from distinctly feminist care for pelvic exams and diaphragm fittings. Finally, self-help had proved especially useful for routine gynecological examination, assessment, and treatment. Because reproductive health care focused largely on healthy women and offered a limited array of services, it was especially suited for lay health workers trained through self-help clinics.

Clinics extended the reach of feminist health politics beyond the gynecological self-exam. Yet for many health activists, clinical services often proved inhospitable to their political goals. As Hannah Dudley-Shotwell described it, "Moving gynecological self-help to a clinic setting meant compromise."[38] If they believed that women's health should be returned to women's hands, if they promoted self-help as a transformational tool for female empowerment, how did health services provided by others—sometimes men—fit with their agenda? Were they fomenting social change, or were they providing social services? These questions vexed many of the women who founded feminist health clinics.

To explore these tensions, let us now examine two women's health collectives as they enacted their version of feminist health care. Both groups created independent women's clinics, but they also developed other programming to increase women's investment in their health. The Santa Cruz Women's Health Collective, committed to self-help as a political tool for women's liberation, struggled mightily with the compromises direct services seemed to require. In contrast, the women of the Northcountry Clinic for Women and Children, who always sought to provide woman-centered health care by women, were thrilled to meet the health needs of women in their community.

Santa Cruz Women's Health Collective

Santa Cruz, California, located seventy-five miles south of San Francisco on the northern edge of Monterey Bay, was in decline. Once economically dependent on lumber and railroad money and then on tourism dollars, by the early 1960s, it had become a rundown beach and retirement town. When the Board of Regents of the University of California System announced the development of a new University of California campus, business interests in Santa Cruz lobbied hard for the city, seeing a new university as key to economic growth in the area. Their efforts paid off, and in the fall of 1965, 650 students attended the University of California, Santa Cruz.

The University of California, Santa Cruz (UCSC), was not exactly the campus that economic boosters had envisioned. The campus focused on the liberal arts rather than fields proven to support technological innovation and economic growth. It also eschewed many of the hallmarks of collegiate life that made college attractive to mainstream tastes. It sponsored no intercollegiate sports and supported no fraternities and sororities. Classroom achievement was graded pass/fail. It recognized no school mascot until 1981, when the banana slug became the school's unofficial symbol. In 1969, it developed a pathbreaking program in community studies, one that provided college credit for studying and engaging with local communities and their needs. This program encouraged community involvement while providing students with academic tools to understand and evaluate their experiences.

Energized by the escalation of the Vietnam War and the continuing fight for civil rights, young people across the country threw themselves into political battles for increased freedoms and against oppression. By the end of the 1960s, students at UCSC were among the most left-leaning in the nation. In 1970, for example, a survey of students at more than five hundred colleges found that 41 percent considered themselves liberal or Far Left in their political views. Nearly 83 percent of UCSC students, by contrast, identified as left-leaning. UCSC students were even more politically radical than their compatriots at the allegedly liberal bastion UC Berkeley. In 1974, 77.2 percent of Santa Cruz students identified as liberal or Far Left, compared to 49.1 percent of Berkeley students.[39]

The left-leaning university politics attracted other radicals and liberals to Santa Cruz, making it a hotbed for progressive politics of various stripes. Movements to increase the rights of farmworkers, support environmental activism, and eliminate nuclear energy all found a supportive home in Santa Cruz. Business interests and growth advocates, however, remained active, setting up significant town-and-gown conflicts so common in college communities.

At the beginning of the 1970s, women in Santa Cruz, like women across the nation, hoped to learn more about their bodies and make informed decisions about their health and their reproduction. Some had gotten ahold of a publication out of Boston, *Women and Their Bodies* (1970), and were sharing it among their friends. They used this "course" to educate themselves and each other. Other women in the area—including nurses working in prenatal care and midwives attending homebirths—came together and founded the Santa Cruz Birth Center (SCBC), which opened its doors in March 1971. The SCBC provided education, support, prenatal care, and, most controversially, assistance to women giving birth at home.[40]

In April 1971, word of Carol Downer's performance in Everywoman's Bookstore had reached Santa Cruz, and a group of women headed to Los Angeles to see a self-exam for themselves. They both discovered the wonders of their bodies and felt "an incredible well of rage" at the patriarchal forces that kept them ignorant and ashamed. They returned inspired by the potential power of self-help and eager to foment a self-help revolution in Santa Cruz. They created the Santa Cruz Women's Health Collective (SCWHC) to serve their revolutionary cause.[41]

Armed with a bag full of plastic specula and a determination to "empower" women, the SCWHC organized self-help groups. In these groups, women learned about their bodies, discussed their experiences with their bodies, and bonded with other women. They also developed a critique of the medical system, arguing that medicine profited from illness and ignorance and guarded access to information. Women, they discovered, were especially vulnerable to medical influence because physicians controlled most methods of reproductive control and childbirth practices. According to Kater Pollock, one of the early participants in the group, the intimacy of self-help and the dawning outrage fostered "a special feeling of sisterhood" among the women as they shared their joy, disappointment, and anger.[42]

As women in self-help groups learned about their bodies together, they vowed to do more to restore knowledge about women to women. Pregnancy screening proved vital in this process. Linda Bennett, whose experience with self-exam "was so mind bogglingly amazing . . . it became my life's work," resolved to find a way to circumvent medical control of pregnancy tests. Rejecting medical gatekeeping, Bennett acquired the equipment and knowledge needed to perform the tests and interpret the results. To round out their efforts, the women shared reviews of local doctors to warn women away from especially sexist or troubling physicians, and they staffed a "hotline" to answer health questions.[43]

Some of these women also served as community resources for information about and access to abortion in the years immediately before *Roe*. In 1967, California enacted the Therapeutic Abortion Act, which authorized abortions, pending approval from a hospital committee, in cases where "pregnancy will gravely impair the physical or mental health of the mother."[44] Because both hospitals in Santa Cruz were affiliated with religious groups, therapeutic abortions were not available within the city.[45] Bennett, who had navigated the process on her own behalf, helped other women find options elsewhere. She explained to historian Kline: "I would talk to people. . . . They would let me know what they wanted, I would show them what options there were for them and then if they wanted a ride I would pick them up."[46] The demand for counselors and rides to the Bay Area for abortion outstripped Bennett and other collective members' capacity to meet them. In the summer of 1972, they recruited other women to provide "sympathetic rides" to the Bay Area to prevent desperate women from hitchhiking.[47]

After the Supreme Court struck down state prohibitions of early abortions in 1973, self-help projects declined in Santa Cruz and abortion advocacy and counseling efforts intensified, attracting new women to the cause of bodily self-determination. These activists, most of them working outside of the established SCWHC, successfully lobbied the county health center to provide abortions and volunteered to provide counseling. Two Santa Cruz physicians also furnished abortions in their offices; feminist health advocates served as counselors in both settings. But these access points to abortion still failed to meet the local need. Health activists continued to transport women to the Bay Area for abortions, headed to the newly established Feminist Women's Health Center in Oakland, a 150-mile round trip.[48]

Although their work met crucial needs, some of the women grew tired of primarily guiding women through their individual health crises. They aspired to provide more comprehensive health services and information that increased women's control over their bodies and their lives. In the spring of 1973, the remaining members of the SCWHC and the women who had devoted themselves to abortion work came together to envision a feminist model of women's health under their control. They rededicated themselves to gynecological self-help, but they envisioned a broader and more ambitious program of educational outreach.[49]

By the fall, the reinvigorated SCWHC of about fifteen members (and growing) began in earnest the work of defining their project and their process. Primarily, they hoped to provide the tools to help women "take more control of their own health and lives in general." To make this possible, they sought to abolish "male-domination of both health institutions and society as a whole." In addition to ridding society of male domination, they also aimed to sever health care "from the profit-oriented economic system." Self-help and health education promised to move the SCWHC toward these goals.[50] By the end of the year, however, at least some of the members had grown frustrated by the limits of self-help and its inability to meet the health care needs of the women who sought their assistance. Self-help (at least, as they practiced it) had limited tools for contraception, for example, and it could not treat a sexually transmitted infection. At some point, one of the planners wondered aloud, "Why don't we start a clinic?"

Initially, most of the membership responded skeptically. Pollock recalled, "We were barely past being teenagers."[51] But eventually, their skepticism turned to excitement as they began to believe they could make it happen. They vowed to create a feminist gynecology clinic and an abortion clinic for the women of Santa Cruz. Robin Baker, an early member of the collective, said that they relied on the power of the "beautiful arrogance of youth" and the connection to a larger movement. As Baker described it, they believed women had a right to responsive and competent health care, even if they had to build it themselves. "So we'll just do it," they agreed. In retrospect, collective members remembered feeling "afraid we could never pull such an undertaking together, and at the same time unaware of the actual difficulties we would encounter."[52]

To better envision what feminist health services might entail, some of the Santa Cruz women spent time at the Oakland Feminist Women's Health Center (Oakland FWHC) learning about its gynecology and abortion clinics. The Oakland FWHC, founded in 1972, was closely associated with Carol Downer and the Southern California Feminist Women's Health Centers. (One of the founders of the Oakland FWHC was Carol Downer's daughter, Laura Brown.) Intrigued, the SCWHC considered joining forces with Oakland to create one organization with two clinics. Over time, however, they became increasingly skeptical of the politics of the Oakland organization. According to the Santa Cruz women, the Oakland FWHC women were too committed to seeing abortion as "no big deal" and too invested in the abortion "business."[53] They struck out on their own.

Designing Feminist Health Praxis

Even before they committed to creating a health clinic, the women of the collective believed that their goal—women's self-determination—required careful attention to the group's structure and process. As they put it, "The impact of social change institutions is measured not only by the direct work they do, but also by the working and personal relations between the people in them."[54]

They aimed to abandon traditional workplace models that valued competition, power differentials, efficiency, and specialization. After they reaffirmed their collective identity, they agreed to consensus-based decision-making because it provided an alternative to administrative hierarchy and the abuses of majority rule. Indeed, the SCWHC believed that "the *means* of reaching a decision [were] as important as the decision itself" because it allowed members to recognize and exercise power in a way that benefited everyone without "hierarchies and mystifications."[55]

Although former members of the SCWHC recalled that the collective process required meetings that went long into the night, filled with "talk talk talk talk," some of them nevertheless remember the process quite fondly.[56] Jody Peugh, for example, a member from early 1974 through 1983, found consensus-based decision-making "so equalizing" because members were "all involved in some kind of process together. There was something just so right about it."[57]

Collective members were also committed to the practice of criticism/self-criticism. Criticism/self-criticism was a process, frequently adopted by American groups on the Left, of holding movement people accountable.[58] Feminist groups frequently employed it as a vehicle for feedback, reflection, accountability, and praise. The SCWHC put it into practice by reserving time at the end of each meeting to debrief on the process and content of the meeting, to attend to the ambiguity and negativity produced, and to provide support for and criticism of individuals and the group.[59] According to Peugh, the process was "actually amazing [because it] kept things more honest." It gave people a pathway and a forum for sharing their admiration for each other and for airing grievances. As Peugh recalled, "[if someone] really hurt my feelings" and it was in some manner "holding me back . . . I'd say it in front of the group so that [they] could hear it. People would all know about it. It wasn't like this little secret. . . . That might have been a part of the secret of our longevity."[60] Other members found less to admire in the process. Some found it threatening and hurtful; sometimes it was merely "superficial and useless."[61]

The SCWHC's commitment to relationship-building extended beyond work. Ultimately, they hoped to reimagine relationships among women. They viewed themselves as woman-identified women. They described this position in 1976: "Our prime energy in our lives goes into women and/or women's struggles: we work with women, get a lot of our life support from women, often live with women." Women of the collective did not reject men as a group or necessarily eschew relationships with individual men. They did, however, reject much of what was understood as male and masculine in society.[62]

The term *woman-identified women* was coined by the Radicalesbians in 1970, in part to challenge straight-identified women's commitment to women's liberation. In the famous publication "Woman-Identified Woman," the Radicalesbians argued that "it is the primacy of women relating to women, of women creating a new consciousness of and with each other which is at the heart of women's liberation."[63] For the Radicalesbians, women's primary attachments to men in the midst of a culture of male supremacy indicated self-hate, an internal assessment that women were less than men. In contrast, women would be freed from male oppression and domination only by turning their energies away from men—the oppressor—and toward other women. Woman-identified women—those truly fighting for the liberation of women—needed to form their primary relationships, sexual and otherwise, with other women. A woman-identified woman in this concept was not synonymous with a lesbian; it did, however, require withdrawing sexual and emotional energies from men. Not all the Santa Cruz women identified as lesbians, and some continued relationships with men. But their embrace of the woman-identified woman construct suggests their commitment to politicizing their personal lives and devoting their lives to the liberation of women.

To facilitate their commitment to each other, some of the women structured their living arrangements to reflect their politics, organizing their personal lives to reflect their political aims. They sought to "spend time and energy" in each other's lives beyond running the collective.[64] "We consider how we live to be an on-going, changing process which we want to integrate with our theoretical development."[65] To this end, by the spring of 1974, nearly half of the then twenty-nine women in the SCWHC lived with at least one other collective member; one household included six collective members. SCWHC members also frequently explored a variety of relationships with each other, including sexual connections. Pollock noted, "On a variety of different levels we shared incredible love for each other."[66]

Their commitment to love preceded a more particular political vision: they developed a feminist politics and a vision for how they wanted "things to change" through a collective process of study and discussion. By April 1974, they had labeled their political framework "socialist feminism." Precisely what this meant to the individual collective members probably varied significantly. The label provided the flexibility to accommodate a variety of political commitments that focused on the need for women's liberation and an end to capitalist oppression. To the SCWHC, it signaled a political awareness of the structures of oppression within and beyond patriarchy. Pollock wrote, "It helped us see that our struggle as women was linked to the struggles of blacks, Chicanos, people of Third World countries, workers and other oppressed peoples." The feminist aspect of socialist feminism validated the SCWHC dedication to a woman-centered politics. Again, according to Pollock, "feminism was . . . a very personal way for us as women to work against all oppression; it was the most basic, powerful way to fight against our own oppression." In practice, this designation signaled political aspirations beyond feminist health care, connected the SCWHC with a larger feminist movement, and provided a syllabus for further political education.[67]

This political commitment to socialist feminism lacked a clear theoretical foundation. Nevertheless, it demonstrates the collective's commitment to feminist praxis. Because each member entered the SCWHC with different political views and goals for the collective, the process of education, discussion, and negotiation brought them together in a shared political and personal process of discovery and commitment. In the end, it signaled their desire for social change rather than an alignment with any particular strategy for revolution. As Pollock described it, "[We] took the name and vowed to make it continue to mean what we wanted it to."[68]

Feminist Self-Help and Embodied Education

In the beginning and throughout the SCWHC's first decade, its membership was remarkably homogeneous. Almost all the members were young, white, middle-class women with at least some college education. Many were college graduates, hoping to find a way to stay in Santa Cruz. Only a few were mothers. Nevertheless, they joined the SCWHC for a variety of reasons. Some brought a keen interest in health and health care; others sought a feminist cause and a feminist community. Robin Baker joined in 1971 when she was still in college. Her eyes had been opened by an early edition of *Our Bodies, Ourselves*, and she was outraged by how little control women had over their reproduction. She eagerly sought self-education initiatives, and she embraced the shift to providing woman-centered health care. When Colleen Douglas graduated from UCSC in 1975, she was looking to join something "political, a change movement," and she thought the "women's health collective was pretty much the main exciting thing going on at the time." Linda Wilshusen, who joined in 1974, wanted to be part of the feminist effort to give women information about and control of their bodies. She wanted to "work with women on something that was meaningful." Jody Peugh joined the SCWHC because she wanted to explore her identity as a woman. Some were especially focused on rejecting medical care as usual and creating alternative health institutions. Others saw abortion access and provision as their primary political goal. Still others embraced the feminist politics at the heart of the women's health movement.[69]

The members' interests influenced their work assignments within the

SCWHC. Their distinct but complementary concerns and priorities guided the organization of separate "working groups" within the larger collective, devoted both to areas of service (e.g., abortion, clinical services, and outreach/ education) and to particular tasks within each area (e.g., newsletter production, self-help facilitation, and clinic scheduling). These working groups, sometimes understood as mini-collectives, allowed members to engage with different kinds of health activism while furthering the SCWHC's larger goals. While these groups encouraged intergroup bonding, significant tensions also developed among groups, as members of each mini-collective felt overworked and undervalued by members of other groups. These groups changed over time as the priorities and budget of the SCWHC changed.

Politically if not always in practice, self-help remained the guiding principle of the SCWHC, even after it began to offer clinical services. In a document written in 1974 to support the Santa Cruz Birth Center after the arrest of three midwives, the SCWHC explained self-help and its significance:

> Self-help means that instead of turning our bodies over to professionals for diagnosis and treatment in which we take no part, we look to ourselves for knowledge and we make our own decisions about how to care for our bodies. This is a revolutionary concept in American medicine, a medicine that is built on profit, hierarchy, and mystification. We refuse to be consumers, even informed consumers any longer; health care is not a product to be packaged and sold. Healthy bodies are our human right; medical knowledge and skills should be freely accessible to every person, whether or not she or he has a license from the state. Self-help means that we share all knowledge and skills with each other and all women.[70]

This dense statement presented key problems with medicine—its embrace of profit, mystification of knowledge, and alliance with the state—and proposed self-help as a "revolutionary" challenge to medical prerogatives. Self-help encouraged women to be curious about their bodies, share their knowledge with others, and fully participate in their bodily care. Self-help galvanized many of the Santa Cruz women into lives of activism, and it guided many of the projects, at least for the first few years.

The goal of the self-help education group was to bring self-help into the community, to "proselytize," as Wilshusen put it. The health center offered drop-in self-help workshops, which generally lasted six or seven weeks. In addition to demonstrating self-exam, the very popular classes also covered a variety of political and health-focused topics. At one point, there were more than one hundred women on the waiting list for these classes.[71]

Wilshusen was especially grateful for the opportunities these classes gave women to reflect on their lives and to share their own stories. As she put it, "A lot of us had our own . . . personal experiences of not knowing what was going on with our body," and that ignorance sometimes resulted in pregnancy or an aversion to sex. "You know, everybody had their own personal story and . . . part of these groups was people telling their story." For Wilshusen, then, these courses provided women an "opportunity to reflect" on their relationship with their bodies, share their stories about their bodies, and consider alternatives. These experiences bonded women together and empowered them to change their lives. After Peugh saw her own cervix in a self-help group, she immediately understood self-exam as a tool for demystifying women's bodies and for encouraging women to take a more active role in their health. She just kept saying to herself, "Oh, my God! Everybody needs to do this." Her enthusiasm for self-help was infectious. She "loved" teaching self-help classes including self-exam because it enabled her to help "people get over being afraid of themselves." (Efforts to convince her mother, however, were rebuffed.) Overall, the women of the SCWHC saw self-exam and self-help as intimate tools for political action.[72]

The self-help/education group also developed and disseminated feminist health materials. One of its first projects was a self-help booklet. This 1974 project began as Robin Baker's senior thesis as a community studies major.[73] The self-help/education group subsequently published pamphlets on the gynecological checkup (1975), herpes (1976), pelvic inflammatory disease (1978), and, most famously, lesbian health (1978). It also established and sustained a newsletter, running from 1976 through the summer of 1986, providing information about the SCWHC and its process, local health care stories, and political commentary on the medical-industrial complex.

WomanKind Health Clinics

The effort to promote self-help and develop educational materials encouraged creativity and exploration. The women involved did not have to worry about billing, licensing, or the bureaucratic demands of nonprofit organizations. Starting a health clinic, on the other hand, was a completely different undertaking, requiring skills and know-how that the collective members initially didn't have. Indeed, they had very little sense of where to start. Find a building? Raise money? Hire physicians? Incorporate? It all felt overwhelming to this group of young women. But they persevered. They spread a wide net to secure funds, applying to both the UCSC and the progressive Vanguard Foundation for grants, appealing to their friends and families for loans, and selling T-shirts, pancakes, and dance tickets for donations.[74]

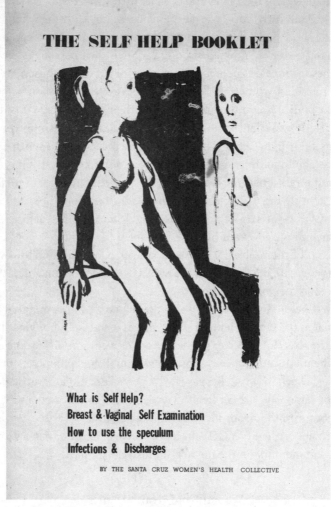

FIGURE 2.1. The original SCWHC self-help publication began as a senior thesis in the Community Studies Program at UCSC. Permission by Santa Cruz Community Health.

Becoming a legal entity created another set of hurdles, both practical and political. Although the women of the SCWHC legally needed to create a health center to operate the clinic, they resented the mandatory relationship with the state. Their resentment grew after an initial consultation with a lawyer who informed them that incorporation as a nonprofit required a hierarchically arranged board of directors; they could not incorporate as a collective. In the end, the collective created a titular board composed of SCWHC members. While the board would provide legal cover, the collective itself would govern the Santa Cruz Women's Health Center, incorporated in March 1974.[75]

Becoming a legal entity also required licensing. The health center had two options: it could become licensed as a medical clinic, a multistep and time-consuming process; or it could work under a physician's license, treating the clinic as the medical office of the physician. The SCWHC choose the latter option in the short term, hoping to eventually acquire a clinic license. Both options required medical participation. With this decision, the SCWHC compromised—perhaps abandoned—an early guiding belief that working with physicians compromised their position as an "alternative" to the medical mainstream.[76]

Now a legal entity, the Santa Cruz Women's Health Center scrambled to make final arrangements for a June opening. In May, the SCWHC signed a five-year lease on office space at 250 Locust Street in Santa Cruz.[77] Despite the odds, in June, the center opened WomanKind, offering general gynecological care one day a week.

The women of the SCWHC understood WomanKind as an extension of their political work. They envisioned a clinic space that enacted the principles of self-help and furthered women's empowerment and bodily autonomy. According to Pollock, "We had the idea that women should participate in their own health care as equals. And that the woman who was the patient would be fully respected and have control over the decisions that were being made for her body." To encourage a deprofessionalized, egalitarian approach to health care, the SCWHC planned to use lay health care workers to provide routine gynecological screening and basic reproductive health tasks (e.g., fitting a cervical cap). This reflected the practice of many feminist and free clinics of the moment. Indeed, for some feminist health clinics, the provision of health care by lay health workers—modeling the democratization of medical knowledge—served as a lynchpin to avoid re-creating the very power differentials typical of medical care as usual.[78]

And yet, the women of the Santa Cruz Women's Health Center abandoned their plans before WomanKind even opened, rattled by a "bust" of home-birth midwives working through the Santa Cruz Birth Center. An undercover sting operation in March 1974, led to the arrest of three midwives for allegedly practicing medicine without a license. Over the next three years, the courts considered women's ability to choose where they wanted to give birth and with what assistance and midwives' right to provide assistance at birth without state licensure.[79]

The women of the health collective understood the relevance of the case to their work and to the women's health movement more generally. They issued a position statement:

> The Birth Center arrests represent a grave threat to the work of the Santa Cruz
> Women's Health Collective and the feminist health movement. . . . If selective
> enforcement of these laws continues, we could be prevented from opening our
> clinic and providing services which the community greatly needs. . . . These
> are not just three individual women; it is the entire feminist health care move-
> ment on trial.[80]

The state's action created a crisis for the SCWHC, which discovered in the aftermath of the arrests that it, too, had been infiltrated by state agents. The group understood that the state was invested in "maintaining a hierarchal medical model and preventing women from controlling their own lives"[81] and that they risked arrest if they enacted their vision. After a series of wrenching meetings, the SCWHC chose to avoid arrest and closure by toeing the legal line. They would not use lay health workers without medical oversight. The SCWHC understood that this position "compromised" their ability to demonstrate women's capacity to gain the skills and exercise their right to control their own health care. Without this exercise of self-help, the SCWHC struggled to find the political value of their clinical services.

The women of the SCWHC had always agreed to bring health care professionals into the clinic, seeing it as a necessary concession to the state. They understood that without "[health] professionals, the Collective would not be able to offer alternative services in any form at all, and the conservative medical establishment would remain in firm control." In fact, they hoped that they would gain "legitimacy" from their association with medical professionals.[82] So they tried to hire physicians and nurses and other midlevel health care workers who shared their vision and politics. Their efforts to recruit women physicians failed; the SCWHC eventually located a local male doctor to provide gynecological care and an out-of-town male physician to provide abortions.

Although the SCWHC had hoped to employ health professionals who shared their political ideals, here, too, they largely failed. The doctors and nurse practitioners (and eventually physician assistants) generally supported the clinic's emphasis on preventative care and believed that clients should learn from their medical encounter. They sometimes "disagreed sharply" about other issues, however, including the socialist-feminist politics of the SCWHC and its critique of the health care establishment.[83]

By their own assessment, the SCWHC felt that by hiring health care professionals, they "acceded to the medical establishment's control over who provides diagnosis and treatment."[84] To compensate, the collective members tried to find other ways to demonstrate their commitment to women's empowerment. To that end, they established a policy of shared clinical decision-making where the physician or nurse, the SCWHC health worker, and the patient shared power equally. This commitment, too, was short-lived, as one clinical encounter challenged the practicality of their vision. At the gynecology clinic, a woman who had recently been diagnosed with gonorrhea asked to be fitted with an IUD. The health worker explained that an IUD was contra-indicated because it would likely cause reinfection. Nevertheless, the "woman remained adamant." The health worker agreed but insisted that the women sign a waiver acknowledging the risks and agreeing not to hold the clinic responsible if infection ensued. The doctor, however, refused. According to Pollock, "At that moment, a certain clarity of vision dissolved. . . . We couldn't say either we're empowering women or we're harming women. We began to see how you could make a wrong decision while empowering a woman." They realized that their current analysis was not yet "sophisticated enough" to understand how to weigh women's rights to make decisions about their body against the SCWHC's responsibility to avoid causing harm. In the aftermath of this incident, the SCWHC concluded that clinical power could not and should not be shared equally when expertise was not equal. They also realized that they could never force professional health care workers to provide care they viewed as medically irresponsible. As a result, the SCWHC returned medical decision-making more fully to professional health workers.[85]

Within months of opening WomanKind, the women of the SCWHC realized that their dreams for providing clinical services infused with feminist politics had fallen short. They had abandoned their vision for lay health workers and shared medical decision-making, and they realized that the clinic's limited scope could not meet women's diverse health needs. In turn, some of the women grew dissatisfied, sometimes wondering what the point was.[86] They continued nevertheless, looking for opportunities to provide a feminist health care experience.

To showcase their vision of health care, the SCWHC instituted a monthly Participatory Annual Gyn Exam Clinic, later referred to as the Well-Woman Clinic. Presumably modeled on the participatory clinic developed by the Los Angeles FWHC, the Santa Cruz version welcomed two groups of four women for a hybrid self-help workshop and gynecological exam. In addition to learning and performing some basic procedures—breast and vaginal self-exam, Pap smears, bimanual pelvic exams—the participants also received political education about reproductive oppression, medical abuses, and profit's perversion of health care. Physicians were present for these clinics, but SCWHC members generally kept them out of sight. (Curious or bored doctors apparently sometimes wandered into exam rooms uninvited.)[87]

Participatory clinic helped the women of the SCWHC deliver politics in a clinical or quasi-clinical setting, and they believed it helped align Woman-Kind with their vision for it. But it did not eliminate their "dissatisfaction" with the clinic. Pollock said, "We were beginning to feel that women just saw us as another doctor's office. Many of them simply handed their power over to us rather than the doctor."[88] This reflection captures the difficulty of enacting self-help politics within a health services model.

In November, members' dissatisfaction had reached a breaking point. Running a clinic with a largely volunteer staff, most of whom required intense on-the-job training, proved stressful and exhausting. Deferring to medical judgment proved politically unfulfilling. These difficulties loomed especially large because many SCWHC members were increasingly unsure that "service work" furthered the SCWHC's political goals; they wondered "what was so revolutionary about a groovy, woman-run gyn office." The SCWHC closed the gynecology clinic in December 1974 to evaluate the clinic's protocols, reassess the SCWHC's ambitions for the clinic, and consider the clinic's ability to meet its goals.[89] Although this was intended as a short-term shutdown, licensing problems kept the gynecology clinic closed until December 1976, when it reopened under the medical license of a local doctor, Peter Nash.[90]

Providing Abortions at WomanKind

WomanKind opened its gynecology clinic in June 1974. The abortion clinic opened a few weeks later, in early July. Abortion provision had always been a goal of the women involved with the SCWHC, many of whom had launched their activism by guiding women to safe, affordable, and respectful abortion care before and after *Roe*. Their vision for WomanKind, then, included abortion provision for both political and practical reasons. The SCWHC's political commitment to women's autonomy, empowerment, and self-determination and its practical need to generate income led the SCWHC into the abortion marketplace. Despite their denigration of the Oakland FWHC on just this point, abortion paid the bills.[91] Bringing this vision to life, however, proved more difficult than they had anticipated.

Finding physicians to perform abortions at WomanKind posed the first obstacle. The Santa Cruz medical community was generally hostile to abortion, and the two local physicians who provided abortions in their offices refused to work at the SCWHC. Because no local physician would provide

abortions at WomanKind, the SCWHC hired a physician from the San Francisco Bay Area, seventy-five miles away. While this solved the immediate
problem, the SCWHC also struggled to secure local backup care in case complications arose after the abortion provider left town. Eventually, two local
physicians agreed to provide backup care unofficially; they stipulated that
they not be called often.[92]

To make medical abortion provision consistent with their commitment to
self-help, the women of the SCWHC tried to control abortion protocols. Like
many other feminist health clinics, they treated the abortion-providing physician "as a technician," discouraging him from even speaking to the client.[93] As
you might imagine, this caused significant friction between the SCWHC and
its physician. The SCWHC felt a great deal of pressure to avoid any abortion
complications, however minor, so the women frequently lashed out at the
doctor, questioning his skill and demanding that he be perfect. Unsurprisingly, he frequently threatened to quit.[94]

Despite the SCWHC's efforts, within months of opening, one of the abortion patients at WomanKind experienced a significant complication.[95] This
gave the State of California the ammunition it needed to deny WomanKind
a clinic license, citing lack of medical backup for the abortions. The abortion clinic closed in March 1975.[96] For at least a year, the SCWHC scrambled
to find a local doctor to provide backup, even reaching out to physicians in
neighboring counties. They tried to recruit newly graduated physicians to
move to Santa Cruz to work at the clinic. After searching for a year, they
gave up, blaming medical hostility to both abortion and feminist health care.
Womankind never resumed its abortion service. As a result, abortions could
be secured at only three locations in Santa Cruz County: the county STOP
(Selective Termination of Pregnancy) clinic and two general practitioners'
offices.[97]

The SCWHC did not abandon abortion work entirely. Indeed, abortions
remained crucial to the financial health of WomanKind. Beginning in the
spring of 1975, women from the SCWHC again began escorting women to
abortion clinics in the larger San Francisco Bay Area.[98] For providing the referral, transport, and counseling, the SCWHC received $45 per patient.[99] The
members tried to put a positive spin on their diminished involvement with
abortion care. As Robin Baker described it, "Providing access [to abortion]
in a very Catholic-dominated community that absolutely barred it . . . felt like
a very political act . . . more than a service act."[100] Baker's comment suggests
that while the distinction between politics and service worried these women,
the division on the ground became hard to maintain.

Financing the Clinic, Paying the Workers

The Santa Cruz Women's Health Center kept afloat its first few months on individual grants. After the clinics opened, the center came to rely on Medi-Cal reimbursements and fees charged on a sliding scale for clinic services. The center also charged for its ovulation method of fertility awareness classes and, after WomanKind's abortion clinic closed, for abortion referrals and counseling. Eventually, the SCWHC also received county revenue-sharing funds for their educational projects.[101]

By the fall of 1974, the clinical services began to cover their own overhead, allowing the SCWHC to consider paying wages to its members as accounts receivable exceeded accounts payable. Members of the collective had always hoped to pay themselves for their labor, especially because they recognized that women's work was "consistently underpaid and undervalued." They also understood that financial inequity left women with less social and personal power. Still, the health center never brought in enough funds to pay all the members, so the SCWHC embarked on a frequently revised and often contentious effort to develop criteria for deciding which members received payment for their labor.[102]

Three basic proposals emerged to guide which SCWHC members should be paid. Some members argued that women who provided the most "value" to the collective—determined by their seniority, commitment to the collective's future, and level of responsibility—should be rewarded with payment. Other members objected, claiming that all members were equally valuable to the organization and that wage decisions should be determined by political goals rather than by ephemeral contributions to the collective. They suggested that wages might be paid based on financial need or to meet diversity goals. Still others argued that all members be paid and that surplus funds be divided equally among the membership. This proposal drew little support, because it would have afforded token payments for everyone rather than providing a living wage for any.[103]

None of these suggestions were codified into policy. In practice, decisions were made on a case-by-case basis as members requested wages. The decisions were always contentious—wages in the SCWHC became conflated with value. The de facto policy that the clinic workers deserved wages more than the educational workers proved especially divisive. Clinic workers tended to work more hours than those in the education groups and were therefore less likely to hold other jobs. They also contributed to the clinic's income. But the education group believed they were primarily responsible for maintaining the SCWHC's political work and therefore resented their lack of compensation.[104]

Paying some but not all the members of the SCWHC wages created unforeseen problems. Unsurprisingly, resentment grew between paid and unpaid members, as paid workers could afford to dedicate more time to the organization and gain more responsibility and (unrecognized) power. Unpaid workers felt underappreciated by the collective because they were not remunerated. The members also discovered that their new identities as "workers" sometimes conflicted with the needs of the organization. This emerged most intensely over the issue of job security. Receiving wages for SCWHC work allowed some members to quit other jobs to dedicate themselves the collective, yet their wages were available only when the clinic was thriving.[105] Would members be subjected to layoffs as finances weakened? The answer proved to be yes.

The Rise of the Clinic and the Decline of Self-Help

From the time it resumed clinical services in December 1976 through 1978, the Santa Cruz Women's Health Center continued its gynecological services and its educational outreach. It established a newsletter and developed new educational pamphlets addressing herpes and pelvic inflammatory disease.[106] The health center also sponsored self-help clinics and workshops and launched a lecture series on a variety of topics of interest to women. In addition, it offered a monthly fertility awareness training to give women and couples a noncontraceptive method of fertility control.[107]

By the end of 1978, the SCWHC suffered a drastic cut in funding that reshaped its services. In June, California voters passed Proposition 13, a form of property tax relief that decimated state funding for education and a variety of other programs.[108] A conservative shift on the Santa Cruz County Board of Supervisors channeled increasingly scarce resources away from radical causes.[109] In anticipation of the funding cuts looming with the passage of this law, the SCWHC scrambled to reorganize its services.[110] It increased its medical services, including abortion counseling, and broadened the kinds of health issues that could be brought to the clinic, including ear, nose, throat, and skin problems.[111] This gave the clinic access to more funds, both from fees-for-service and from increased access to Medi-Cal reimbursement.

While support for clinical services increased, educational programs suffered.[112] In August 1978, the Santa Cruz County Board of Supervisors withdrew all its funding for the Women's Health Education Project, which had supported the educational mission of the health center.[113] This cut of nearly $25,000 from its budget essentially gutted the educational programming.[114] The self-help programs were eliminated (perhaps also reflecting decreased community interest), and other projects, including the pamphlets and the newsletter, were significantly curtailed.[115]

This loss of funds required a careful audit of their finances. The health center's bookkeeping had been fairly loose, but the financial emergency required a disciplined approach. Linda Wilshusen took over the books and found that the SCWHC had been on a "completely unsustainable" trajectory: "We were paying . . . something like fifteen, eighteen people, and we could afford to pay like six."[116] This led to drastic cuts. In February 1979, the majority of the SCWHC (sixteen members) received wages (up to $360 a month to work up to thirty hours a week); in the aftermath of the funding cut from the county and the financial reckoning, the SCWHC began paying four members $5.15 per hour.[117]

These budget cuts—shrinking the SCWHC's involvement with educational projects and drastically reducing the collective's ability to pay its members a living wage—marked a turning point in the SCWHC's history. Members who had brought to the collective their hopes for institutionalizing self-help, educational outreach, and abortion access wondered what had happened to their vision. Throughout the organization's history, the women of the SCWHC struggled to bring their political mission of female self-determination into clinic spaces. They worked creatively to retain their focus on self-help and feminist health education as tools for social change and women's liberation. By the end of 1978, the Santa Cruz Women's Health Center provided health care; but for many collective members, health care had never been enough. From this moment of mission uncertainty, further challenges—this time to their collective structure—were on the horizon.[118]

The Santa Cruz Women's Health Collective created a health center and a health clinic to bring feminist health politics, education, and services to the women of Santa Cruz. Committed to the power and promise of self-help as an embodied feminist practice of knowledge creation and transmission, the women of the collective developed courses and materials to give women more understanding of their bodies and more control of their lives. Some of their educational materials represented milestones in the women's health movement. Ambitions for feminist health services, however, were frequently thwarted by some of the very elements animating their critique of medicine. Although women of the collective aimed to democratize medical knowledge and skills, as they sought to deprofessionalize health care, as they tried to give women more decision-making power, state supports for medical prerogatives intervened.

Their project, however, was never exclusively about pamphlets, specula, or reproductive health care. It was never exclusively about health. The women of the SCWHC strove to live woman-identified lives, enacting policies and processes that valued all members' perspectives. Their commitment to the collective, to consensus-based decision-making, and to their entwined lives marked their dedication to feminist praxis within and beyond their health movement goals.

Health Activism in California's Far North

In Arcata, California, a college town 350 miles north of Santa Cruz, a different group of women launched their own feminist health care experiment, first at the Humboldt Open Door Clinic and later at the Northcountry Clinic for Women and Children. The women in Arcata shared with the Santa Cruz Women's Health Collective a desire for social change and a commitment to returning women's health to women's hands. They, too, had seen their cervices and encouraged women to shed their bodily shame. But if the women in Santa Cruz saw clinical services as a means to an end, the women in Arcata viewed feminist health care as an end in itself. They created a lay health worker training program and a health clinic that supported women's self-determination while also meeting local health needs.

In the early 1970s, Arcata was a small town of nine thousand people, known for its hippies, its college, and its marijuana—hallmarks that occasionally caused friction between the city and other communities in the rest of this rural, largely working-class area in the far northwestern part of the state.[119] Arcata embraced, and sometimes led, many of the countercultural projects of the moment. By 1973, it boasted a grocery co-op, a nonprofit recycling center, and an environmental center.

It also supported a variety of health care experiments. In the late 1960s and early '70s, the city of Arcata and other communities in Humboldt County nurtured, for example, a loosely aligned home-birth midwife community. These midwives came to the work through a variety of avenues. Some learned midwifery in the aftermath of finding themselves unexpectedly at a birth. Another had been on the margins of the community of midwives in Santa Cruz. Still others were trained by and worked with former Vietnam War-conscientious-objector-medic-turned-midwife William Fisher. Fisher, who both inspired admiration and condemnation from the women midwives in the community, ran a midwifery school out of his house in Arcata. Although Fisher usefully publicized midwifery and home birth and provided strong technical training, several of the local midwives denigrated his approach to midwifery as "reactionary and male" and "too alternative groovy."[120] Local law enforcement and the medical community also had issues with Fisher. In 1975, he was charged and recharged with multiple counts of practicing medicine without a license and possessing obstetric drugs with the intent to distribute.[121]

Activists also developed innovative care for the many Native American people from several nations in the area. After federal termination in the mid-1950s, many Native communities in California were left without federal health resources. Not surprisingly, health surveys conducted after termination documented deteriorating health conditions among California Indians. In response, the California Department of Public Health initiated in 1968 a Rural Indian Health Demonstration Project to document and address the health needs of Native Americans at nine different locations. In 1969, this project gained independent status under the direction of the California Rural Indian Health Board. Although this organization became a crucial resource to Native communities throughout California, its initial projects left Northern California Indians significantly underserved.[122]

Even before the Department of Public Health began its demonstration projects, individuals from the Yurok, Karuk, Tolowa, and Wiyot communities in Humboldt and Del Norte Counties envisioned a collaborative, inter-tribal approach toward meeting the health care needs of Northern California Indians. In 1969, this group partnered with the Center for Community Development at Humboldt State College, an organization to provide services and outreach to Northern California Indian communities, to create an intertribal model of health care provision. They applied for funding through the Regional Medical Programs (one of President Lyndon Johnson's "Great Society" programs) to train community health workers, organize transportation for health referrals, and establish a medical and dental clinic staffed by local providers, "Flying Samaritans," and community volunteers.[123] In 1970, in part to apply for newly available federal money, the group incorporated as the United Indian Health Services (UIHS).[124]

These health projects document the region's comfort with health care experimentation, especially in the context of intense need. They also suggest that Humboldt County's geographical isolation from urban centers may have encouraged a health politics, including a feminist health politics, unbeholden to any particular party line. Health activists in Arcata, while clearly part of a larger women's health movement, enacted a feminist politics influenced by local possibilities, circumstances, and needs.

Women's Health at Humboldt Open Door Clinic

In 1971, members of Arcata's "young idealistic counter-culture" decided to put into practice their belief that "all people had the right to healthcare, not just those who could afford it," and founded Humboldt Open Door Clinic.[125] The clinic was designed for "people with problems who feel they might be 'turned down' or 'turned off' elsewhere."[126] The founders envisioned a clinic that addressed a full range of medical, psychological, and economic problems; but in the early months, it served largely as a referral service "where people could get information about anything from pregnancy testing to food stamps."[127] By 1973, the clinic had recruited a few local physician volunteers, allowing the clinic to expand the range of its services. In addition to providing legal advice and welfare counseling, it also offered a full range of medical services including clinics that provided prenatal and well-baby care, pediatric care, drug abuse treatment, and various gynecological services.[128] For a while the clinic even offered obstetrics.[129]

The clinic staff came from a variety of backgrounds, linked perhaps by radical politics but little else. Suzanne Willow was one of the clinic's early volunteers. She had started her work in health care by volunteering at the Humboldt County Health Department. Willow had very little initial interest in health, but she signed up to spend time with the mother of a recently deceased friend. At the health department, she assisted the physicians, especially in gynecological exams, serving as both a chaperone and a helping hand. She joined Open Door while it was still an idea when Richard Casey, one of the physicians at the health department, invited her to participate in the planning. She eventually became Open Door's clinic manager. Susan Riesel was also an early volunteer. Riesel had moved from New York City to San Francisco in the late 1960s with increasingly radical politics and a desire "to become a hippie." After a few years, Riesel and her boyfriend moved to Humboldt County, eager to be "in nature" and looking for a political cause. After a stint working at a local alternative school, she learned that the new Open Door Clinic was seeking volunteers. Riesel joined up, administering pregnancy tests and contraceptive counseling. She even began to provide therapy. "I did lay therapy. People who just wanted to talk. Any bartender can do that, right?" Deborah Sweitzer also worked at the clinic in the early years. Sweitzer, an almost-graduate of University of California, Santa Barbara, found herself stranded in Humboldt County when her car broke down during a road trip. She learned about Open Door Clinic through her car mechanic, and she quickly joined the staff as a VISTA volunteer.[130]

Gena Pennington, a 1970 graduate from St. Louis University Medical School, was one of the early physician recruits. One of fifteen women students in her medical school, Pennington remembers hearing repeatedly that she "took a good man's place." To combat this hostility, she and several of her female classmates "got really rebellious," taking on a variety of causes,

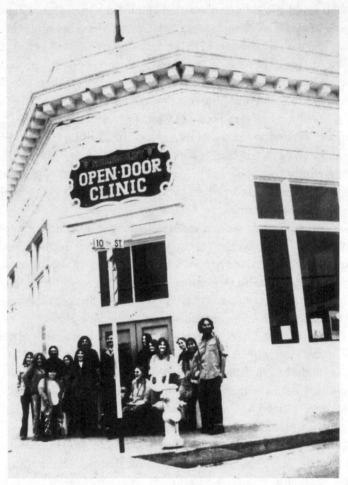

FIGURE 2.2. An early image of the Humboldt Open Door Clinic in Arcata, California. Note the countercultural presentation. Permission by Cheyenne Spetzler, Open Door Community Health Centers.

including protesting the Vietnam War and wearing pants to a Saturday lab
class. After she graduated, friends and acquaintances continued to denigrate
her achievement, insisting that she must have "slept her way through medical
school. . . . They *told* me that's what I did!"

After graduation, Pennington moved to the Berkeley area. Irritated by her
experiences with sexism, Pennington was receptive to the feminist politics
of the moment. She read Shulamith Firestone's *Dialectic of Sex* (1970) and
remembers thinking, "Whoa. This is good! . . . I'm a liberated woman." While
Pennington did not immerse herself in feminist theory, she nevertheless believed that women approached problem-solving differently than men: "You

put a bunch of women together, they work together. You put a bunch of men together, somebody has to be boss."[131]

She had started her medical career working as a resident at Kaiser Permanente in Oakland, but she soon decided she could not stand "four more years getting screamed at all night long, every other night." She took a year off from her residency and came to Humboldt County to visit her sister and "never left." She found part-time work at the Humboldt County Health Department staffing its women's clinic. Looking for additional work, Pennington apparently "wandered into" Open Door and asked whether she could be of use. Initially, Pennington was unsure about the clinic's atmosphere. Like so many other health clinic projects of the time, Open Door was inspired by the Chinese Revolution and the "barefoot doctors." As Pennington, who was not enamored with communism or collective decision-making, described it, "People were wearing these Mao jackets . . . and walking around with Little Red Books."[132] Nevertheless, she wanted to be of use, and she needed a job.

Because she was a woman and a doctor, Pennington was immediately pegged as someone who could attract female patients to the clinic. Clinic personnel asked her to lead a new initiative, running a state-sponsored family planning clinic. Pennington, although she had no formal training in "women's health" beyond her work at the county, gamely agreed.[133]

Many health institutions, including Open Door, relied on Title X funds. Established in 1970, the federal Title X Family Planning Program, otherwise known as the Family Planning Services and Public Research Act, funneled federal funds to health clinics to provide "family planning" services. Funded services included contraceptives as well as breast and pelvic examinations, blood pressure screenings, and Pap tests. Federally funded contraceptive health services provided the gateway for basic health care for many women and enabled many clinics to survive.[134]

Pennington's arrival and the development of a family planning clinic—a clinic that also provided basic gynecological screening—inspired the creation of a Women's Health Collective within Open Door. Over time, women in the collective asked for more training in women's health care so that they could help provide services. Perhaps the impetus came from Suzanne Willow. Willow had learned some women's health basics while volunteering at the county health department. One of the doctors there had said to her one day, "Well, why don't I teach you?" He showed her how to do various procedures, teaching her how to do breast exams, Pap smears, and speculum exams, but he drew the line at bimanual exams. "It's just too hard to teach you bimanual exams," he said without offering further explanation. When Willow and some other women at Open Door asked to learn more, Pennington didn't see why they shouldn't. She, too, had needed to be trained to perform bimanual exams and other procedures after she began seeing women patients. Consequently, she started providing a "crash course in office gynecology," teaching the interested women how to perform pelvic and other examinations. "We had pelvic parties. We would have a potluck, and then someone would lay down on the kitchen table and everybody would do a pelvic on 'em—including me."[135] At some point, the women who had been trained at these pelvic parties began performing health screening exams in the clinic.

Legitimating Lay Workers: Women's Health Care Specialists

In the beginning, no one appeared too concerned that laywomen performed pelvic exams in the family planning clinic. Eventually, however, an administrator, worried about the legality of the practice, suggested that they protect themselves and the clinic by taking advantage of California's Experimental Health Manpower Act, Assembly Bill 1503.[136]

California's Experimental Health Manpower Act responded to the alleged shortage of physicians in the state, especially in rural areas and among poor communities. Too many patients were demanding too many procedures from too few doctors. In 1966, the National Advisory Commission on Health Manpower concluded, "There *is* a crisis in American health care."[137] To cope with the crisis, physicians and hospitals reconsidered which health care procedures required a physician's expertise. Informally, physicians and hospitals began to assign nurses technical tasks that had once been understood as medical. More formally, physicians, hospitals, and medical schools established experimental training programs that shifted or expanded the roles of people with some health care experience.

Developed in 1972 and enacted in 1973, California's Experimental Health Manpower Act simultaneously confronted the shortage of medical professionals in the state and addressed the large number of midlevel health professionals who routinely worked beyond their scope of practice. The act approved the training and licensing of a variety of midlevel health workers and provided a "legal umbrella" over a range of current practices that were technically illegal (or at least ambiguous) when performed by trainees in or graduates of those programs.[138] These programs created new midlevel positions and gave other, more established positions (e.g., nurses, nurse practitioners, physician assistants, and dental professionals) expanded responsibilities and opportunities. Although the Experimental Health Manpower Act invited creative and innovative alternatives to medical practice as usual, its reach was limited.

Individuals who trained under the programs enjoyed relaxed rules and wider practice boundaries, at least during their training and apprentice years; but they remained constrained, legally speaking, by state laws dictating practice.[139]

Some of these programs focused on training practitioners to meet the routine needs of well women. The physicians Donald Ostergard and Duane Townsend at Harbor General Hospital in Los Angeles, for example, founded a pathbreaking program for training women's health care specialists (WHCSs) in 1969, even before state sanction. Ostergard and Townsend imagined the WHCS as the "first-line provider of patient care to well women." WHCS trainees, who included registered nurses, vocational nurses, and women with no prior health care education, learned to conduct breast and pelvic exams, insert IUDs, fit diaphragms, and perform other routine, well woman, and prenatal tasks. The program's founders argued that WHCSs could provide "total or nearly total care for the well or worried well patients." According to their proponents, WHCSs addressed key social and medical problems by meeting the health care needs of otherwise underserved women and containing health care costs. They also helped physicians steer medical reform rather than become its "unhappy, passive recipients."[140]

Some proponents of WHSC framed their creation as a concession to the women's health movement. Richard Briggs, for example, founder of the Gynecorps project in Washington State, acknowledged that "much of the impetus in women's health care [had come from] the women's liberation movement." He agreed that women deserved to know more about their bodies and conceded that physicians had withheld information. He also understood that many women dreaded pelvic exams and discussing sexual issues with male physicians. He posed the WHCS program as a legitimate compromise, addressing feminist demands, patients' discomfort, and medicine's need to control health care.[141] By design, however, this compromise left WHCSs under medical control. They were "not independent practitioners." They functioned under the authority delegated to them by physicians.[142] Furthermore, architects of these programs insisted that WHCSs could discover "abnormalities," but they were not authorized to diagnose disease, treat illness, or prescribe medications.[143]

The Women's Health Collective of Open Door Clinic drew inspiration from this model. Rather than sending interested women to Harbor General for training, Pennington, Nancy Henchell—a nurse practitioner who came to Open Door from the United Indian Health Services—and other clinic staff created their own training program. This move was unprecedented. In 1974, there were only eleven "para-medical" training programs in women's health in the country; most of these accepted only trainees who were already nurses or nurse midwives, and nearly all were connected to universities or

hospitals in major cities.[144] By contrast, the Open Door program had no hospital or university support, and desire for training was its only requirement
for admission. "[Harbor General] had a bunch of people and lots of teachers and lots of money, and there was us. And we were in this decrepit bank
in California." According to Willow, "everyone was a little shocked" that a
tiny community clinic in rural California would take on such a big project.
"How could this little thing" aim so high?[145] Current clinic workers, including
Willow and Sweitzer, filled half the initial class; informal community health
workers, including at least two lay midwives, rounded out the cohort.[146] Pennington provided most of the didactic teaching, but Henchell did the bulk of
the organizational and logistical work (bringing in guest speakers, devising a
curriculum, organizing the classes, winning state approval).[147] The program
ran through three cycles, graduating about seven or eight students each time.

The women at the Open Door Clinic embraced and employed legal—
though clearly cutting-edge—efforts to gain legitimacy for their otherwise
lay health care providers. Their willingness to seek state approval highlights
their generally friendly relationship with the medical profession rather
than their antagonism to it. Indeed, medical doctors supported the WHCSs
in their attempt to gain more health care power and authority. A formal training program and the state approval it conferred allowed and encouraged these
women to learn and to do even more.

The Women's Health Care Specialists Training Program at the Open Door
Clinic enacted the goals of self-help in ways different from, and perhaps antithetical to, the women of the Santa Cruz Women's Health Center. On the one
hand, it failed to give women direct control of and responsibility for their
own well bodies, it acceded to state regulatory demands, and it created another category of female caregivers under hierarchical control of the male-
dominated medical profession. On the other hand, the program developed by
the Women's Health Collective of Open Door Clinic remained under feminist
control, run by women who challenged male medical prerogatives. They developed a curriculum that honored the experiential knowledge of clients and
health care workers alike. It created more women health care workers, thus
giving women in the community more access to health care by women. And
it gave a small group of women access to careers in health care that bypassed
the professional acculturation foundational in traditional medical education.

Breaking Away: Northcountry Clinic for Women and Children

In the midst of this remarkable success, the Women's Health Collective
found its continuing relationship with Humboldt Open Door Clinic unten-

able. The precise reason for the split is unclear, but things started to fall apart in 1976 when Norman Bell was hired as the clinic's first full-time physician and medical director. Bell believed that his medical training and his official position at the clinic earned him significant deference from the other clinic staff. This was not immediately forthcoming, especially from the members of the Women's Health Collective. According to Bell, they saw him as "another symbol of male dominance."[148]

Tensions also arose because the Women's Health Collective ran as a somewhat autonomous unit within the larger clinic. When the nurse practitioner Nancy Henchell came to work at Open Door, her partner, Carol Ervin, became the family planning clinic's administrator. Because it received Title X funding for the family planning clinic, the Women's Health Collective also provided major funding for Open Door. As one former collective member described it, "I think a lot of people resented the fact that the women were . . . not running the place, but we were supporting the place pretty much exclusively."[149]

The idea of a separate women's clinic began to take shape in 1976 after Bell's arrival. The Women's Health Care Specialists Training Program required a capstone project. Two of the first trainees, Suzanne Willow and Christine White, developed a plan to open their own "pie-in-the-sky" clinic as their culminating project. At some point, some members of the WHC began to take the idea seriously. Ervin, who saw her herself as person who could turn other people's dreams into reality, began to say aloud, "I wonder if we could actually do that."[150]

Most of the founders and early participants in Northcountry Clinic credit Ervin with its early success. Henchell and Ervin met in the early 1970s through their work at the United Indian Health Services. Of Yurok and Karuk heritage and a member of the Trinidad Rancheria, Ervin worked as a community health representative for the UIHS. She visited Indian homes, connected them to economic and health care resources, and assessed their various needs. Henchell was her boss. Henchell was eventually fired from the UIHS—perhaps in the wake of a contentious board election and recall attempt—and after some time "politicking and raising hell," they found themselves in Arcata, where Henchell worked at Open Door as a nurse practitioner through the VISTA program.[151]

Many of the women who worked with Ervin in the family planning clinic regarded her as an administrative genius. Bell, however, viewed her as a "human adversary" unlike any he had ever encountered. Financial disputes likely increased the tensions. The Women's Health Collective saw the family planning clinic and the funds that came from it, as well as the Women's Health Care Specialists Training Program, as theirs, while Bell, as medical director of Open Door, viewed them as his. As soon as his "honeymoon" at the clinic subsided, Bell realized that the Women's Health Collective was "not going to coexist with me."[152]

To gauge the level of community interest in a women's clinic, Willow and White set up a table at one of the many local fairs housed on the Arcata Plaza.[153] They had posters and pamphlets describing a possible women's clinic and circulated a questionnaire to gather community input. Felicia Oldfather, a longtime resident of Arcata, came by the table and was taken with the idea. "What they were doing appealed to me. I mean, I . . . don't consider myself a big feminist or anything—maybe I was. . . . It just seemed like a good idea to me." Within a few days of the fair, Oldfather decided to give the clinic $5,000, considered "a fortune" at that time. According to Oldfather, "They had the people ready to do it, and they just needed a little push and shove to get started." This gift, and Ervin's administrative skills at fulfilling big dreams on little money, brought the pie-in-the-sky clinic to life under the name Northcountry Clinic for Women and Children.[154] It opened in early December 1976.[155]

Northcountry Clinic was an immediate success. Within its first year, it had already opened a stand-alone children's clinic and expanded its staff from seven to twenty-four. Within two years, the clinics reunited in a larger building down the street. Northcountry Clinic's outreach to poor women and their families and its acceptance of Medi-Cal, California's Medicaid program, drove its popularity. At a time when few physicians accepted Medi-Cal, 65 percent of Northcountry Clinic's clients relied on it. Ervin speculated that the clinic served about "80 percent of the community residents who received MediCal."[156] But economic accessibility did not entirely explain Northcountry Clinic's appeal. The founders had committed to providing health care that treated clients with respect and educated them about their illness and bodies. This service model, provided largely by nurse practitioners and women's health care specialists, likely attracted clients who sought an alternative to medicine as usual.[157]

The founders of Northcountry Clinic originally envisioned it as a place where an all-woman staff provided health care for women and children, including obstetrics.[158] They took with them the family planning clinic, but they did not perform abortions. (Abortions were available at the health department.) As Pennington joked, "Even our janitor was a female."[159] But eventually, women clients asked if they couldn't also bring their partners to the clinic for health care. By 1978, the Northcountry Clinic for Women and Children also saw men.[160]

The women who built the clinic from nothing were proud that their hard work and vision brought respectful, woman-centered medical care to women who had few health care choices. They were also delighted that they had bested their doubters. Henchell described the attitudes of the skeptics: "Our goal from the beginning has been to reach low income women and children. . . . A lot of people said we'd never make it . . . either because . . . we were going to be seeing poor people or because we're women." Henchell proudly celebrated Northcountry Clinic's achievements, but her bitterness at the sexist and classist medical system clearly shined through.[161]

Northcountry Clinic for Women and Children took the Women's Health Care Specialists Training Program with them, and it ran for two more sessions. When the program came to the end of its two-year term, none of the principals appeared to be interested in seeking renewal. As Suzanne Willow put it, "There wasn't enough energy to continue it"; after a while, it became "not so fun." There may have also been ideological differences between members of the second and third classes and the founders and initial trainees of the program (many of whom were associated with Open Door or women's health more broadly). According to Willow, a few women in the subsequent classes subscribed to a notion of feminism that insisted that the instructors and the students in the classes should share power equally. And yet "they knew nothing about women's health care." Exhausting power struggles ensued.[162]

The title of women's health care specialist provided legal cover and professional legitimacy to a handful of women, some who were already providing health care and others who hoped to do so. Still, those who trained as women's health care specialists remained in a professionally precarious position: trained, skilled, and "certified" but without a regulating body or an advocacy group like their physician assistant or nursing counterparts. WHCSs also may have found it hard to secure employment that valued and used their skills. Indeed, too many trainees in the Experimental Health Manpower Act program more broadly were "unable to secure employment utilizing their training," in part because of physician resistance to the erosion of medical prerogatives.[163] The rise of physician assistants and nurse practitioners who could provide roughly the same services added to the WHCS's precarity. To address these professional problems, the WHCS program at Harbor General developed a women's health care physician assistant (WHC-PA) and created a onetime examination that allowed all WHCS who passed it to become WHC-PAs. Many of the women trained in the Arcata clinics believed they needed to take advantage of this opportunity or "fade into history."[164] In the summer of 1980, they traveled to Harbor General in Los Angeles. After a week or so of written and clinical exams, these women then became licensed (and a bit later, board-certified) physician assistants.[165]

One of the goals of the Experimental Health Manpower Act projects was to increase occupational options for individuals from "socially or economically disadvantaged backgrounds" and to increase the number of underrepresented minorities in health care careers.[166] While all the women trained as WHCSs in Arcata were likely white, many of them were economically marginalized. As Willow put it, "We were all very poor, you know, young hippie girls." This training led some of them to parlay their countercultural lives as lay midwives and political activists into legal health care careers. At the end of 2010, at least five were still providing health care.[167]

Most of the women who founded and sustained Northcountry Clinic for Women and Children in its early years viewed themselves as feminists and their work with the clinic as a feminist project. They did not interrogate their efforts, however, to bring their policies and practices into line with a particular feminist politics. They did not prioritize political education projects, and they explicitly rejected collective decision-making. Their feminism was primarily visible from their commitment to serving the health needs of women and their families, their affinity for working together as women, and their impatience with sexism in medical settings and beyond.

In accord with the larger feminist health movement, the Northcountry Clinic aimed to democratize access to information and to demystify women's bodies. Because the Arcata clinics were founded by health care professionals, however, they did not design the clinic as a rebuke to medicine. Still, the Women's Health Collective of Open Door Clinic and the women staffing the Northcountry Clinic believed that physicians and nurses should not have exclusive access to providing basic health care to women. When the state opened the door to a variety of new health care practitioners, these women embraced the idea. Nevertheless, they did not relinquish their training to strangers' hands. Instead, they created their own training program to ensure that it remained feminist and met the needs of the women in the local community.

In the early 1970s, women across the country—many already involved in movements for social change—began to focus their energies on increasing access to and changing the nature of health care. They believed that people had the right to health care regardless of their ability to pay. They believed that people should learn about their bodies and make decisions about their health care based on that knowledge. They believed that women should oversee their own reproduction. They worked as midwives, in hippie-run free clinics, for Indian Health, against medical domination. They developed a critique of medical gatekeeping and protested medical paternalism. They peeked at their cervices, and they taught others how to find theirs.

In Santa Cruz and Arcata, some of these women joined other health activists across the country and founded health clinics focused on the needs of women. They hoped to develop and nurture a model of woman-centered care and to meet the health needs of women in their communities. Women in both cities strove to return women's health to women's hands, but their specific commitments differed. Women in Santa Cruz saw self-help—enacted through cervical self-exam, woman-centered knowledge production, and lay health workers—as an important tool in the struggle for women's liberation, a cause they also championed in the structure of the SCWHC and the styles of their lives. The women in Arcata, by contrast, never romanticized the speculum, but they nevertheless believed that women should take control of their own medical decisions, could learn from other women how to be caretakers of their bodies, and deserved care free from medical paternalism. They provided women's health with women's hands.

The greater aspiration of the members of the Santa Cruz Women's Health Collective led perhaps to greater disappointment when they failed to precisely enact their vision for health services and had to jettison their educational programs. Their belief in the promise of self-help could not—or at least did not—fit into a system that required state licensure, federal funding, and medical cooperation. Many of the most prominent members of the SCWHC left soon after its clinic services increased and its educational mission shrank. By contrast, the women who founded Northcountry found in the clinic work that sustained them, some for years, others for decades. Because they had always focused primarily on health care, their work serving the health needs of the women—and, eventually, the people—of their communities provided an outlet for their political visions. Although each clinic took a different path, reflecting different political relationships with medicine and the state, and somewhat different political goals, they both enacted a feminist politics of woman-centered health.

Creating a Feminist Politics of Abortion

Let us return to Everywoman's Bookstore in Los Angeles in April 1971, where Carol Downer first demonstrated cervical self-exam. Women attended this event to discuss how to better control their fertility. More specifically, they had gathered to discuss the feasibility of opening their own illegal abortion clinic. While most descriptions of the origin of self-help end with a beam of light hitting a cervix and the simultaneous discovery of a tool for liberation, Lorraine Rothman has described what happened next:

> Carol showed us this plastic flexible straw-like device [cannula], and said she had seen this used to do suction abortion in an illegal clinic. . . . The [cannula] is simply attached to the end of a syringe . . . and with [the cannula threaded through the cervix into the uterus] the contents of the uterus can be suctioned out. Well everyone was really excited about how simple this was. "Of course!"[1]

When Downer launched cervical self-exam, she also debuted the idea of menstrual extraction, a woman-centered method to control the timing and duration of menstrual periods, including periods that were "late."

This chapter links the philosophy of the self-help movement to the construction of a feminist politics of abortion. In particular, it highlights the importance of menstrual extraction, a practice developed and honed in self-help clinics that similarly met a variety of feminist needs. Menstrual extraction emerges as the ultimate self-help tool for bodily control, providing women — at least, a few women — with the ability to control their reproduction, outside the oversight of legislators, judges, and physicians. Still, Downer, Rothman, and other feminists invested in self-help understood the practical limits of menstrual extraction, so they developed a broader abortion politics, informed by feminist self-help, but not constrained by it.[2]

Rothman and Downer championed the potential of feminist self-help including menstrual extraction, as a political philosophy and a technological method for securing women's liberation and empowerment. They spent much of the fall of 1971 touring the country to publicize the possibilities of self-help and recruit women to the cause. In December 1971, Rothman, Downer, and a few other women inspired by the potential of self-help and the need for feminist health care established a home base for the promotion of self-help clinics and an abortion referral service in the Los Angeles Women's Center. In February 1972, these activities were brought together and rebranded as the Feminist Women's Health Center, later known as the Los Angeles Feminist Women's Health Center (Los Angeles FWHC).[3] Within the year, two other Feminist Women's Health Centers formed: the second in Santa Ana, founded by Eleanor Snow, and the third in Oakland, founded by Laura Brown, Carol Downer's teenage daughter. In the years and decades ahead, the Feminist Women's Health Centers helped define feminist abortions and identified agencies and individuals whose reproductive politics disempowered or endangered women.

Abortion and the State

Prior to the mid-nineteenth century, abortion before "quickening"—before a woman could feel movement in her uterus—had generally been unregulated in the United States. Doctors led the movement to criminalize abortion, largely as a way to discredit women health practitioners who supplied the overwhelming majority of abortions and to strengthen physicians' position in the crowded medical marketplace. Social anxieties concerning the allegedly robust birth rates of immigrants, Catholics, and women of color and the declining birthrate among white, middle-class women who appeared to be shirking their maternal duties bolstered their efforts. By 1880, abortion was illegal in every state. Physicians, however, could provide "therapeutic abortions"—those deemed necessary to save the life or preserve the health of the pregnant woman. The requirements to qualify for a therapeutic abortion and their general availability varied by state and changed over time.[4]

In the mid-twentieth century, several forces encouraged a reassessment of the prohibitions against abortion. Women's educational opportunities and economic needs surely played an important role. After World War II, women increasingly enrolled in and graduated from college, and their participation in the paid workforce also grew. Probably in response to these changes, women frequently delayed marriage. These developments intensified women's need for reproductive control. As the political scientist Rosalind Pollack Petchesky put it, "Changed social conditions for young women created a need and a demand for more readily available abortion and contraception."[5]

Many organizations saw a role for fertility control beyond the needs of individual women. Many of these groups—including the International Planned Parenthood Foundation and John D. Rockefeller III's Population Council—had formed in the 1940s and '50s in response to the specter of "overpopulation" in the "Third World" that threatened political and economic stability and, of course, US interests. By the '60s and early '70s, federal and state governments also feared unrestricted reproduction at home. In 1970, for example, Congress under the Nixon administration passed the Family Planning Services and Public Research Act to provide contraceptive "services on a voluntary basis to every wanting woman."[6] Although this law excluded funding for "any program that included abortion as a method of family planning," elements of the population-control establishment lobbied for abortion reform.[7]

Finally, women who had needed an abortion, and those who understood that other women would, agitated for the repeal of all laws against abortion or their reform. Patricia Maginnis, a military veteran turned activist, founded the abortion rights organization the Citizens Committee for Humane Abortion Laws in 1962 while a student at San Jose State College (later San Jose State University). In 1963, Maginnis moved to San Francisco, met compatriot Rowena Gurner, and renamed the organization the Society for Humane Abortion. By 1965, Lana Phelan had joined Maginnis and Gurner, forming the Army of Three. These white women advocated for the repeal of all abortion laws, insisting that women had the right to safe and legal abortions for whatever reason without harassment. According to historian Leslie Reagan, this group was the first American women's organization to frame "the problem of abortion in terms of women's right to control their reproduction."[8]

Maginnis, Gurner, and Phelan employed two separate strategies. On the one hand, they provoked authorities by publishing and disseminating information on self-abortion and providing referrals to safe and affordable abortionists.[9] They hoped for arrest to provide a test of the California abortion laws they regarded as sexist and immoral. On the other hand, working through the Association to Repeal Abortion Laws (another organization Maginnis founded), they provided transport to abortion providers in Mexico.[10] These California women led the way, but they were followed by women working both within the feminist movement and independent of it.[11]

Responding to demands for change, state governments in the late 1960s and early '70s considered reform or repeal of their abortion laws. Colorado led the movement in 1967, decriminalizing abortion in cases of rape and incest, and in March 1970, Hawaii became the first state to legalize abortion

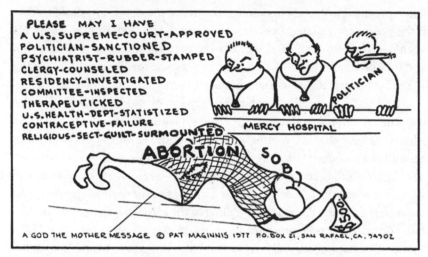

FIGURE 3.1. In this cartoon, Patricia Maginnis captured the despair and humiliation women felt when forced to beg men for permission to terminate their pregnancies. Image by Patricia T. Maginnis. Courtesy of patmaginnis.org.

for Hawaii residents on request. A month later, New York State passed the most liberal abortion law in the country, legalizing abortion up to twenty-four weeks for all women. Washington State followed quickly, legalizing early abortion by referendum in November 1970. In Washington, DC, a 1969 court decision found the district's abortion law unconstitutional, sidestepping the need for legislation.[12]

In the 1960s, California's abortion laws were among the most liberal in the nation. Still, until 1967, abortions were technically restricted to those necessary to preserve a woman's life. Approval for abortions relied on physicians' judgment working through abortion review boards. Some review boards prided themselves in rejecting nearly all the applications for abortions that came before them. While abortions necessary for preserving the life of the mother were generally approved, those that argued for abortion to preserve the woman's health, physical or mental, proved less persuasive. In the aftermath of a rubella epidemic in the mid-1960s, however, physicians had largely agreed that abortions to prevent the likely birth of a severely disabled child were legitimate under therapeutic abortion law. Still, the legal basis for those abortions was uncertain. Consequently, some physicians joined the effort to redefine the boundaries of and authority over therapeutic abortions in California.[13]

In 1967, the California legislature passed the Therapeutic Abortion Act. Theoretically, the act loosened the restrictions on abortion by abandoning life preservation as the only explicitly legitimate justification. It allowed abortion when pregnancy "gravely impaired" a woman's mental or physical health or if the pregnancy resulted from rape or incest.[14] Although the legislation had been designed to clarify and increase the medical indications for abortion and thus broaden women's access to it, in practice, the Therapeutic Abortion Act failed to dramatically change the abortion marketplace. The law restricted abortion to "accredited" hospitals, required approval by a hospital review committee, and left ambiguous the mental health indications for abortion. Abortions were allowed in cases of rape or incest, but only after the applicant submitted an affidavit "attesting to the facts" of the assault to the district attorney. Although the age of consent in California was eighteen for women, only women under fifteen could apply for an abortion under the statutory rape provision of the act. Perhaps most galling to the physician champions of abortion reform, the act did not allow for abortion in cases of "substantial risk" of "grave physical or mental defect" in the fetus. Governor Ronald Reagan had refused to sign a version of the bill that allowed abortion in these situations.[15]

Critics of the new law understood the limits of its reach, noting that less than 5 percent of abortion-seeking women would qualify for a legal abortion. They claimed that some hospitals failed to provide abortions because the law's ambiguity appeared ripe for lawsuits.[16] According to Reagan, "Hospitals and doctors did not feel freed by the new law—they felt more enchained."[17] As a result of these continuing barriers to abortion access, abortion advocates noted that illegal abortion had likely not decreased after the Therapeutic Abortion Act became law.[18] For those whose support for abortion was tepid, the law's limits increased its appeal. A supportive Los Angeles Times editorial, for example, considered the legalization of abortion in "strictly circumscribed conditions" as a step forward for "free choice" while applauding the act for preventing the "misuse" of abortion as "an instrument of birth control."[19]

Poor women experienced the continued barriers to abortion most intensely. Even before a woman seeking an abortion could bring her case to a hospital abortion committee, she needed to convince a doctor—and perhaps a psychiatrist or two—that her pregnancy posed a physical or mental risk to her health. And these consultations required payment. In addition, the cost of the abortion itself could pose a financial hardship. While Medi-Cal would pay for "medically indigent" women, others could expect to pay between $500 and $600 for a legal, hospital-based abortion.[20] As one woman noted with frustration, "You have to be rich, crazy, or a victim of rape to get an abortion legally in this state." Abortion advocates agreed, noting that the Therapeutic Abortion Act was "not a poor women's law." Poor women of color seem to have been particularly discouraged by the process; 91 percent of the women who applied for abortion under the act were white.[21]

Proponents of reform and repeal pressed for more access to abortion, increasingly turning to the courts. In 1969, the California Supreme Court ruled in *People v. Belous* that the state's pre-1967 statutes criminalizing abortion were unconstitutionally vague because they required physicians to decide whether any particular abortion was "necessary to preserve the life of the woman." Childbirth always posed risks to women's lives, the court argued, and the right to avoid those risks, "the right to life," was a bedrock American principle.[22] Consequently, the court ruled, physicians could not assume authority over the right to life by forcing women to put their lives at stake. This ruling also delineated on constitutional grounds a woman's right "to decide whether or not to bear children." *Belous* challenged a doctor's competence to determine whether any particular abortion was necessary to preserve life given that by 1969, abortion was safer than childbirth. Moreover, by articulating a woman's right to decide whether to bear children, *Belous* questioned *any* restriction to abortion. As a result, some interpreters believed *Belous* eliminated the need for hospital abortion committees altogether by challenging the foundation for denying women's requests.[23]

Even though some activists and lawyers argued that, in the aftermath of *Belous*, California law allowed abortion for any woman up to twenty weeks in her pregnancy, many women still struggled to secure legal abortions in a timely fashion.[24] Young women without independent income and poor women who often faced time-consuming bureaucratic hurdles to qualify for state funding under Medi-Cal found the gauntlet particularly daunting. Activists alleged that wealthy women could often "arrange for an abortion literally overnight, while the hard-core indigent woman, who may need medical attention more desperately, is forced to wait in line for a frustrating and often dangerous period of time at a county hospital."[25] One woman who sought an abortion at the Los Angeles County–USC Medical Center, the hospital that handled the bulk of the low-income abortion clients, was informed that her name would be put on a waiting list to be seen by a review board "and some shrinks" in a month or two. "I was already seven weeks pregnant, which is about as early as you can be sure, and if I waited that long, I would be given a saline injection and be sent home to miscarry." Wanting to avoid "that scene," she borrowed money and found a competent physician willing to perform a vacuum aspiration. She found the procedure "simple, quasi-legal, and relatively painless."[26]

As this example shows, the market for "quasi-legal" and illegal abortion remained strong and profitable in the wake of the Therapeutic Abortion Act. One physician, arrested in 1970 or 1971 for performing illegal abortions, claimed to have grossed about $30,000 a month from his practice. He estimated that somewhere between eighty thousand and one hundred thousand women in California received illegal abortions each year—about twice the number performed legally.[27]

In 1972, the California Supreme Court cleared two remaining obstacles in the path of abortion on demand. In November, the court struck down requirements that it found too vague and ambiguous: the need for approval by a medical committee—without ever establishing the criteria for that approval—and the need to find "substantial risk" that carrying the pregnancy to term would "gravely impair the physical or mental health of the mother."[28] As described by the *Los Angeles Times*, "The effective result of the court's action will be to allow any woman who wants a hospital abortion during the first 20 weeks of her pregnancy to obtain one, simply by requesting it."[29] By November 1972, women in California with ready cash and willing abortion providers nearby could receive an abortion in a hospital. The financial and geographic obstacles, however, remained unsurmountable for many women.

Two decisions announced by the US Supreme Court in January 1973 eliminated the need for state-by-state action. In *Roe v. Wade*, the court affirmed that family planning decisions, including pregnancy terminations, were protected by a right to privacy, originally framed as a right to marital privacy for contraceptive decisions in the Supreme Court's 1965 decision *Griswold v. Connecticut*. *Doe v. Bolton* overturned a set of logistical requirements variously in place across the country mandating that women gain permission—from hospital boards and impartial physicians—and that abortions be performed in hospitals. By overturning the hospital requirements, *Doe* made clinic-based abortions a legal option.[30]

As the historian Johanna Schoen and other scholars have pointed out, neither *Roe* nor *Doe* established a right to abortion. Instead, they authorized physicians to provide abortions within the first trimester of pregnancy without state interference. The decisions allowed the state to restrict abortion in the second trimester but left untouchable abortions necessary to preserve a woman's health or life. Although the Supreme Court struck down early state efforts to restrict abortion access post-*Roe*, it rebuffed efforts to establish any state or federal obligation to pay for abortion. As a result, women seeking abortions had to find willing providers and money to pay for their services.[31]

Even without framing abortion as a right, the *Roe* and *Doe* opinions dramatically increased the availability of abortion for women who could pay. The number of physicians offering abortions, for example, increased 76 percent between 1973 and 1979. Initially, most of these physicians worked out of hospitals, especially public and university-based hospitals. But the rise of freestanding abortion clinics over the same time period truly reshaped the abortion landscape. In 1973, 81 percent of abortion providers were tied to hospital practice, but by 1979, that number had dropped to 56 percent. Freestanding abortion clinics provided physicians, entrepreneurs, and feminist organizations with a self-sustaining vehicle for expanding women's access to abortion and other reproductive health services.[32]

Because of the comparatively open access to abortion in California, some predicted that Roe and Doe might have little effect on the abortion marketplace in the state.[33] The loosened venue restrictions, however, clearly changed the abortion landscape. Now women could, at least in theory, terminate a pregnancy at a doctor's office or in a freestanding abortion clinic.[34] Reflecting this change, within days of Roe, the Los Angeles Feminist Women's Health Center announced their intention to open a clinic to provide first-trimester abortions.[35]

Self-Help Politics and Illegal Abortion

Carol Downer's abortion activism began in 1969, after abortion law had been "liberalized" but before Roe and Doe, both decided in 1973. When she joined the Los Angeles NOW's Abortion Committee chaired by Lana Clark Phelan in 1969, she began a relationship with one of the most radical abortion activists in the state.[36] Downer was inspired by Phelan's passion and commitment, and she threw herself into feminism and the women's movement through abortion politics. Downer, Phelan, and Mary Petrinovich, a third member of the Abortion Committee, spoke to civic groups, organized demonstrations, wrote policy papers, and transported women to abortion providers. As part of this work, Petrinovich invited Downer to visit various abortion clinics, and during one of these visits, Downer saw her first cervix; the experience was formative. By the end of her first self-exam demonstration just weeks later, Downer recalled, "we had seen several cervixes and had plans to provide abortions underground."[37]

To better understand what it might mean to open an essentially illegal abortion facility, Downer, her friend and fellow NOW member Lorraine Rothman—a white schoolteacher with four children—and a few other women toured the country in 1971, observing various abortion clinics, both legal and illegal, to get a sense for the kind of clinic they wanted to develop. They had many models to choose from. In Los Angeles, they observed Harvey Karman, an extralegal abortionist, and John S. Gwynne, a physician, performing vacuum aspiration abortions. They visited Jane, the feminist-run abortion collective in Chicago, where they viewed laywomen providing abortions without medical oversight.[38] They traveled to Washington State, where they observed dilation and curettage abortions (D&Cs) provided by the physician Adriaan Frans Koome and trained paramedic women.[39]

Downer and Rothman returned to Los Angeles inspired. After mulling over what they had witnessed, they concluded that women—some of them recruited off the abortion table—could provide better abortions than men because of their own history as abortion patients or potential abortion patients. Rothman noted after visiting Koome's clinic, "The entire procedure takes place along a wave of womanly closeness where the patient is free to talk . . . during the procedure. Guilt feelings were generally lost very quickly, especially when they were told that the para medics [sic] had themselves undergone this same procedure."[40]

Ultimately, Downer and Rothman decided against opening their own extralegal abortion clinic, believing that the increasingly liberal interpretations of California's Therapeutic Abortion Act made underground clinics less necessary. Still, the tour provided significant information that guided much of their future work. First, it demystified the abortion process and allowed Downer and Rothman to imagine that abortions could be more fully controlled by women. Second, by exposing them to various abortion technologies, the trip led the women to embrace suction abortion as the best early abortion method, both because it was the least traumatic procedure for the aborting woman and because it was easily mastered by trained laypeople.[41] Finally, the abortion technologies they viewed in their travels also led to Rothman's development of Del-Em and the self-help practice of menstrual extraction.

Menstrual Extraction: Inspiration

The Del-Em was a technology that allowed women to remove the lining of their uteri, including a fertilized egg that might be embedded there. Fashioned from a Mason jar, aquarium tubing, and a syringe, the Del-Em gave women the opportunity to control their menstrual periods and, within limits, their reproduction. The inspiration for Del-Em came from Downer and Rothman's early visit to John Gwynne's illegal abortion clinic in West Los Angeles. Gwynne, a 1967 medical school graduate of the University of Southern California, began performing abortions immediately upon graduation. Perhaps as early as 1966, he had partnered in the abortion business with Karman, an abortionist with sketchy credentials and a checkered history. During their abortion fact-finding tour, Rothman and Downer had witnessed Karman performing very early suction abortions. These abortions used a syringe to provide the suction and a small (4- to 6-millimeter) flexible cannula (Karman cannula) to remove the tissue.

Suction abortions were new at this time. Before the 1970s, most first-trimester abortions in this country relied on dilation and curettage, or D&C, in which the abortionist dilated the woman's cervix and scraped the uterus with a curette. These abortions posed significant risks to the patient—hemorrhage, perforation of the uterus, and infection—and various difficulties for the abortion provider.[42] In 1968, American physicians, inspired by colleagues in Europe, began to experiment with aspiration abortions, facilitated by a vacuum aspiration machine. This technology revolutionized the provision of early abortion, turning it into a relatively simple procedure posing very little risk. It was quickly adopted. Between July 1, 1970, and June 30, 1971, 93 percent of all first-trimester abortions used suction.[43] Karman's cannula, allegedly invented by Karman while he was in jail in the aftermath of an arrest for an illegal abortion, was also new.[44] Plastic and flexible when most cannulas were metal and rigid, it drastically reduced the risk of uterine perforation.

Karman's use of a syringe and a very small, flexible cannula promised a new approach to very early abortion. The use of a syringe instead of a machine vastly simplified the equipment needed. The small cannula could be used without dilating the cervix, thus eliminating the need for local or general anesthesia. In medical circles, this procedure came to be known under a variety of names, including menstrual regulation, menstrual extraction, and minipump abortion. Karman did not invent this approach out of nothing—he had borrowed the blueprint from older techniques in Russia and China—but he repackaged and promoted it as a revolutionary approach to abortion provision.[45]

Rothman and Downer also believed this technology could be revolutionary because its ease allowed them to imagine abortion in women's hands and a method for women to control their menstrual bleeding. If suction could empty the uterus of a recently impregnated women, they thought, surely it could empty the uterus of a woman who wasn't pregnant. The idea of menstrual extraction—a feminist method for women to control the timing and duration of the menses—was born.

While both Downer and Rothman understood the potential power of menstrual extraction, Rothman took responsibility for developing and revising a suitable device. She borrowed the basic technology (a flexible cannula, a manual source of suction) from Karman. Nevertheless, Rothman worried that the plunger on a syringe could move both ways, thus potentially introducing air into the uterus. Rothman's version added a valve so that the

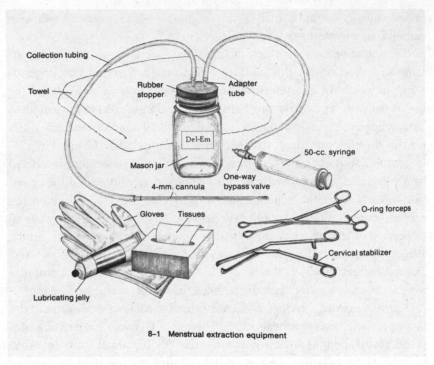

Collection tubing

Towel

Rubber stopper

Adapter tube

Del-Em

Mason jar

4-mm. cannula

One-way bypass valve

50-cc. syringe

O-ring forceps

Gloves   Tissues

Cervical stabilizer

Lubricating jelly

8–1   Menstrual extraction equipment

FIGURE 3.2. The Del-Em, designed by Lorraine Rothman and promoted by the Feminist Women's Health Centers, allowed women to extract their menses. Women could also use it to perform early abortions. From the Federation of Feminist Health Centers, *A New View of a Woman's Body: A Fully Illustrated Guide* (Simon and Schuster, 1981), 122. Permission given by Suzann Gage.

syringe worked in only one direction, thereby making the procedure safer.[46] Rothman also attempted to domesticate the components of the Del-Em. She recommended, for example, "the long-reliable mason jars our mothers and grandmothers used for canning" as the most suitable vessel for capturing the contents of the uterus. She thus connected the technologies of menstrual extraction with women's traditional work in the home.[47]

Menstrual Extraction: Rationale

Although the inspiration for menstrual extraction came from watching an abortion, Rothman and Downer insisted on promoting its value through a wider frame. They maintained that menstrual extraction could benefit women by increasing their control over aspects of their bodies that constrained—or at least inconvenienced—them. Feminist advocates of menstrual extraction argued that the technology (a syringe, aquarium tubing, a Mason jar, and a cannula) and the context (a group of supportive women) served women in several ways: it allowed them to dictate the time and the place of their periods, it provided them the means to discontinue a pregnancy, and it gave them the opportunity to learn about their own bodies and those of their "sisters."

Menstrual extraction advocates offered many reasons why a woman might want to extract her menses. With menstrual extraction, a woman need not "wait passively" for her period to begin or end.[48] Perhaps she was planning a camping trip and didn't want to worry about menstruation. Perhaps she experienced debilitating menstrual cramps throughout her period and she wanted to get through them quickly. Perhaps she wanted to gain more information about her menstrual periods or menstruation in general.[49] These scenarios provided practical reasons for women's participation in menstrual extraction. But for the women of the FWHCs, menstrual extraction was foremost an act of control. It gave a woman a mechanism to extract her menses simply because she could.

Of course, many women had another compelling reason to employ menstrual extraction: it allowed them to avoid the sometimes-frantic worry associated with "late" periods. Before Rothman and Downer, publishing for the

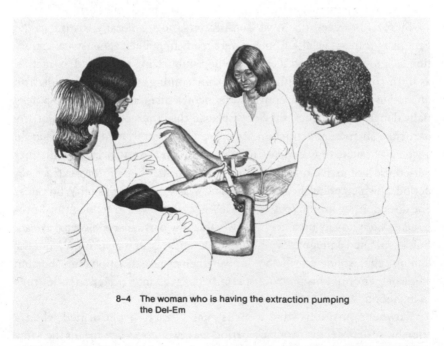

8-4 The woman who is having the extraction pumping the Del-Em

FIGURE 3.3. This illustration of menstrual extraction emphasized the active role of the woman extracting her menses in collaboration with other women. From the Federation of Feminist Health Centers, *A New View of a Woman's Body: A Fully Illustrated Guide* (Simon and Schuster, 1981), 124. Permission given by Suzann Gage.

moment as the West Coast Sisters, began to publicize menstrual extraction, they suggested that the self-help clinic had discovered and "perfected success-ful methods of starting late periods. These methods are based on self-help. To date they are 100% safe, and 100% effective."[50] Here the architects of self-help relied on a longstanding code to announce that feminist self-help had devel-oped a means to terminate early pregnancies.[51]

The West Coast Sisters connected the ability to induce periods with men-strual extraction only tentatively. Their oft-reprinted publication *Self-Help Clinic Part II*, which first described the use of menstrual extraction in ad-vanced self-help groups, does not mention its utility in reproductive control, and the authors initially denied that menstrual extraction was a euphemism for abortion: "When the Self-Help Clinic means abortion we refer to it as abor-tion."[52] They insisted that their position was not "coy or cute."[53] They claimed that menstrual extraction differed from abortion because most women used it when pregnancy was not suspected and certainly not confirmed. The possi-bility that a menstrual extraction might suction out a fertilized egg with the lining of the uterus did not fundamentally change the nature of the procedure. Indeed, they argued, because it eliminated the chance of pregnancy posed by a late period, menstrual extraction "reduce[d] the need for abortion."[54]

By 1972, however, the West Coast Sisters, now generally writing as the Feminist Women's Health Centers, were ready to publicize menstrual extrac-tion as a method of contraception. When publicizing menstrual extraction as birth control, they highlighted the shortcomings of other methods. Too often, they argued, contraceptives were inconvenient, ineffective, and poten-tially dangerous. Further, they downplayed the contraceptive effects of any particular menstrual extraction. As one publication framed it: Why should a woman hesitate to use menstrual extraction on the few occasions that her period did not arrive on time? "Her group meets; she and they extract her period, at which point she is not pregnant. Was she or wasn't she? Who cares? She does not; the group does not."[55] Downer even claimed that feminist pro-ponents were "totally unconcerned" whether any particular menstrual extrac-tion terminated a pregnancy. She argued that it was "the male mind," not the feminist, that wondered whether "a given menstrual extraction is an abortion and whether or not his precious sperm [would] be interrupted in its journey to manhood."[56]

Downer's position—that a menstrual extraction performed when a straight, sexually active woman's period was two weeks late meant the same thing as if it were performed when a woman could not be pregnant—rings false. Clearly Downer understood women's often desperate need to control their reproduction. Women experiencing the stress of a delayed pregnancy appreciated the different meanings of menstrual extraction at different moments in their lives. Still, by refusing to privilege the possible presence of a fertilized egg, Downer kept the focus on women and their ability to control, rather than be controlled, by their bodies.

By 1978, the women of the FWHCs extended their promotion of menstrual extraction as a means of reproductive control; indeed, they claimed that some women viewed menstrual extraction as "an ideal contraceptive technique or back up method" because it did not interfere with sex, alter a woman's hormones, or depend on medical oversight. When women's access to abortion shrank in the wake of the 1976 Hyde Amendment denying federal funds for abortion, the women of the FWHC became increasingly bold in their promotion of menstrual extraction as a tool for reproductive control.[57]

Nevertheless, the women of the FWHCs still insisted that menstrual extraction was not merely abortion by another name. According to Rothman, "Its [sic] not a medical procedure performed by a physician as a service to women who request an abortion, and it is not a do-it-yourself abortion technique. Menstrual extraction is a home health care procedure developed by Self Help Clinic women who saw its potential for regaining control over our reproductive lives."[58] Menstrual extraction as a feminist practice depended on women's ability to control the process and the context. Menstrual extraction was done by women with women; it was not a service or a commodity.[59] At least, not usually.

Clearly, conflating menstrual extraction and abortion inaccurately narrowed its meaning and use as practiced by women in self-health groups. Politically and practically, menstrual extraction and abortion were not identical. Nevertheless, legal concerns may have also led the FWHCs to differentiate abortion from menstrual extraction. Embracing menstrual extraction as a woman-controlled abortion technology might have attracted attention to the legal gray zone it occupied. Abortions performed outside hospitals by non-physicians were clearly illegal in California. The legal status of a procedure that might or might not slough out a fertilized egg was less clear cut.[60]

Menstrual Extraction: Protocols

Initially the West Coast Sisters and later the women of the Feminist Women's Health Centers guarded the details of the menstrual extraction process, likely to avoid a do-it-yourself approach and legal complications.[61] In 1971, in *Self-Help Clinic Part II*, the West Coast Sisters insisted that it would be "irresponsible . . . to give step by step instructions. . . . Just as in learning to sail a boat, it can't be done just by reading a book. It takes a seasoned sailor along to instruct with a carefully outfitted vessel."[62] Rather than provide specifics, they promoted "SISTERHOOD," and they dismissed the private use of the Del-Em as "anti-sisterhood and anti-woman's liberation."[63]

Instead, they insisted that menstrual extraction be used within self-help clinics—particularly, advanced self-help groups—by women who already trusted each other and who understood their own and each other's bodies. The group was critical to menstrual extraction for many reasons. First, advocates noted that the group made the procedure safe by providing a wealth of knowledge about women's bodies in general and each other's bodies in particular. Second, the procedure itself was designed for multiple participants. Some proponents even claimed that women alone could not perform menstrual extraction unless they were "gymnastic geniuses."[64] Most important, the politics of menstrual extraction required a group setting because it was part of a larger effort to generate woman-centered knowledge and strengthen trust between women. Laura Punnett, an activist with the Oakland FWHC, explained, "Menstrual extraction is not done by a woman on herself, which would be difficult and dangerous; this common misconception implies an individualistic solution which entirely misses the importance of the group in the self-help movement."[65] Another menstrual extraction advocate insisted that "as much as we advocate every woman having a speculum in her bathroom, we do not advocate that every woman have a Del-um [sic] in her bathroom."[66]

Although menstrual extraction advocates never abandoned their insistence that menstrual extraction required a group of women familiar with each other, they eventually shared details of the procedure. They recommended that it be performed at the beginning of a menstrual period or within a few days of a period's expected arrival. They noted, however, that menstrual extractions had been safely and successfully performed "up to eight or nine weeks after the last period."[67] In a 1978 publication, Rothman described the process in further detail: "Three women are the key people involved with the extraction: the woman who is to have the extraction . . . a woman who observes the equipment for proper functioning, and a woman who inserts and moves the cannula."[68] She also described the content of the conversation surrounding the extraction:

> The woman inserts her own speculum, examines her own cervix and talks with the group; has others in the group look at her cervix; and then decides whether or not she wants to have the extraction. She talks about her past experiences and purposes for extracting her period, such as relief of menstrual pain. If she suspects she is pregnant, she will discuss her subjective signs and these signs will be evaluated in light of her previous experiences with pregnan-

cies, amount and frequency of exposure to sperm, and her fertility at the time of exposure.[69]

This passage emphasized the importance of menstrual extraction as a learning experience for a group of women and highlighted its role in teaching women about their bodies and how to read their signals.

Menstrual extraction was also meant to be a reciprocal experience, with all members in a self-help group eventually playing all the roles. According to one author, "There is no distinction between 'subject' and 'object,' since each woman has both roles in, literally, caring for her sister's body as she does for her own."[70] This construction heralded menstrual extraction as an explicit challenge to the typical doctor-patient relationship. Women in self-help groups were not acted upon by other women; they acted with and for their "sisters."

Despite the FWHCs' insistence that they did not offer menstrual extraction as a service, sometimes they did. On at least a few occasions, women associated with the FWHCs used menstrual extraction to provide early abortions to desperate women. Francie Hornstein, for example, described how in 1971 a "friend of a friend" needed an abortion in Iowa City. Rothman and Downer had recently been in town on their self-help tour, so Hornstein asked if they could return. Rothman "flew back" and "helped us do a menstrual extraction on this woman."[71] These cases were likely rare, but they occurred frequently enough to cause consternation among FWHC activists. At a leadership meeting of the Los Angeles, Santa Ana, and Oakland FWHCs in 1973, Laura Brown, a director of the Oakland FWHC, insisted that everyone recommit to the policy that menstrual extraction was "done in a group setting and not as a service." Downer protested that they had only "deviated" from the official line "for good reason." Brown didn't disagree that good reasons might emerge, but she wanted the policy to remain clear and the FWHCs' adherence to it firm. This conversation suggested that advocates working within the FWHCs struggled to control the practice of menstrual extraction and its messaging. Nevertheless, they all agreed that promoting menstrual extraction as a do-it-yourself abortion misrepresented its political value and left its practitioners vulnerable to state crackdown.[72]

Feminist Reaction to Menstrual Extraction

The feminist response to menstrual extraction was decidedly mixed. A few feminists, excited by its potential, proclaimed menstrual extraction "the most exciting discovery of the women's health movement."[73] But many were unconvinced about the value of menstrual extraction. In particular, feminists worried that the promoters of menstrual extraction were recommending a procedure without sufficiently understanding its risks. Barbara Seaman, who rose to feminist fame with her denunciation of the birth control pill in 1969, for example, found the idea of menstrual extraction performed by women for women "exciting," but she wondered whether self-help groups weren't "experimenting" on women and needlessly "tampering with nature."[74] Ellen Frankfort offered a sharper criticism. In her 1971 *Village Voice* article "Vaginal Politics," she described cervical self-exam as "revolutionary," though limited; she found the FWHC's promotion of menstrual extraction politically "naïve," medically reckless, and emotionally "exploitive." Frankfort worried that the physical consequences of "this kind of monthly tampering" were unknown, and she condemned the use of women as "guinea pigs." She warned that Downer and Rothman dismissed the dangers of menstrual extraction, including the risk of infection and incomplete abortions, too cavalierly. Frankfort particularly condemned the confidence Downer and Rothman had in their "discovery" and its potential to liberate women. Frankfort ultimately declared that instead of "pushing the very psychologically appealing but methodologically questionable period extraction method, I would like to see women organize around the institutions where the power lies."[75] Safety also drove Tacie Dejanikus's caution. Writing in *Off Our Backs*, Dejanikus regarded menstrual extraction as a "potentially significant concept and technique," but she was nevertheless unsure that it was safe enough to recommend: "Without adequate research, how can we decide?"[76]

This critique—that until menstrual extraction had been thoroughly "researched," the women promoting it treated women like guinea pigs— frustrated its advocates. They promoted menstrual extraction as a form of woman-centered research, and they argued for a critical distinction between experiments done on women and research done with and by women. Laura Brown pointed out, "As long as menstrual extraction is in the hands of women, we are safe. . . . [O]nly when males use menstrual extraction to their own ends does it become dangerous."[77] The claim that women, and especially feminist women, could not harm each other reflects both recklessness and naiveté. Brown's larger point—that medical research, often framed as treatments and procedures, frequently posed significant risk to women without their consent or knowledge—highlights the irony of calling for more "research" to keep women safe. Menstrual extraction might not be safe, but in the context of self-help, it allowed willing, curious women to use their own bodies for feminist knowledge production.

Menstrual extraction, as promoted by the women of the Feminist Women's

Health Centers, symbolized the ultimate feminist abortion, in part because it was not merely abortion. It also encouraged trust between women, fostered feminist knowledge, and challenged the medical control of women's bodies. It allowed women to control their reproduction outside both medicine and the market. Because it was controlled by women for women, it acknowledged and facilitated women's ability to control their own bodies.

Menstrual Extraction: Physicians

But feminists did not have sole control over the technology of menstrual extraction. Neither did they control its politics. While Rothman and the West Coast Sisters were publicizing menstrual extraction as a feminist tool, a handful of physicians had also taken notice and were imagining how it, or something much like it, might contribute to medical practice. Beginning in 1971 and picking up speed in 1972 and 1973, physicians and other health professionals began considering a procedure to aspirate the lining of the uterus within a few weeks of a late menstrual period. In these early years and beyond, this procedure was known by many names, including menstrual regulation, menstrual aspiration, and menstrual extraction.[78] In addition to the confusing nomenclature, there was some ambiguity about the procedure it described. In general, however, menstrual regulation and its synonyms referred to the "vacuum aspiration of a patient's uterine contents within 14 days of a missed menstrual period."[79] Some practitioners believed that this could be extended to twenty-one days. Most practitioners employed a small (4- to 7-millimeter) Karman (flexible) cannula and a 50-millimeter syringe. In most cases, this procedure did not require cervical dilation.

Proponents argued that menstrual regulation offered many benefits over traditional abortion methods. These included increased safety for the patient, ease for the practitioner, efficiency, and cost.[80] Many medical champions promoted menstrual regulation to avoid abortion, by eliminating a woman's "risk" of pregnancy, echoing the language of the feminist advocates.[81] The key to regarding menstrual regulation as an alternative to abortion rather than an early abortion relied on the absence of definitive markers of pregnancy. In the early years, candidates for the procedure included those whose menstrual periods were less than three weeks late and whose uterine enlargement was clearly not advanced.

Because menstrual regulation was generally regarded as a medically uncomplicated procedure, a handful of doctors, like a handful of feminists, argued that nonphysicians could and should be trained to offer the procedure, especially in medical contexts.[82] Not surprisingly, however, most of those who supported the procedure did not believe it should be performed by paramed-ics. For example, the obstetrician-gynecologist and abortion advocate Jane Hodgson and colleagues insisted, "The role of paramedical personnel in menstrual extraction is dubious, as the evacuation of a nonpregnant uterus may be a difficult procedure."[83] Indeed, some doctors believed it should be reserved for obstetrician-gynecologists. Another set of physicians made the case: "With our failure rate, we are not in a position to encourage the utiliza-tion of this procedure by individuals other than obstetrician-gynecologists who are developing experience with this procedure."[84]

Some physicians acknowledged that women might occasionally use medical regulation as a substitute for contraception. One team labeled men-strual regulation, without apparent judgment, a "postconceptive" form of family planning.[85] Another declared, "Menstrual regulation serves as a logical intermediate step between contraception and abortion."[86] Several physicians who supported the procedure nevertheless found its use as birth control "dis-tressing." One group of physicians, for example, described women coming in for "repeat menstrual aspirations." Some of these women had been seen at this facility before and had been counseled on contraceptive methods but "for a personal or other reason" did not use the recommended method. Although the authors were concerned that so many of the customers were university students, they concluded that "adequate counseling and availability of contra-ceptive methods by themselves will not completely prevent 'unwanted' preg-nancies."[87] This team clearly disapproved of this situation, but they seemed resigned to the need for inexpensive and minimally risky methods of preg-nancy termination.

For a variety of reasons, some women likely did rely on menstrual regu-lation and menstrual extraction as substitutes for other forms of birth con-trol, avoiding the cost, inconvenience, and side effects coincident with other methods. Especially for women who did not plan to have sex and those who had sex only occasionally, menstrual regulation must have seemed like a rea-sonable alternative. Physicians' disapproval reflected their frustration with these women's refusal to comply with medical recommendations and their dismissal of women's choices.

The medical procedure of menstrual regulation and the feminist practice of menstrual extraction emerged at roughly the same time and clearly met some of the same goals. But while in medical hands a syringe and a flex-ible cannula offered primarily, though not exclusively, a simplified version of an already widely used practice, for feminists it suggested something much more revolutionary. Indeed, it promised reproductive control beyond medical agendas and surveillance. As we will see, feminist advocates struggled to retain control of the meaning of menstrual extraction and to keep menstrual regulation, wrapped in the promise of family limitation, from being used to limit women's desires and choices.

Shaping the Abortion Marketplace

According to the self-help activists of the Feminist Women's Health Centers, menstrual extraction was both practical and symbolic. It literally placed reproductive control in women's hands. Nevertheless, its advocates realized that it could not replace all medically controlled abortion provision. The women of the FWHCs understood that they must continue to fight for safe, legal, and affordable abortion beyond self-help. These feminists understood that abortion was not inherently good for women. Abortions could be and often were sites of exploitation, co-optation, coercion, and humiliation. Feminists, at least some feminists, understood that context mattered: the political and personal meanings of abortion were defined by who performed the abortion, on whom, with what tools, and for what ends. As a result, the FWHCs strove to shape the abortion marketplace in Southern California and beyond by creating and enacting a feminist abortion politics that influenced abortion referrals, protocols, and provision.

By the time Downer, Rothman, and the FWHCs entered abortion politics in the early 1970s, a few Southern California physicians had abandoned their earlier trepidation and entered the marketplace with gusto. According to the *New York Times*, by 1971 some physicians acted "like businessmen [who had] discovered a bullish stock that promise[d] to be a good performer."[88] The abortion business, however, was concentrated in just a few hands. In Los Angeles County, for example, it is likely that less than 5 percent of all hospitals performed over 90 percent of the abortions between 1967 and 1972.[89] A mere fifty-six physicians (fifty-five of whom were men) likely performed the majority of these abortions.[90] These physicians varied in the amount of time they spent on abortion provision. Some obstetrician-gynecologists provided abortions in the course of their practice. Other physicians earned the bulk of their income from abortion, frequently owning hospitals and, after *Roe* and *Doe*, freestanding abortion clinics. Still others primarily worked for abortion "entrepreneurs."[91]

Physicians who dedicated their careers to abortion provision understood abortion as a highly desired commodity, and they viewed themselves as experts who could meet the demand. Abortion scarcity and potential profits encouraged these physicians-cum-businessmen to scale up their operations. As one of them noted, "The whole point was to do as many as possible, back to back." Another described his procedure room as an "assembly line. You couldn't slow down or take a break." To maximize efficiency, these facilities, sometimes described pejoratively as "abortion mills," were typically open only a few days a week. Some of them provided hundreds of abortions a day. The sheer volume allowed for considerable profit even while keeping the price low.[92] Eventually a few physicians strove to maximize profits by purchasing small hospitals and hiring other physicians to work exclusively as abortionists. Others offered their abortion business to struggling hospitals eager for a lift in exchange for administrative control.[93]

The women of the FWHCs understood that women's need for abortion could lead to their exploitation, economic and otherwise. They believed that they could improve the abortion marketplace by entering the abortion referral business, under the name Women's Abortion Referral Service (WARS) in November 1971. WARS aimed to guide women to safe and respectful practitioners and publicize the dangers of others.

By providing abortion referrals for a fee, the FWHCs entered a practice with a controversial history. In the years before *Roe* and *Doe* clarified the boundaries of legal abortion, women struggled to find practitioners to perform legal therapeutic abortions or safe illegal abortions. As the journalist Lawrence Lader described it, "The search for a skilled abortionist may be the most desperate period in a woman's life."[94] Abortion providers varied in their moral and political investments and in their skill. Abortion referral agencies—for profit, nonprofit but fee collecting, and free—emerged to funnel women to some providers and away from others. Some of these agencies developed to help women safely navigate the treacherous abortion marketplace. Of these, some (like Jane, the Chicago referral service turned abortion provider) were feminist. Others (most notably, the Clergy Consultation Service on Abortion, founded in 1967) were not.[95] Other referral agencies emerged to lure patients to particular providers in exchange for lucrative fees.

Fee-based abortion referral agencies, both before and after legalization, frequently attracted feminist outrage, in part because the agencies could easily exploit women's desperation and increase the cost of abortion, and because they did not necessarily prioritize women's comfort, safety, and dignity. The author of the *Feminist Manifesto* put it bluntly: "MOST REFERRAL AGENCIES ARE CORRUPT. . . . Even some so-called non-profit agencies get a kick-back, or 'sell' us to the doctor who gives them the best discount."[96] In 1971, a Chicago reporter captured the shadiness of these agencies as she posed as a woman needing an abortion. Nancy Banks described the hard sell she received from an abortion clinic in New York State. Although Banks responded to an ad that promised abortions for $100, the counselor on the phone claimed that the price was $185 and insisted it was a bargain when compared to the cost of raising a child. A representative from Ethical Abortion Service in Philadelphia, also scheduling abortions in New York, repeatedly lowered the price as Banks proposed to go elsewhere. According to Banks, these referral services depended on women's desperation to force quick commitments to abortion at any price.[97]

Women of the FWHCs framed their participation in the referral business as a feminist intervention. They unapologetically charged for their abortion referrals, arguing with pride that their fees took money out of the hands of men—physicians and hospital administrators—and put it into the hands of women for feminist ends.[98] They maintained that their presence in abortion referral networks helped reduce the average price of abortions in the area because they refused to refer to facilities with high fees.[99] They also believed they could affect the quality of abortion care. As they described it:

> We received blocks of time at the hospital during which women could receive abortions from our handpicked physicians. We accompanied women and counseled them every step of the way, making sure they received nontraumatic abortions in a respectful atmosphere. This not only gave us a financial base upon which to open our own health center later, but it also gave us entry into hospitals where we could observe the medical profession at a close range.[100]

They believed that physicians unwilling to meet their standards would "simply find themselves with very few abortion clients."[101]

With referrals from an FWHC, women received the services of a counselor who performed the uterine check, described the abortion procedure, and accompanied the pregnant woman through the procedure.[102] At least one observer appreciated the FWHCs' approach, testifying that "the psychological and physical care given these women . . . surpassed my deepest hopes for good problem pregnancy [c]are for women."[103] Accounts like these provided vivid contrast to the alleged "abortion mills" described in popular accounts of the abortion marketplace.[104]

By providing feminist abortion referrals, the FWHCs influenced the abortion marketplace in Southern California. They referred clients to facilities with reasonable fees and comfortable accommodations, and they helped women avoid clinics and hospitals where abortion providers might demean or exploit them. By escorting their clients through the abortion procedure, activists from the FWHCs demanded respectful behavior throughout. They used their economic relationship with providers and their presence in clinical spaces to shape abortion practice.

Providing Feminist Abortions

After *Roe* and *Doe*, the FWHCs were not content to only shape abortion practice; they wanted to provide feminist abortions. As the historian Johanna Schoen has described, abortion clinics founded in the 1970s fell into two groups, medical and feminist. Medical clinics, owned by physicians or businesspeople, prioritized high-quality medical services, lauded the integration of abortion provision into gynecological practice, and valued medical prerogatives and decision-making. Feminist clinics, owned by businesspeople or feminist organizations of one kind or another, also valued quality health care, but they centered the needs of the woman patient. Feminist clinics were committed to providing women with choices and education and to raising their consciousness. Feminist abortion care also highlighted women's ability to take care of themselves and each other without the need for medical intervention and oversight.[105]

In March 1973, the Los Angeles FWHC led the feminist investment in abortion provision by opening the Women's Choice Clinic, which they claimed was the "first woman-owned, woman-controlled abortion clinic in the country."[106] Over the next few months, the FWHCs in Oakland and Santa Ana also opened Women's Choice Clinics to provide abortion care.[107] In addition to abortions, these clinics offered reproductive health services and education. Over the next few years, feminists founded other FWHCs in Detroit, Tallahassee, Atlanta, San Diego, and Chico, California; most of them included abortion services. In 1975, some of these centers, though not all of them, joined together to form the Federation of Feminist Women's Health Centers.

Providing abortions post-*Roe* posed new dilemmas for the FWHCs. How did providing legal abortions via medical professionals help women claim their well bodies back from the medical profession? How did medicalized abortion empower women? How did health provision promote a politics of self-help? How did it further women's liberation?

From the outset, the FWHCs denied they were merely health providers. They described themselves as "political organization[s] that . . . provide[d] abortion" and other health services.[108] Abortion provision raised money to fund political causes, including self-help. As Barbara Hoke of the Oakland FWHC put it, "Abortion was the economics of it. That was where the money came from. There wasn't any way to make money, other than doing abortions."[109] Abortion provision provided capital to secure women's liberation and wages to support liberationists.[110]

FWHCs did not offer abortion on the cheap. They argued that only cut-rate abortions could be had for cut-rate prices. To preserve the quality of abortions, the FWHCs campaigned for a low price threshold. By their own as-sessment, they offered woman-centered abortions at reasonable prices, which helped fund women's liberation.[111]

Although financial consideration encouraged the FWHCs to enter the abortion marketplace, they sought to model woman-centered abortion care consistent with their self-help politics. The women of the FWHCs hoped other abortion providers might copy many of their protocols, if not their phi-losophy.[112] In the early years, lay health workers, trained only through self-help clinics and on-the-job experience, provided the most visible symbol of their feminist approach. Lay workers performed pelvic exams, diaphragm fit-tings, and pregnancy tests, advised about possible vaginal infections, and edu-cated women about contraceptive options. At the FWHCs and other feminist clinics, laywomen workers symbolized the feminist challenge to the medical domination of women's bodies and the effort to demystify those bodies in a clinic setting.[113]

Despite the FWHCs' commitment to self-help and lay health workers, in California and most everywhere else, legal abortion provision required phy-sicians. The FWHCs therefore hired physicians to provide abortions, but the centers refused to abdicate their own authority in the clinic. The feminist leaders of the clinics made every decision about abortion care. Physicians, famously and infamously, were regarded as technicians, doing the bidding of the clients and the feminist directors of the clinics. Early on, physicians were forbidden to even speak to the patients.[114] This policy diminished the physi-cian's authority and allowed the feminist workers to control all communica-tion with the patients. Two clinic workers accompanied each woman through the procedure, one to attend to the client, the other to supervise the doctor.[115]

The FWHCs also attempted to extend their vision for abortion care through their physician training program. As early as 1974, the Los Angeles, Santa Ana, and Oakland FWHCs together provided a course designed to in-crease the number of physicians willing and able to provide vacuum aspira-tion abortions. Over the course of six days, physicians in training learned to perform abortions and about feminist abortion care. Likely some physicians appreciated the training and rejected the politics. Nevertheless, the FWHCs claimed that these trainings "had a far-reaching effect on the type of abortion care provided at both a local and national level."[116]

By influencing physicians' practice and limiting their power and authority, the leaders of the FWHCs believed that they enacted their political commit-ments while meeting women's concrete needs. Still, Downer believed that a more radical approach was possible. In 1977, she spearheaded an effort joined by two other FWHCs to train laywomen, who already performed bimanual pelvic exams, fit diaphragms, and prepared Pap smears, to perform early abortions.[117]

The idea was not unprecedented. Increased demand for physicians after the establishment of Medicare and Medicaid in 1965 had led to a perceived shortage of physicians, especially in rural areas and among poor communities. In 1966, the National Advisory Commission on Health Manpower concluded that the physician shortage constituted a "crisis" in health care.[118] To cope with the crisis, individual physicians and hospitals began transferring some technical procedures to paramedical personnel. Consequently, a range of experimental projects emerged nationwide, expanding the health care marketplace. As part of this trend, paramedics in Washington and Vermont provided legal abortions in both feminist and nonfeminist institutions.[119]

In 1977, through the provisions of the state's Experimental Health Manpower Act, the Los Angeles FWHC applied to the State of California for permission to train laywomen to provide abortions.[120] In the proposal, they argued that all abortion providers learned through an apprenticeship with a more experienced practitioner. Laywomen, the proponents claimed, were as capable as doctors to learn by watching and doing. Further, the proposal argued that lay workers at the FWHCs already had much of the requisite knowledge.[121]

The state did not approve their application. In a February 27, 1977, memo, Hope Blacker of the Board of Medical Quality Assurance (BMQA) recommended denial. She insisted that while the BMQA did not oppose the idea of "paramedics providing abortions," she found the FWHCs' proposal too thin and some of the "protocols" insufficiently observed. Noting also that the clinic was "unpopular among women-controlled clinics," she feared graduates of the program would not find placement.[122] The Women's Health Collective in Arcata had used the Experimental Health Manpower Act to legitimize their training of laywomen as "women's health specialists," but these paramedics did not propose to perform abortions. To Blacker, the Los Angeles FWHC was not a good candidate for such a radical innovation.

As part of their efforts to model feminist abortion provision, the FWHCs promoted feminist approaches to abortion counseling. Abortion counseling emerged as a routine fixture of abortion practice in the early 1970s as the first legal freestanding abortion clinics—especially the pathbreaking clinics in New York City and Washington, DC—began to provide care. Unlike most patients, women seeking abortions did not rely on providers to diagnose their conditions; nor was the abortion necessarily part of an ongoing medical relationship. According to the sociologist Carole Joffe, physicians struggled to understand their role in this new and unique medical context. Eventually, most abortion-providing physicians came to believe that abortion clients would benefit from a consultation of sorts, but they conceded that it did not require a physician.[123]

Two overlapping models of abortion counseling emerged to fill this role. An "advocacy" model emerged when early abortion clinics partnered with feminist health activists to provide counseling. Advocacy counselors sought to protect the client from mistreatment by the abortion provider, supply basic information, and attend to the patient's physical and emotional needs. Counselors frequently escorted patients to the clinics, accompanied them through the procedure, and provided feedback to the doctor or clinic manager in the case of problems. At the same time, a "professional" model developed, most notably at Washington, DC's Preterm Clinic by Terry Beresford. Beresford, an early counselor and the clinic's first medical director, promoted more in-depth counseling. Seeing abortion as the occasion "of the first important decision" of a woman's life, Beresford fostered abortion counseling that supported "self-exploration" and increased personal understanding. Professional abortion counselors used counseling sessions to encourage introspection and life change. Beresford shared this vision of abortion counseling widely.[124]

The FWHCs adopted an advocacy approach, often described as "information sharing."[125] Information sharing began when women first contacted the clinic. FWHC phone counselors provided information about abortion and described possible alternatives to it.[126] Women with appointments for abortions received further information sharing the morning of the procedure. In groups of ten or so, amid comfy chairs, tasty snacks, and an easy camaraderie, women learned about the procedure, birth control options, and postabortion care. The women became comfortable, at least allegedly, sharing their health care experiences, thus creating a pool of shared knowledge. After the group meeting, pairs of clients and counselors entered the procedure room together. During the abortion, the counselor described the process, explaining the sounds the client heard and the sensations she felt. Through it all, the counselor stroked the client's head, held her hand, and offered reassurance. Finally, the counselor sat with the client after the abortion.[127]

The leaders of the FWHCs resisted psychological counseling about the gravity of abortion or their clients' feelings about it. They treated abortion as a medical procedure, arguing that conversations about ambivalence, conflict, uncertainty, or trauma only increased the stigma surrounding the procedure. In this case, then, feminist care meant not assuming that abortion was more traumatic than other health services. They insisted that abortion could be and should be a positive experience.

Other feminists condemned this approach, arguing that the FWHCs were insufficiently sensitive to women's conflicted feelings about pregnancy and abortion. One observer protested that the Los Angeles FWHC's counseling left women to sort through their conflicted feelings and emotions alone. She believed that clinics should offer compassionate care and political analysis at this critical juncture. As she concluded, abortion counseling provided an opportunity for "some of your best consciousness-raising," and she was frustrated that the Los Angeles FWHC was not taking advantage of it.[128]

Providing information rather than psychological counseling made a political point: women deserved medical procedures without being barraged by intrusive questions or sympathy. The FWHCs' insistence on group counseling also served the political goal of diminishing stigma. But at what cost? Was this approach truly woman centered? Surely not for some women. But by focusing on the atmosphere of abortion care within their clinics, the women of the FWHCs aimed to change the context for abortion everywhere.

Abortion as Exploitation

Although the FWHCs believed that feminist or woman-centered abortion facilities provided the best care for women, they nevertheless recognized that feminist centers could not meet all the demand for abortion. They knew the value of a "nice abortion clinic," as Downer described most abortion facilities—places that provided competent care but were not invested in women's liberation.[129] As a result, the FWHCs tried to help women choose among options in the sometimes-crowded abortion marketplace. They insisted that "your abortion should be a positive experience" and outlined what women should expect from their providers.[130] In addition to advocating for particular procedures, they also urged women to demand a respectful attitude and clear information about the procedure. Most important, they urged women who might otherwise feel vulnerable and overwhelmed to see themselves as legitimate participants in the abortion process. The FWHCs insisted that women should influence the shape and quality of abortion care. As one FWHC worker put it: "Abortionists live off women. We can demand and get quality health care, or we can put the provider out of business."[131] They understood that women, by withholding their abortion dollars from disrespectful doctors, could influence the abortion experience for others.

The FWHCs insisted that some facilities were not at all "nice abortion clinics," and they condemned the offending individuals and institutions by name. Harvey Karman received particular criticism for pretending to work for women while exploiting their vulnerability. Karman began his work with abortion in the mid-1950s while a theater major at the University of California, Los Angeles, when he joined a network of abortion activists connecting pregnant women with abortionists. He eventually began performing abortions himself. In 1955, one of his clients died, and Karman was arrested and convicted of performing an illegal abortion; he served more than two years. Upon his release, he resumed his abortion practice. In the late 1960s and early '70s, he worked with the physician John Gwynne providing underground abortions in Southern California. Karman claimed to have "participated in" roughly fifty thousand abortions between 1957 and 1977.[132]

Rothman and Downer had originally supported Karman's efforts. In more congenial times, Karman's clinic and cannula inspired menstrual extraction. The Los Angeles FWHC had referred women to him, and Rothman and Downer had defended him against police harassment and legal prosecution. As their relationship continued, however, anger and resentment replaced their admiration and support. On one level, the women of the FWHCs resented the accolades charismatic men like Karman received for their "heroic" bravery in the battle for abortion reform while women's need for and right to abortion faded into the background.[133] But their condemnation of Karman also reflected other concerns. In particular, they begrudged how he capitalized on his ties to feminist health activists. The FWHCs highlighted how Karman advertised do-it-yourself abortion kits in feminist periodicals, making it appear as though his product was part of the feminist self-help movement. They also alleged that he intentionally misled the public about his relationship with the West Coast Sisters and Self-Help Clinics.[134]

Perhaps most seriously, they claimed that Karman, working through the International Planned Parenthood Federation, sought to dump do-it-yourself abortion kits in the "Third World," thus serving population controllers while endangering women's lives. On the domestic front, they condemned Karman for experimenting on women while claiming to be their benefactor. Two examples supported the FWHCs' position. In the spring of 1972, Karman and four other abortion experts traveled to Bangladesh at the invitation of the new Bangladeshi government to perform abortions and to train native doctors and paramedics in abortion procedures in the aftermath of the widespread rape of Bangladeshi women and girls—estimates range from two hundred thousand to four hundred thousand—by Pakistani soldiers during the war for Bangladesh's independence. Although raped women in Bangladesh were traditionally considered defiled and shunned, the new government deemed them "heroic" and legalized abortion for these women to give them a fresh start in the new country. During the initial month, the delegation performed an estimated 1,500 abortions and trained a hundred doctors and another hundred paramedics to perform abortions.

This humanitarian crisis afforded Karman a chance to test and publicize two of his abortion technologies that did not require cervical dilation, anesthetics, or traditional metal instruments. For early abortions, he recommended suction abortions with a syringe, and for abortions between three and seven months, he advocated a "supercoil" method that involved the insertion of plastic strips through an undilated cervix into the uterus. The strips coiled inside the uterus and swelled as they absorbed moisture. This swelling caused a miscarriage. According to Karman, "The technique is so simple to administer that we were able to go into outlying . . . villages often with nothing more than a small model of the pelvic area, and teach the technique quickly and on the spot to midwives, village chiefs, young girls—anybody who wanted to learn."[135] For this work, Karman was frequently heralded as a hero, but the supercoil's safety was unproven. In the context of the desperate need—need created by war, gendered violence, the state's desire for a racially unpolluted nation, and the availability of abortion itself—the experimental status of the supercoil method was largely ignored.[136]

Karman's experiments in the United States attracted more notice and scorn. He received widespread attention and condemnation for his involvement in the infamous Mother's Day abortions in Philadelphia. In May 1972, Chicago police arrested seven abortion providers working as the Jane Collective.[137] At least 250 women who had been scheduled for abortions, some fifty or so in their second trimester, were left in seemingly desperate circumstances. The Jane women turned to their networks for alternatives. Merle Goldberg, a sometime collaborator with Karman and head of the National Women's Health Coalition, arranged to bus twenty women, fifteen of whom were in their second trimester, to Philadelphia. There, Karman, flying in from Los Angeles with another abortion provider, Benjamin Graber, would train Graber and the Philadelphia physician-abortionist Kermit Barron Gosnell in the use of supercoil abortions at Gosnell's Women's Medical Society Clinic. (Abortion was still technically illegal in Pennsylvania, but the district attorney's office was prosecuting only "unsafe" abortions.) For transportation and abortions, the women were charged $75.[138]

The politics of abortion in Philadelphia were already tense when the Chicago women arrived, with a clergy-led abortion referral organization called Choice already critical of Gosnell and his operation. Representatives from Choice and women from the Philadelphia Women's Health Collective (PWHC) learned about the plan only shortly before the bus delivered the women to the city. They worried about several aspects: the inadequate facility, the unproven experimental procedure, and the camera crew intending to record the abortions.[139] According to Phyllis Ryan, a representative of Choice, the PWHC offered to make other arrangements for the Chicago women and, when they were rebuffed, arranged to have the women seen, postabortion, by a prominent local obstetrician-gynecologist. Goldberg declined their offers.[140]

The procedures did not go well. Of the fifteen women who had abortions, nine suffered from complications, and three of these complications were major. One of the women had a hysterectomy in the aftermath.[141] Ryan filed a complaint. Karman was arrested, tried in Philadelphia municipal court, and found guilty of two counts of practicing medicine without a license.[142]

At the time and beyond, interpretations of this event have differed sharply. For many feminists, including several women from the FWHCs, it provided clear evidence that Karman was a dangerous, self-aggrandizing rogue who exploited vulnerable women. As they summed up the situation in the *Monthly Extract*, "Karman seeks publicity at the expense of women. . . . [He is] a man who experiments with techniques on very young women from the black community."[143] But other women dismissed this perspective as a gross mischaracterization of the events and a malicious attempt to smear Karman's reputation. Jen BenDor, writing in the Ann Arbor feminist publication *Her-Self*, rebutted the characterization of the Jane women as reckless, the patients as victims, and Karman as exploitive and dangerous. She also disputed the gravity of the complications and Karman's responsibility for them.[144] (A retrospective investigation of this event concluded that the supercoil method "is not without significant risk."[145]) Frances Chapman, writing in *Off Our Backs*, insisted that the anger against Karman had been misplaced. She acknowledged that he and Goldberg were publicity seeking and admitted that Karman's efforts might constitute "an experiment on women." She argued, however, that feminist outrage should focus on the "racist and classist healthcare system" that allowed such experimentation to exist. She also condemned Ryan for relying on the state to resolve the issues. Citing Ti-Grace Atkinson's sneering dismissal of Ryan and the women from the PWHC—"Only a pig calls the pigs!"—Chapman accused the Philadelphia women of "dragging their sisters' vaginas into court."[146]

The women of the FWHCs were not convinced by BenDor's attempt to rehabilitate Karman's reputation, and they defended their outrage. They launched a campaign to publicize the dangers he posed to women. In the aftermath of the Philadelphia debacle, the FWHCs relentlessly described his exploits in the feminist press while also trying to separate themselves from him. They warned that Karman was "being presented as a saviour [*sic*] of women which not only hampers and obscures the very real and important work that is being done by women in many countries and creates a hopeless confusion among us, but also promotes a man that is using extremely dangerous techniques."[147]

The FWHCs targeted institutions as well as individual providers; they cast Planned Parenthood as another foe in feminist clothing. The FWHCs' critique of Planned Parenthood emerged from their condemnation of the population-control movement, a condemnation shared by other health feminists.[148] According to its detractors, the population-control movement, typified by the United States Agency for International Development (USAID), the Population Council, and International Planned Parenthood, served the interests of the "industrial ruling class" and the American imperialist state by promoting anti-natalist reproductive policies, especially in the developing world. Population control institutions promoted global "family planning" to prevent "overpopulation" and the inevitable overconsumption of resources and the political instability it would foment, instability that challenged US political and economic interests. Critics, including the women of the FWHCs, denounced the efforts to solve poverty by reducing the number of poor people rather than redistributing global wealth. They also indicted population policies designed to quell "rebellion of the Third World, whose resources they were plundering" and "revolution" in the US inner city.[149] Feminists further highlighted how population control institutions enacted their oppressive policies on and through women's bodies, either without their consent or by exploiting their desperation in contexts that made consent meaningless. Feminists frequently seized upon the population policies in Puerto Rico that left nearly 35 percent of the island's women sterilized and the drug trials that used Puerto Rican women as experimental material on the effectiveness and safety of birth control pills.[150] These health activists understood that population control agencies frequently co-opted the language of feminism to promote their agendas. According to the feminist activist and historian Linda Gordon, for example, "Imperialist agencies are adopting the slogans of women's liberation to promote population control, particularly in the Third World. We must bear in mind that they are not our allies."[151]

For the women of the FWHCs, Planned Parenthood became a particular target for their rage. Although lumped under one label, the FWHCs condemned as "Planned Parenthood" the practices of two separate but linked organizations, the Planned Parenthood Federation of America (PPFA) and the International Planned Parenthood Federation (IPPF). The PPFA, formed in the late 1930s, had by the '70s emerged as the recognized national leader in the fight for contraception. The IPPF, founded in Bombay (present-day

Mumbai) in 1952, was an international organization composed of member groups devoted to the diffusion of reproductive health care and contraceptive technologies. The PPFA was a founding member of the IPPF. Although the particular goals of the IPPF changed over time, they have clearly been part of the population-control enterprise, hoping to reduce poverty and quell revolution through controlling population growth in developing countries.[152] For the FWHCs, the distinction was irrelevant. As one position paper framed it, "Planned Parenthood is population control. . . . For those who are . . . fighting to control our bodies, we know that as long as population control exists, no woman can control her life."[153]

The FWHCs also had a more particular complaint: the use of menstrual extraction, or a technology very much like it, as a tool for population control. Clearly some physicians and population control advocates saw in menstrual extraction or menstrual regulation a potential tool in the effort to forestall "overpopulation." Early advocates noted that because of "the urgent need to slow population growth, new techniques of pregnancy termination" were in great demand.[154] For proponents, Karman's efforts in Bangladesh demonstrated how laypeople could be trained to use simple abortion technologies, even in locations without electricity or modern medical facilities.

To publicize the possibilities posed by menstrual regulation in December 1973, USAID and the IPPF jointly sponsored the First International Conference on Menstrual Regulation in Hawaii to discuss how menstrual regulation might be used "throughout the world" as a cheap, safe, and simple method of pregnancy termination.[155] Many of the roughly three hundred participants from more than fifty countries were inspired by the technology. One participant suggested with delight, "We have finally found a way to use women's menses for fertility control."[156] A Philippine physician remarked with excitement that "we will be able to bring [menstrual regulation] practically into the rice paddy."[157]

In anticipation of the enthusiasm, Reimert (Ray) Ravenholt, director of USAID's Office of Population, had had ten thousand disposable menstrual regulation kits made and distributed at the conference. In the aftermath of the conference, USAID ordered one hundred thousand more. Although anti-abortion senators quickly passed the Helms Amendment to the Foreign Assistance Act, prohibiting the use of federal funds for abortion and involuntary sterilization, Ravenholt's vision was eventually carried out by NGOs. That menstrual regulation could bypass most legal prohibitions against abortion enhanced its success.[158]

Enraged by the deployment of something that resembled "their" technology for ends antithetical to their politics, the women of the FWHCs aimed their anger at the conference. Laura Brown of the Oakland FWHC headed to Honolulu to confront and disrupt the institutions that aimed to oppress women with the same tools which could support their freedom. At the conference, Brown challenged Ravenholt about his planned dump of one million menstrual regulation kits in the developing world, and she shared the feminist promise of menstrual extraction with the women participants.[159] This confrontation between a young feminist health activist—Brown was nineteen or twenty years old—and the institutions of Western imperialism became an often-deployed symbol of the FWHCs' fight to empower women against Planned Parenthood and other population control agencies' effort to control them.

The FWHCs' complaints against Planned Parenthood were not limited to IPPF. They understood that many feminists might unknowingly side with Planned Parenthood, particularly on the local level, seeing it as a strong voice against antiabortion forces. Indeed, the health centers warned that Planned Parenthood had "a plan to defuse and co-opt the grassroots feminist movement" by supporting abortion rights with tools consistent with a right-wing ideology. The federation accused Planned Parenthood of "coloniz[ing] women's bodies . . . through population control and . . . by trying to derail the women's health movement that is fighting for the right of all women to control their lives."[160]

Finally, the FWHCs condemned Planned Parenthood's local politics. Planned Parenthood was slow to enter the domestic abortion marketplace, composing only 5 percent of all abortion clinics in 1983; they only invested significantly in abortion provision in the 1990s.[161] As a result, the federation and other independent abortion providers alleged that Planned Parenthood routinely moved into communities only after Feminist Women's Health Centers had gained community support for abortion and other reproductive services. In effect, by making the terrain safe for abortion, FWHCs laid the groundwork for their economic and political competition. Consequently, Planned Parenthood competed in the same community for client and state dollars while leaving many communities unserved by any abortion providers.[162]

In their critique of Planned Parenthood, the women of the FWHCs highlighted how birth control policies, including abortion policies, were always political but not always empowering. They stressed how anti-natalist agendas encouraged women to "choose" family limitation as a vehicle for liberation instead of demanding social and economic support for families, including non-nuclear families, of all sizes.[163] Abortion, *without* feminist politics to support all women's choices, did nothing to set women free from medical or state control.

The FWHCs developed out of the struggle to secure safe, woman-centered abortion and from a desire to free women from the medical control of their bodies. The women who founded these centers viewed access to abortion and freedom from medical domination necessary precursors to women's liberation. As they forged an abortion politics, they did not aim to create nice abortion clinics. Instead, they distinguished abortion provision that furthered women's oppression and dependence on medicine from one that encouraged women's freedom and empowerment. Only menstrual extraction—as a political challenge to medical and biological vulnerability, and as a technology of feminist connection and knowledge production—truly liberated women. It encouraged women to consider and embrace their bodies as their own and to assume responsibility for them. When we add the cannula and the syringe to our reconstruction of the events at Everywoman's Bookstore, we understand that feminist self-help was from its beginning intimately connected to the desire for reproductive control.

But the women of the Feminist Women's Health Centers understood that most women would never experience the power of menstrual extraction. For many women, abortion would remain a medical procedure for sale in a marketplace of health services. For others, abortion would be offered as the price of restored social status, access to education, or sufficient food and clean water. Given these realities, activists strove to improve abortion provision for women by modeling feminist abortion care and shaping the abortion marketplace in their communities. They also challenged the forces that endangered and oppressed women with the same tools that promised relief, if not liberation. The women of the FWHCs understood that not all abortions—not even all safe, legal, and affordable abortions—benefited all women equally, and they struggled create a politics of abortion that depended on self-help and female autonomy for its foundation while acknowledging women's varied needs and circumstances.

4

"Will We Still Be Feminist?":
Abortion Provision at the Chico
Feminist Women's Health Center

In the mid-1990s, directors of the Chico Feminist Women's Health Center weighed their options. After nearly two decades of struggle to keep their reproductive health clinic open, they wondered aloud whether their continued survival justified yet another concession, another loss of their original vision for feminist health care. They feared that they were "helping construct a health model [they didn't] even believe in." They wondered if they would "still be feminist health centers."[1]

The Chico FWHC, founded in 1975, sought to provide abortion and other reproductive health care within a feminist framework to the women of Northern California, southern Oregon, and eastern Nevada. Its directors saw the center as an alternative to medical care as usual, a clinic where female lay workers and women patients called the shots, directly challenging medical authority. At their most ambitious, the women who led the Chico FWHC strove to empower women, enabling them to secure their liberation. Over time, however, feminist health praxis proved hard to sustain, even hard to imagine; the activists at the helm of the Chico FWHC struggled to protect their political principles within an institution reliant on state funding, subject to state regulation, and vulnerable to antiabortion violence.

And yet, the founders of the Chico FWHC, and the scores of women who followed them, built and sustained an institution with staying power, providing Pap smears, abortions, and other gynecological services into the twenty-first century. Its survival makes it exceptional. Most of the health centers founded during the peak of feminist health activity folded over the years or sold out to other, non-woman-controlled vendors. Still others struggle mightily to remain open.[2]

From the beginning, the women of the Chico FWHC were committed to providing abortions—indeed, the clinic emerged because of the need for abortions in far Northern California—but resisted becoming mere health service providers. Instead, they vowed to offer abortion within a context that encouraged women's knowledge about and control over their own bodies. Their commitment to abortion within a woman-controlled, feminist space attracted attention from a hostile medical community, state politicians and regulators, and antiabortion activists. This attention and scrutiny left the clinic vulnerable on many fronts. Despite these difficulties, the women behind the Chico FWHC remained committed to providing woman-centered, feminist abortions and other gynecological health services both to fund the larger health center and to meet the intense community need for reproductive control. The founders considered abortion provision in a feminist clinic to be an essential tool for women's liberation.

This chapter examines the founding and survival of the Chico FWHC to explore how one group of women enacted feminist abortion provision and how they responded to state and medical attempts to control the policies and politics of their practice. The founders and sustainers of the Chico FWHC struggled to meet the legal requirements of state-regulated health care while challenging the medical profession's authority over women's bodies. From its founding, the Chico FWHC faced generalized opposition and targeted attacks from a variety of sources: state regulators, physician groups, and antiabortion activists. These challenges frequently asked the women of the center to balance the value of the clinic's survival against the loss of some of their foundational practices—particularly the use of lay workers and the participatory clinic. Although the directors of the clinic did not abandon these practices without a fight, they eventually acquiesced to keep their doors open. These concessions led them to wonder repeatedly whether their clinic continued to serve feminist goals.

These capitulations took place, however, within a changing political context. The model of feminist abortion provision imaginable at the beginning of the 1970s was no longer possible at the beginning of the 1980s. By the end of the 1990s, antiabortion activists had decreased access to abortion on several fronts. As a result, the political significance and value of abortion provision changed.[3]

Initially imagined as a mobile abortion clinic in 1975, the Chico FWHC struggled over the years to survive as a feminist institution promoting the empowerment and liberation of women as increasingly conservative regulatory and political forces challenged its approach to women's reproductive health care. The women of the clinic developed a flexible feminist approach to abortion as abortion itself became increasingly endangered, changing the political meaning of the procedure and the political significance of access to it. The women of the Chico FWHC reconsidered what it meant to provide feminist abortions—indeed, any safe, legal abortion—in an environment increasingly hostile to women's control over their own bodies. In many ways, the continual threats to abortion changed the clinics' focus from a broad-based effort to empower women in all aspects of health care to a narrower but crucial focus on access to abortion and other reproductive health services. They abandoned some practices and cultivated some once-repugnant relationships, but they never lost their enduring belief that women's bodily autonomy remained foundational to self-determination.[4] They never abandoned their commitment to feminist health care, even as the tools they used to secure it changed.

The first part of this chapter describes the origins of the center and examines how the founding women struggled to imagine and create a feminist institution that simultaneously provided health information and services and fomented revolutionary change. The second part explores how the Chico FWHC was tested over the years, examining four developments that forced its directors to reconsider its mission, practices, politics, and survival. These developments—local medical antagonism, increased regulatory scrutiny by state funding agencies, intensified antiabortion campaigns, and the rise of managed care—each threatened to close the center. The center, however, led by determined directors, strenuously resisted outside attempts to shut them down. On occasion, however, in what may have felt like a Faustian bargain, the directors loosened their commitment to a founding value in order to continue their work, accepting that the nature and shape of that work changed with each decision.

Entering Health Politics

In 1975, Chico was a small town of eighteen thousand at the north end of California's agriculturally rich Central Valley. In general, this largely rural area of the state has long leaned distinctively to the political right. Nevertheless, Chico, influenced by its California State University campus, also had a history of progressive politics and radical protest. Not easily reduced to town-versus-gown conflicts, the city and its surrounding communities frequently became a "battleground" of Far Left and Far Right politics.[5]

One sign of the progressive impulses in the area was the neighborhood health center—Your Clinic—known by its partisans and its detractors variously as the socialist clinic, the neighborhood clinic, and the "hippie-free-clinic."[6] The birth control services were run by a group of feminist or feminist-leaning women who had volunteered their time and effort because they wanted to make a difference in the world, because they wanted to put their progressive—or, in some cases, radical—politics to work, and because they saw health care as a worthy outlet for their passions. The culture of the clinic, however, proved frustrating and disillusioning to some of the women, as they confronted the sexism of their coworkers ("just too many blah blah leftist men") and discovered the drawbacks of collective decision-making (power incommensurate with effort and dedication). A few of these women started wondering whether there were better outlets for their political energies.[7] The local landscape and politics of abortion allowed them to imagine a tantalizing alternative.

Although the California Supreme Court significantly loosened restrictions on abortion in 1969, California women's access to abortion remained curtailed.[8] Women still had to plead their case to hospital review boards, and hospitals remained the only site for legal abortions. Only after *Roe v. Wade* in January 1973 did women's access to legal abortion in California improve dramatically. Even after *Roe*, the women of far Northern California were largely denied easy access. In 1973, there were no walk-in abortion facilities available north of the San Francisco Bay Area, and in Chico, only two obstetrician-gynecologists performed an occasional abortion in the local hospital. Most women seeking abortions in Chico and the surrounding counties had to travel to the Bay Area. Because abortion was generally not an option locally, the women of Your Clinic referred clients who needed an abortion to the Oakland Feminist Women's Health Center, 150 miles away. Eventually inundated by the number of referrals coming from Chico and points north, Laura Brown of the Oakland FWHC asked the Chico women whether they would be interested in starting their own abortion service—an abortion mobile—in conjunction with the Oakland center.[9]

Many of the women were excited by the prospect of founding their own health clinic, but it sounded too ambitious, too big. Further, some of the women wondered how running a health clinic, even a feminist health clinic, fit with their larger political vision; they wondered how they could simultaneously provide health services and effect social change. Significantly, these women did not want to become mere providers of alternative health services, cogs in a medical hierarchy. They wanted to spark a revolution. Despite these seeds of doubt and apprehension, Dido Hasper and Janice Turrini traveled to Oakland to see the FWHC facility and to hear more about an abortion mobile.[10]

What they saw in Oakland dispelled Hasper and Turrini's doubts by demonstrating the radical possibility of a health center. The Oakland facility did not merely offer medical services; instead, the center challenged medicine as usual by providing lay- and women-controlled health care and information, thus simultaneously empowering the health workers and the clients. In this setting, health services overlapped with political action. As Hasper described it in 1975, "I went down and went to the Oakland FWHC and was just knocked over dead. . . . To me it was a reality that I had never seen before and [I] got totally hyped." With an outburst of optimism, Hasper assured Brown that Chico would be ready for the abortion mobile in about two weeks: "We'll get a building. We'll get a doctor. We'll have the abortion [mobile]. . . . We'll put it together in three days." The reality, of course, proved more complicated.[11]

Convincing the other women in Chico that establishing a health center was both desirable and feasible was the first of many obstacles Hasper and Turrini faced. To replicate their own conversion experience, Hasper and Turrini invited two of the Oakland women to Chico to explain what FWHCs were all about. About fifteen women gathered to hear the Oakland women's pitch: "They brought out the slide show, brought the Del-em, brought the speculums, brought everything. . . . We were just totally amazed. I mean[,] we couldn't believe it. We couldn't understand it all. You know, it was all way too much for us."[12] Nevertheless, the revolutionary potential and promise of cervical self-examination, menstrual extraction, and lay health workers began to appeal to some of the women, and the conversation about founding a women's clinic in Chico began in earnest. They asked themselves whether they wanted to open a health center, whether they wanted to be an FWHC, whether they could make it financially. Despite some lingering doubts, by the summer or fall of 1973, a group of nine women—some who had worked at the community clinic, others who joined the effort along the way—agreed to open a Feminist Women's Health Center in Chico.[13]

Women's health clinics emerged in the 1970s as institutional centers of the larger women's health movement. They varied widely in the scope of their services and the length of their survival. Some only offered pregnancy tests, while others provided a range of reproductive health care. Only rarely did they offer comprehensive health services. Although abortion care occupied a central role in many of the feminist health clinics that survived into the twenty-first century, most early feminist health centers did not provide abortion.[14] In most states, abortion provision required medical participation and state oversight, and it invited community and medical pushback.[15] These requirements and pressures discouraged most feminist health centers from pursuing abortion care. Others, like the Santa Cruz Women's Health Center, briefly offered abortions, but licensing problems forced their abortion clinics to close. Still others, like the women of Northcountry Clinic, considered offering abortions but concluded that the need was met through extant facilities.[16]

Feminists looking to open abortion clinics had several models to consider. Many health activists launched independent feminist abortion clinics. Although these clinics generally shared a commitment to challenging medical authority, providing health education, and respecting women's choices, feminists in Iowa City; Chicago; Seattle; Gainesville, Florida, and elsewhere developed abortion clinics with management structures and clinical practices consistent with their local feminist politics. Other feminists owned or managed for-profit clinics across the country. These women sought to create "woman-friendly" institutions, though they were frequently thwarted by physicians committed to medical hierarchies and male prerogatives.[17]

By agreeing to open a Feminist Women's Health Center, the Chico women aligned themselves with a network of clinics and a feminist mission articulated in part by Carol Downer and Lorraine Rothman. When the Chico center opened, FWHCs existed in Los Angeles, Oakland, Santa Ana, Detroit, Tallahassee, Salt Lake City, and Ames, Iowa. After 1975, some of these clinics joined the Federation of Feminist Women's Health Centers. (Over time, surviving FWHCs varied in their formal and informal connections to the federation and to each other.)

From the outset, the FWHCs insisted that they were not merely providers of health services. Instead, they sought to give women the power to control their lives. In particular, they focused on the way medicine and other institutions oppressed women by controlling their bodies and the information about those bodies. In response, FWHCs aimed to return women's health and women's bodies to women themselves. Key features of their strategy included the exclusive use of laywomen to perform all the health services other than abortions, the direct disruption of traditional medical institutions, the creation and diffusion of knowledge about women's bodies, and, perhaps most crucially, the global spread of self-help.[18]

The women involved with FWHCs insisted that not all abortion provision benefited women equally; not all abortion providers put women's needs at the center. At worst, some abortion providers threatened women's health, while others threatened their reproductive autonomy. Health activists also differentiated feminist abortion provision from "nice abortion clinics."[19] Feminist abortion clinics provided right-priced, destigmatized, and woman-centered abortions. For the FWHCs, abortions were not different in kind from other attempts to control fertility. Therefore, feminist abortion provision was necessarily delivered in the context of more general women's reproductive health services. Feminist abortion, then, existed within institutions that met women's health needs, encouraged their bodily autonomy, provided information, and fought for their participation in the world. The women of the

FWHCs provided access to abortion within institutions that sought to secure bodily autonomy and liberation for all women.[20]

Although the women of the FWHCs argued that abortions were theoretically indistinct from other methods of fertility control, in practice, abortions required specialized tools. In particular, in California and most other states, legal abortions required physicians. Because these health activists understood that apprentice-trained women could perform menstrual extraction and provide abortions (demonstrated so clearly by the women of Jane[21]), the required use of physicians to perform a relatively safe and routine procedure rankled. Consequently, for the women of the FWHCs, lay control and oversight of most of the health care, and especially the abortion procedure, was key to feminist abortion provision.

These working- and middle-class white women had traveled to this moment in their lives along various paths. Turrini had recently finished her degree in nutrition at Chico State and was working at a local convalescent hospital. Hasper had long been involved in community and feminist action; when still in high school, for example, she helped women secure safe abortions in Mexico. She moved to Chico in 1972 and quickly became involved in local politics. Judy Rutherford, having recently left a commune and a women's health collective in Eugene, Oregon, was looking to continue her feminist health work. Betty Szudy found Marxism, feminism, and a vocation in a women's studies classroom. While some of the founders were inspired primarily by feminism, others were moved initially by other left-leaning causes. Gayle Sweigert, née Flaggert, for example, began her activism in the antiwar and prisoners' rights movement. Most of them understood their work with the clinic as an extension of their larger progressive causes.[22]

Although united around the founding of the clinic, these women did not share a single political vision. For example, Szudy was inspired by Marxism and Marxist feminists and saw her work at the Chico FWHC as one part of her larger fight on behalf of oppressed people. By contrast, Turrini primarily wanted to "demystify medicine and get it in the hands of women" and to make health care accessible to poor and rich women alike. Indeed, she worried that the health aspects of the clinic might get lost if the directors became too involved in "extraneous" political causes.[23] At least one of the women was ambivalent toward feminism, both as a label and as a cause.[24] This suggests that the political goals of the center were more ambiguous and contested than its association with other FWHCs might suggest. From the beginning, the importance of providing direct health services to the needy women of the community existed in productive tension with the desire to overthrow the forces of oppression.

Connecting with a Movement

Committing themselves to establishing and running a health clinic had been a grueling process, but the founders of the Chico FWHC soon realized that transforming their vision into a reality required skills, resources, and perhaps a unity of purpose that they didn't possess. They traveled frequently to Oakland to learn both the political philosophy guiding the FWHCs and the ins and outs of running a health care facility. (They learned only later that individual FWHCs differed in their political positions.) At the same time, they wondered aloud how they could ever pull this off while many of them still worked full time, and they wondered how they could support themselves if they left their jobs. As they came to realize what running a center involved, their resolve got shakier. Before it evaporated completely, they rented a one-room office above a Chinese restaurant as their home base, and two women without regular jobs, Rutherford and Sweigert, began working for the center full time. Eventually their savings gave out. They realized that more women needed to leave their jobs and work full time for the center while others continued to earn and share their wages with the group. Although this seemed like their only option, the process took a significant toll. One woman noted, "The process was unbelievable. It was horrible. I mean[,] there were some things that were real good about it. But I can remember sitting around in this 110° heat and saying, 'OK, here's this 110 dollars here that we've all put together. Who's going to take it?' And nobody being willing to take it. 'I can make it. I can make it. Yeah. I can make it another week.'" In the end, each woman who had any surplus income would give it to one person, who then distributed it "on a regular basis" to the women who were no longer working. But by November 1974, all the women were working full time for the clinic, anticipating a February 1975 opening.[25]

Pooled income helped the women support themselves until the clinic began earning money, but it was not enough to also fund the clinic itself. The women rejected grant money and instead relied on individual donations from the community, a loan from the Feminist Federal Credit Union, and, most important, a payment from a student group at Chico State. The Associated Students for Chico State University provided $2,500 worth of supplies because the clinic offered services that the university health center did not.[26]

The center found some financial support from the local community, especially students from Chico State. Still, they regarded the Oakland FWHC as their lifeline. The Chico staff trained in Oakland. When their attempts to get a clinic license were rebuffed, the Chico women met with the Oakland women and brainstormed a strategy. When Chico's aspirator arrived looking "like a

Waring blender," the Oakland women rented a car and brought them a new one, along with other supplies. These interventions helped the Chico center open. They also demonstrated to the Chico women that they were not merely creating a health center for their local community. Their connection to Oakland and the other FWHCs demonstrated that their efforts were a response to a widespread popular need and thus helped them see themselves as part of a larger social movement.[27]

The Chico FWHC founders struggled over financial issues; they also disagreed about the center's structure and leadership. When they signed on as an FWHC, they agreed to an organizational structure that challenged conventional notions of feminist workplaces. Most important, the FWHCs were not, strictly speaking, collectives.[28] Instead, they were organized on two levels: the contract workers who had little or no say in governing the centers, and the staff who made the day-to-day and long-term decisions. The staff, in turn, were divided into part-time workers, full-time workers, and directors, with the directors assuming most responsibility for the center. Advocates defended this clearly hierarchical structure, insisting that all staff members could and should become directors by increasing their involvement with the center. At the director level, the health centers did work as collectives, or at least as "democratically based organizations."[29]

At other FWHCs, this organizational structure was denounced as exploitive and antifeminist by some disgruntled workers because, they alleged, it forced the women who were least connected to the decision-making process to do all the grunt work while reserving the "glamour jobs" for the directors.[30] The Chico women, however, tentatively accepted the structure, having seen how collectivity at the "hippie clinic" rewarded aggressive personalities rather than commitment to the cause and hard work on its behalf. They also agreed philosophically with the position articulated by the Los Angeles FWHC director, Francie Hornstein, who argued in a 1974 *Quest* article that collectivity itself could be seen as an antiwoman position. "The women's movement has weakened itself by refusing to recognize leaders among our own people," she argued. Indeed, she claimed it was antiwoman to punish women for exercising leadership skills. Defining leaders as "people who help groups achieve their goals," she claimed that a demand for collectivity and a rejection of leadership played into the power structures that promoted women's oppression.[31]

Although the nine founders generally agreed with this position, they initially believed that until the center opened, the structure did not apply to them. But as the deadline for opening drew closer and the obstacles remained daunting, some of the women reconsidered the organizational structure. Four of the women—Dido Hasper, Wendi Jones, Rutherford, and Szudy—believed that they had been more committed to the center than some of the other women, and therefore they deserved recognition for their work. Relying on the organizational structure and process of the other FWHCs, they "evaluated" themselves to the larger group and argued that they had earned the right to be "directors."[32] These self-appointed directors became increasingly discouraged that they might ever get the clinic open. In their despair, they "took off" for Oakland, seeking advice and consolation. This decision was not well received by the rest of the staff. Indeed, it caused a "mutiny" of sorts. Turrini described her reaction: "We were just bananas because . . . up until then, we had all been working right along, all equally. There hadn't been any structure. . . . Certain women were more committed and were taking control and being strong women. It just wasn't recognized was the problem." The nondirectors also felt betrayed that the other women had just "gotten up and split." According to Turrini, "It was the first time not everybody had been involved and known everything. And it was very frightening. It was a readjustment, and it was very heavy for everybody."[33]

This episode suggests that while the women agreed in theory to the idea of a hierarchy, the reality of the situation—the implicit claim that some women were more committed, perhaps more politically engaged, than others—came as a tougher sell. As the center evolved, the process of evaluation, criticism/ self-criticism, and leadership criteria became frequent nodes of conflict and dissatisfaction.

Providing Feminist Health Care

The women of the Chico FWHC sought to further women's liberation by changing women's relationship with their bodies. This was key to their conception of feminist, woman-centered health care. They also modeled feminist politics through their management choices as well as their approaches to health care provision.

The founders of the center discouraged volunteer labor, and they promoted its "no volunteers" model as an expression of their feminist vision.[34] They believed that women's labor had long been extorted as the obligation of women, and they highlighted the class and heterosexist assumptions undergirding women's volunteer efforts. They insisted that women needed to be paid for their labor (including their political labor), to internalize an identity as "worker," and to make possible a life independent of family ties and romantic relationships.[35]

Prioritizing women's control within their feminist approach, laywomen rather than physicians called all the shots in the clinic, developing the "politics, policies and philosophies" that guided the clinic forward. According to Szudy, "woman control" afforded them "power to give women medical care in the most supportive and most feminist way we can." Like other FWHCs, Chico named their clinic a "Women's Choice Clinic" as a way to signal it as a place that honored women's right to make decisions about their health care. Lay health care workers provided information to help women make up their own minds. When publicizing their new center, the founders highlighted its role as a women's gathering place, providing health education to "de-mystify" medicine and to encourage woman-centered, woman-guided health research to promote self-discovery and to counterbalance the claims of the medical profession and the drug companies that endangered women in the interests of profit or population control.[36]

The clinic offered a variety of reproductive services, including pregnancy screening, birth control clinics, and well-woman gynecological clinics. These services also reflected their commitment to feminist health care. Most significantly, all the well-woman and contraceptive services were performed by lay health workers rather than nurses or physicians. These health workers received in-house training (or, in the case of the original nine, training in Oakland) over the course of six months. They learned a variety of procedures (e.g., bimanual and breast exams, Pap smears, and sickle cell screening) and researched medical and alternative views of women's bodies. The use of lay health workers challenged the medicalization of women's bodies, insisting that through practice, women, or at least well women, could learn to take care of themselves and each other.

The use of lay health workers demonstrated, at least to some self-help activists, that health services could also affect social change. The "participatory clinic" offered another challenge to both medical care as usual and the cultural view of women's bodies. The participatory clinic, providing gynecological services in a group setting, brought the methods and politics of self-help into the clinic environment.[37] Promoted as an antidote to the medical model wherein the "physician uses her/his knowledge and instruments to . . . arrive at a diagnosis of any malfunction," the group setting of the participatory clinic "insure[d] a more egalitarian process." Women, in consultation with other women, would learn to value their own subjective experiences of their bodies, along with objective measurements, in order to "make educated decisions regarding their own health care." In addition, the participatory clinic sought to diminish the shame women had been taught to feel about their bodies. By experiencing in a group the sights, smells, and secretions of their own bodies and the bodies of other women, women would come to understand the power and beauty of their bodies and reject them as sources of shame and betrayal.[38]

Although similar in approach, the participatory clinic differed from the self-help clinic in at least three ways. First, the participatory clinic was a one-time event, bringing together women who were strangers to each other for a quick self-assessment and some basic health education. By contrast, a self-help group typically met at least four times, and each meeting built on the information and experiences gained from the previous exchange. Second, while self-help clinics provided education, the participatory clinic provided health *services* by lay health workers. Women received gynecological care (such as Pap smears, pelvic exams, and pregnancy tests) in their groups. Third, because women received health services in the participatory clinic, the center billed the women for those services. Indeed, in a move that eventually caused considerable trouble for the Chico FWHC, it even billed Medi-Cal for services rendered in the participatory clinic.

The Chico FWHC directors saw the participatory clinic as a major innovation that highlighted their feminist, woman-centered approach. At least some women clients were less enamored; some were outright repelled by the concept. In October 1976, for example, when the clinic scheduled a student family planning clinic, eight of the thirty-two women scheduled to attend canceled after learning that they would receive care in groups.[39] The participatory clinic for pregnancy screening similarly failed to "go over very big."[40]

In addition to well-woman care, the center offered abortion services. Although the initial inspiration for the center came from the need for abortion services in Northern California, and although its provision of abortion services became the catalyst for much of the controversy surrounding the center, the women involved during the early years did not see abortion as the centerpiece of their political project. They understood that women needed the option of abortion in order to control their fertility, but initially, providing a setting for physicians to provide a legal procedure did not seem like a fruitful path to profound social change. As Hasper put it, the early clinic "was not about abortion. The first effort was to provide lay health care to women like us."[41] Nevertheless, some of the women saw abortion services as crucial—as providing the financial base for the health workers and for the center's larger political goal of social transformation.[42] Abortion, then, provided a means to at least two ends: reproductive control for the center's clients and funding for the center's broader objectives. Still, abortion became an increasingly important service of the center. In 1975, for example, only 14 percent of the women who received clinic services had an abortion; by 1979, that percentage had reached 36 percent. The absolute number of abortions also increased significantly, from 460 in 1975 to 1,912 in 1979.[43]

Although abortion may not have been at the center of the clinic initially, the directors of the Chico FWHC nevertheless strove to provide abortion consistent with their political goals. The clinic's approach to counseling, for example, reflected their conviction that abortion was just another medical procedure and not a personal milestone that required particular forms of emotional or psychological counseling. The Chico clinic followed the lead of the other FWHCs and focused on "information sharing."[44] As a result, while the clinic provided clear descriptions of the abortion process and what the client could expect from the procedure, Chico FWHC abortion counselors refrained from offering support in ways that affirmed abortion as an emotionally fraught event. To destigmatize abortion, clients met as a group before their procedure to learn more about postabortion care and birth control options. Ideally, the group atmosphere—stressing the normality of abortion—encouraged women's comfort with their decision and discouraged feelings of guilt.

But clearly this approach to abortion did not meet the clients' needs. One woman described her dissatisfaction in the aftermath of an abortion. After the procedure, she had broken down in tears and felt that the women of the clinic "weren't sympathetic."[45] This was likely not the only such complaint. In discussion, the Chico FWHC's directors struggled to balance their fervent political beliefs with their awareness that they failed to meet some of their clients' emotional needs. As they discussed in a February 1977 medical policy meeting, "Sometimes we either feed into women's fears or ignore it which is interpreted as being cold," but they were committed to creating an atmosphere in which everyone felt that "abortion is [a] normal, routine procedure." They acknowledged that some women might feel depressed after abortion, so they considered ways to address their clients' depression—explaining it as hormonal or the result of "social pressures" without conceding that women might feel personal anguish about their decision.[46] The women of the Chico FWHC wanted to support their clients, but they rejected the position that aborting women needed counseling.

The women running the Chico FWHC also demonstrated their woman-centered approach to abortion by diminishing the authority and the involvement of the physician-abortion providers. The clinic directors hired doctors to provide vacuum aspiration abortions, believing them to be the safest and best for women. Indeed, FWHC clinics, including Chico, often trained the doctors who performed the abortions.[47] Women involved with the clinic frequently boasted that they hired physicians to serve as "technicians," recalling the physician-technician model used by the Santa Cruz Women's Health Collective. Again, the physician-technicians were discouraged from interacting with the clients.[48] We have no documentation about how the clients felt about this approach, but we have ample evidence that physicians found it unacceptable. Orsel McGhee, for example, a newly minted MD from Howard, found working at the clinic intolerable because the laywomen directors "would not allow him to make professional diagnoses of the medical needs." Instead, he claimed, "management tended to instruct him as to needs."[49] During a 1980 site visit to the Chico FWHC, the noted abortion provider Warren Hern was similarly appalled by the lack of deference to medical authority. He fumed that the physician was "completely subservient" to the lay health workers and suggested that the physicians were "strongly discouraged" from interacting with the patient at all. He dismissed as dangerous the clinic's requirement that "intra-operative medical decisions" be discussed with the lay health workers and the patient. Hern concluded that such policies increased medical hostility toward the clinic, which in turn endangered patients.[50]

Because the Chico FWHC aimed to return women's health to women's hands, medical *oversight* during these clinics was nil. Medical *involvement* was similarly slight. For licensing reasons, the center always had a medical director, at least on paper; but this person had very little input regarding the direction of the center or its policies. Initially, the Chico FWHC worked with a doctor who agreed to order prescriptions, but he didn't want to be involved in the clinic, which suited the women from the center fine. Allegedly he was happy to show up and "write out the prescription for whatever [they] told him." A second doctor, a resident from Sacramento, "wanted total involvement." He left after he discovered that lay health workers planned to remain in charge of the medical exams and the health education. By September 1975, the Chico FWHC had hired a nurse practitioner, Brenda Hanson, who worked under the license of a physician 150 miles away.[51]

When the founders of the Chico FWHC imagined their clinic, they envisioned it as a feminist institution that delivered reproductive health care, encouraged knowledge gathering and information sharing, provided key tools for bodily self-determination, and offered a challenge to mainstream medicine. These health activists hoped to provide reproductive health care that empowered women. By downplaying medical authority and valorizing women's experiential knowledge, the women of the Chico FWHC sought to change the way women saw themselves and their bodies.

"Way Too Much into Services"

When the Women's Choice Clinic of the Chico FWHC opened in February 1975, it filled two pressing community needs: it provided the only abortion clinic north of Sacramento,[52] and it offered reproductive health services

to low-income women. None of the physicians in the Chico area accepted
Medi-Cal. Further, there was no county hospital. To highlight the importance
of their services, the Chico FWHC declared that "the only place Medi-Cal
recipients can receive care outside of the Chico Feminist Women's Health
Center is at the emergency room of the local hospital."[53] The center's unique
services and its accessibility to poor women translated almost immediately
into overwhelming client demand.

From its second month of business, the clinic struggled to keep up with
the community's needs. The women scrambled to get through each day,
learning new skills, solving new problems, encountering new situations. The
pace of the work was intense; center staff regularly worked more than sixty
hours each week. They often felt like they were just getting by. Consequently,
some of the women worried that the broader political work of the center—the
self-help groups, the public outreach, the political education on topics beyond
health care—had taken a back seat while the staff struggled to provide the
health services they promised. As they committed themselves to increasing
the number of women served, improving the quality of their services, and
streamlining their business, they found themselves "really, really wrapped up
in the service end of it." They were constantly tempted to add more services
and more clinic hours to meet the community demand and to raise more
money for the center and the women who staffed it. (Meeting payroll was
an issue on and off for much of the center's life.) At the same time, they de-
spaired that they had become exclusively health care workers. Indeed, within
six months of opening, some of the women worried that they had created
what they had initially resisted, a social services organization. One of the directors admitted in September 1975, "I'm getting really scared. I personally
feel that we're way too much into services and way out of self-help."[54]

The fear this woman expressed points to an unresolved tension at work in
the center from the beginning: How revolutionary could health services, by
themselves, be? While the founding women never intended to be exclusively
health services providers, they had still seen the revolutionary potential of
providing health services and promoting a health care philosophy outside the
medical model. Clearly, the center, through the use of lay health workers and
the participatory clinic, succeeded on this level. And yet, at least some of the
women believed that it wasn't enough.

The opening months took an enormous toll on the founders. Within six
months of opening, four of them had left the clinic. For some, the internal
structure of the clinic, with some women serving as "directors" with decision-
making power and others working as staff, became untenable.[55] Others lost
interest in direct service work and left to seek out projects that were more

clearly political.[56] Other founders stayed longer, but most of them also left within two years, "spent" by the workload, anxious to try new things, and ready to leave Chico.[57] By the beginning of 1977, only one of the founders, Dido Hasper, remained.

The founders of the Chico FWHC channeled their varied political commitments into the creation of a feminist clinic providing reproductive health services. They built it with grit, passion, and the belief that their efforts could make a difference. And yet, most of the nine women who willed the clinic into being found that its political intervention or its physical work did not match their vision. They left the Chico FWHC to a new generation of health activists. Some of the replacements left quickly, but a few found their life's work, devoting more than four decades to the center. Hasper worked at the Chico FWHC from its founding until her unexpected death in July 2004. Shauna Heckert started at the Chico FWHC in 1976 and worked at the center for over four decades before she retired as executive director of Women's Health Specialists (the rebranded name of the former Chico FWHC) in 2017. Eileen Schnitger began in 1983 and worked at the Chico center through 2017. Hired in 1977, Maureen Pierce and Thora DeLey also committed more than ten

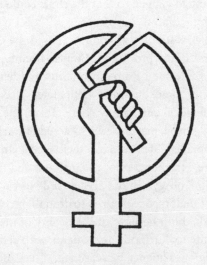

Chico Feminist Women's Health Center

FIGURE 4.1. The Chico FWHC added the speculum to the omnipresent upraised feminist fist. Many other feminist health clinics created similar logos that melded the symbols of medicine and liberation. Chico FWHC collection.

years to the center. They faced near-constant threats—from medical hostility, state regulators, abortion opponents, and managed care, among others—and so the leaders of the Chico FWHC continued to contemplate the political value of their work even as the form and context of their work changed. They struggled to survive, and they questioned the political value of their compromised survival.

Medical Antagonism

The relationship between the medical community in Chico and the Chico FWHC was strained from the beginning. Indeed, some local doctors opposed the center before it even opened. For example, at the Butte-Glenn Medical Society directors' meeting in 1975, an influential physician allegedly blustered that the center would open "over my dead body." The medical society responded, perhaps with more significance, by recommending that its members not refer patients to the clinic.[58] In addition, none of the local physicians agreed to work at the clinic or to provide backup for its abortion clinic in cases of emergency.[59] Still, publicly, members of the medical profession generally kept their views of the Chico FWHC to themselves, choosing to sit back and wait "for something to happen so that the clinic could be shut down."[60] In October 1978, something did.

On October 4, 1978, Katherine Romano came to the Chico clinic for an abortion. In the course of the procedure, Bonita [Bonnie] Palmer, an intern from San Francisco, perforated Romano's uterus and left the abortion unfinished. Romano went home, but a few hours later, bleeding, feverish, and scared, she went to the local emergency room. There, the attending ob-gyn, detecting a perforated bowel, performed a hysterectomy, claiming that it was necessary to save Romano's life. Romano then sued Palmer and the health center for malpractice.[61] In the wake of the incident and the lawsuit, Jerome Weinbaum, the "senior" ob-gyn in the area, urged Norcal Mutual Insurance Company, the center's malpractice insurer, to drop their coverage because the clinic was a "poor risk," both because of the quality of medical care and the propensity of the clinic to "turn off" its patients with self-exam. ("Turned-off" patients were litigious patients, he reasoned.) The Chico FWHC claimed that Weinbaum also reported the clinic to the Board of Medical Quality Assurance, but he denied this repeatedly.[62]

On July 23, 1979, the Chico FWHC received notice of the impending cancellation of their malpractice insurance policy by Norcal. Norcal gave the two major justifications for the cancellation: the use of "unlicensed health care workers for examinations and the absence of an established local medical relationship for direction, backup, and emergency care of patients." Norcal also cited the lack of privacy inherent in the "participatory clinic," the use of "volunteers" to staff the clinics, and the "significant potential claims" against the center.[63]

The Chico FWHC appealed the decision but lost. Its new insurance carrier charged them roughly twice as much money for significantly less coverage. The directors, however, had been working on another strategy to challenge the medical profession's power over them. The day after they received the cancellation notice from the insurance company, the directors began researching and building a case for an antitrust suit.[64]

On January 22, 1981, the eighth anniversary of the *Roe v. Wade* decision, the Chico FWHC and Lorene Reed (on behalf of the class of women harmed by the defendants' actions) filed a federal antitrust suit against eight local obstetrician-gynecologists, a nurse practitioner, N.T. Enloe Memorial Hospital, the Butte-Glenn Medical Society, and Norcal Mutual Insurance Company.[65] The complaint alleged that the defendants, in violation of the Sherman Antitrust Act, conspired to restrain trade by limiting the activities of the health center. More specifically, the plaintiffs claimed that the defendants had interfered with the center by refusing to work there or to provide backup medical services; refusing to give their medical director hospital admitting privileges; dissuading local physicians and nurses from working there; defaming the center to current and potential clients; refusing to refer clients to the center; and urging the cancellation of their malpractice insurance. This suit followed in the footsteps of a similar case filed by the Tallahassee FWHC in 1975 and settled in 1980. In the Florida case, the defendants agreed to refrain from "monopolistic practices" and paid the plaintiffs $75,000 (an amount that did not even cover the center's legal fees).[66]

Research for the lawsuit uncovered the depth of local medical resistance. A December 1979 survey of local doctors by the Chico FWHC revealed that only one local ob-gyn was willing to refer women to the center for abortions. One group of doctors didn't refer abortion cases "locally" (presumably to the Chico FWHC) because of "too many problems that we've had with them."[67] The doctors at the university health center also declined to refer patients to the Chico FWHC, having heard from their ob-gyn colleagues that the center had high rates of postabortion infection and no medical backup.[68] It was not lost on the women of the FWHC that local physicians had created the very situation that they blamed on the center.

Some of the local doctors clearly believed that the center should be shut down, but the reasons for the medical hostility varied. Some physicians seemed to be antiabortion and would be hostile to any abortion provider.[69]

Others may have been threatened by the idea of self-help and a woman-controlled clinic run outside of medical control.[70] Indeed, the Chico FWHC conceded no power to medical authority. Overwhelmingly, however, the medical opposition seems to have been inspired by the perceived hubris of the center's directors, who dared to challenge the medical establishment and who did so boldly and without apology. For example, Richard MacDonald, speaking as chairman of the Public Relations Committee of the Butte-Glenn Medical Society, chided the directors of the center for alienating the medical community.[71] Another physician suggested that the center's staff might try to be "nicer to the doctors" because their present attitude alienated the center from the local doctors rather than establishing a "good relationship."[72] Yet another physician characterized the women who worked at the FWHC as "demanding, pushy, unrealistic and abrasive," and noted that they "were really turning off the medical community" with their attitude, demands, and anti-medical bias.[73] Finally, a local physician, Gary Cooper, complained that the clinic was run by a "group of aggressive, macho, females" that he just "didn't like." He found them "notoriously critical" of the local medical community. Tellingly, he also disliked treating women referred to him by the clinic because "the patient would always be accompanied by at least one worker from the clinic who would insist on accompanying the patient into the examining room and watching everything [Cooper] did."[74] Even the support from the center's allies was sometimes surprisingly shallow. Hans Freistadt, for example, who agreed to provide medical backup for the abortion clinic, admitted that he was "not terribly sympathetic" to the idea of self-help.[75]

The Chico FWHC never presented this evidence of "medical conspiracy" to a jury. Instead, in May 1983, after an out-of-court settlement, the center dropped the suit against all but two of the local physicians and Enloe hospital. Both sides seemed to get something from the settlement. The health center received an undisclosed cash payment from Norcal, backup care from local doctors when clinic doctors were unavailable, and assurances that clinic patients referred to local doctors could bring with them a "client advocate" for office appointments. On the other side, the center agreed to hire a medical director "to provide on-going, on-site physician care for center patients" and promised that no local doctor would "be required to engage in medical procedures which, because of training, or experience limitations, or personal convictions, he does not ordinarily perform." The press release issued jointly insisted that "the settlement is not an admission of guilt or wrongdoing by any party but was achieved in a good faith effort to avoid the burden and expense of continuing litigation and to meet the medical needs of the Chico community."[76]

On balance, this looks like a victory of sorts for the Chico FWHC. The lawsuit forced a cash settlement from Norcal, which the Chico FWHC used to build a new clinic in Redding, California, seventy-five miles north. The settlement also brokered a deal to create a more formal system for emergency backup. But the agreement "to provide on-going, on-site physician care for center patients" represented a further incarnation of a compromise the center had been forced to make a year before.

State Regulation

From its inception in 1975, laywomen ran the Chico FWHC and provided most of the health services. The center hired physicians only to perform abortions. Laywomen provided health education and counseling, performed pelvic exams and pregnancy tests, looked for yeast infections, and recommended interventions. These practices, followed by all the FWHCs, embodied their philosophy that the natural functioning of women's bodies need not be controlled by the medical profession. Repeatedly, this policy came under attack. Most famously, two women in the Los Angeles clinic were arrested in 1972 for practicing medicine without a license in the Great Yogurt Conspiracy. One of the women pleaded guilty in return for a suspended sentence; the other, Carol Downer, was found innocent.[77] Although this early victory encouraged optimism, eventually state regulatory authorities, armed with financial threats, wore the centers down and diminished the role of lay health workers.

The Chico FWHC's reliance on state funding forced this diminished role for lay health workers. Since it began in 1975, the Chico clinic, along with other California FWHCs, had received a significant percentage of its revenue from the state Office of Family Planning (Title XX funds). Securing these funds, however, had always been a struggle. Although Governor Jerry Brown publicly supported innovative approaches to health and health care delivery, the Department of Health and the Office of Family Planning (OFP) proved more resistant to funding nontraditional programs—at least, the nontraditional programs and policies of the FWHCs.[78]

Many FWHC practices blatantly contradicted the policies set forth in the Standards for Family Planning Services, and others fell into a legal gray area. But initially, the state focused its critique of the center on small details rather than challenging the distinctive policies at the heart of its mission, such as the use of lay health workers and the participatory clinic.[79] In April 1977, Barbara Aved, a nursing consultant within the OFP, visited the California FWHCs, including Chico, to determine whether the clinics met the legal standards of care. Although not hostile to medical innovation, Aved concluded that the clinics both violated Standards for Family Planning Services and broke the law by using lay health workers who "practiced medicine without a license." Beginning in May 1977, Aved required that the Chico FWHC make significant changes to qualify for continued funding. She asked the center to hire a medical director who would have an active role in "setting medical policies, writing standing orders, and assisting with the procedure manual," and she insisted that lay health workers could no longer provide "direct patient services," including pelvic and breast examinations. Aved recommended that the Chico FWHC apply for state-sanctioned training through the Experimental Manpower Act if its directors objected to employing physicians or nurse practitioners to provide basic gynecological services.[80] In response, Shauna Heckert and Dido Hasper explained that because the Chico FWHC strove to challenge the medical control of women's bodies, it would not abandon its commitment to woman-controlled care in a "well-woman clinic." Hasper and Heckert refused to relinquish women's right to diagnose and treat minor ailments, even within a clinic setting, and they rejected the "professional separation between women and their health care" required by the state.[81] Not surprisingly, Aved was not moved. In August, she reiterated her position that the lay workers provided the "majority of direct medical services without proper licensure to do so." She insisted that the funding from the OFP would not continue until the situation was "resolved."[82]

In the fall of 1977 and through 1978, the Chico FWHC and the other California FWHCs appealed to and negotiated with several state agencies to find a compromise that would allow the clinics to retain their political commitments while receiving state funding.[83] The clinics had some support. Jerome A. Lackner, outgoing director of the Department of Health, for example, believed that some mechanism should be found to "legally allow state funds to speak to the objectives of health care through a variety of different processes which may range from the very traditional to the very unconventional."[84] Thelma Fraziear, chief of the OFP, also seemed sympathetic, but she worried about spending taxpayer funds on activities prohibited by the state. By the beginning of 1979, this support apparently yielded a short-term compromise: in February, the Chico FWHC received a waiver from the state that allowed funding, pending further negotiations.[85]

By midyear, however, complaints from physicians in the wake of the Romano case and an alleged client complaint put the Chico center and all the other California FWHCs under increased scrutiny.[86] For example, concern about the quality of care at Feminist Women's Health Centers led the Office of Preventive Services to perform a site visit at all the FWHC clinics. The investigators, two women physicians, evaluated the centers positively, suggesting that the clinics—particularly Chico—provided first-rate care that required only minor tweaking to make it superior to that provided in most medical settings. Further, the investigators defended the centers' nontraditional approach, arguing that "clients have the right to choose their care provider," even if that provider was a lay health worker. Nevertheless, their medical training seemed to get the best of them in the end. In their May 1979 report, the investigators suggested that if these clinics were to remain eligible for state funding, they must have a nurse practitioner *or* a physician present at, though not involved in, the clinics.[87] Although this ruling seemed punitive given the conclusions about the quality of care, the directors of the FWHCs reluctantly agreed. They decided that this requirement did not challenge their central structure or mission.[88] By July, however, the requirements had become more stringent, requiring a physician present on-site when family planning services were provided. The FWHCs protested; they eventually acquiesced.[89]

By 1981, even this compromise was no longer enough for the state, reflecting perhaps the conservative mood of the country and the increased power of Mike Curb, the Republican lieutenant governor.[90] On several fronts, state agencies acted to close the FWHCs. In March of 1981, representatives of the Medi-Cal Fraud Division made an unannounced visit to the Chico center, asking workers and clients alike about the health care and billing procedures of the clinic. Investigators focused particular attention on clients funded by Medi-Cal, showing up at their homes, asking them who performed their abortions, and threatening them with court appearances to coerce answers. Although the fraud investigation was ultimately dropped, the Office of Family Planning notified the Chico center in April that its funding would be cut because its "methods" thwarted the Standards for Family Planning.[91]

This reversal of state policy caused a crisis among the health centers. What remained of their mission if they turned over routine well-woman examinations and care to the very medical professionals they hoped to displace? How could they weigh the relative importance of their ultimate political goals and their immediate health services? At the time of this demand, the Chico FWHC remained the only Medi-Cal provider of reproductive services in the community; it was still only one of two abortion clinics north of Sacramento.[92] With much despair, the Chico directors decided that providing urgently needed health services was, at least for the short term, more important than standing by principle and risking closure. In July 1981, Dido Hasper wrote a carefully phrased letter to Aved, who by then had become chief of the OFP, explaining the center's new policy: "We have had many discussions about how . . . we can still maintain the integrity of the well woman clinic concept and at the same time come into compliance with the *Standards for*

Family Planning. We have implemented a new clinic format that utilizes mid-level practitioners and physicians for all examinations, diagnosis and treatment while still using trained lay health workers in the health education aspects of the clinic." In an optimistic tone that covered the deep resentment and disappointment the women likely felt, Hasper concluded, "Now when a woman comes into the well woman clinic she has the advantage of both group participatory information sharing and learning self-examination, as well as an examination by a medical professional with a trained patient advocate to insure the woman receives the best possible care and gets all of her questions answered."[93] Although it required a few more bureaucratic changes, the Office of Family Planning eventually restored Chico's funding, but role of lay health workers remained diminished.[94]

Antiabortion Onslaught

Strings attached to state funding demanded the move away from lay health workers; antiabortion forces challenged the center's very survival. In the late 1980s, the antiabortion movement began a multipronged assault on women's access to abortion services. The strategy was partly legal, and in two landmark Supreme Court decisions, the antiabortion forces successfully chipped away at women's reproductive options.[95] In *Webster v. Reproductive Health Services* (1989), the court ruled that it was constitutional for the state to place restrictions on abortions and upheld state laws that prohibited the use of state funds for abortion services. In *Planned Parenthood of Southeastern Pennsylvania v. Casey* (1992), the court upheld *Roe v. Wade* but introduced a new standard for judging the validity of abortion laws: "undue burden." Under this standard, states could restrict a woman's access to abortion—by requiring a waiting period or parental consent, for example—as long as the restrictions did not place an "undue burden" on the woman.

Not content with the legal approach, however, factions of the antiabortion movement also organized a personal campaign of harassment and threatened violence.[96] In 1993, this campaign turned deadly when the physician David Gunn was shot and killed by an antiabortion zealot in Pensacola, Florida. In that year alone, abortion clinics across the nation experienced twelve arsons, one bombing, and sixty-six blockades.[97]

The Chico center and one of its spin-off centers in Redding were particular targets. The harassment began in earnest in January 1988 when antiabortion protesters first appeared at the Chico clinic, passing out literature and harassing clinic clients and workers. Nearly every day for the next five years, antiabortion protesters descended upon at least one of the Chico

FWHCs, denouncing and damning "baby-killers" and "butchers," blocking doorways, harassing clients and workers, and displaying images of allegedly aborted fetuses. The assault quickly turned more violent, and in October 1989, the Redding clinic suffered its first of four arson attacks.[98] John Steir, an itinerant abortion provider, received written and verbal death threats. He considered Redding a "war zone."[99] Vandals also employed less explosive but similarly damaging tactics. For example, in September 1992, a woman doused the Chico clinic with butyric acid. The attack and the horrible stench it left behind closed the clinic for five days and forced more than $15,000 in cleanup costs.[100]

The FWHCs fought back aggressively, using all the judicial, legislative, and law enforcement tools at their disposal. They lobbied state and national legislators to offer more protection for clinic clients, they sued protesters for harassment, and they prodded local police to enforce existing laws. Their biggest victory came in 1995, when the California Supreme Court affirmed the "free speech zone" (a twenty-foot swatch of protected space around clinic entrances that was off limits to protesters) and ordered the offending hecklers to repay the Chico FWHC nearly $100,000 to cover the center's court costs.[101] Women from the Chico center were likewise gratified that their lobbying efforts on behalf of FACE, the Freedom of Access to Clinic Entrances Act, paid off. President William Clinton signed the bill into law in 1994.[102] On the way to these victories, however, the Chico women also became all too familiar with the procedures for filing a temporary restraining order, the details of a safe clinic evacuation, and the phone numbers of sympathetic law enforcement officials.

The siege of the centers exacted a tremendous toll from the health center staff. Indeed, across the country, many woman-controlled health centers, including several FWHCs, closed in the early 1990s in response to the constant harassment and the threats of more serious violence.[103] The women at the Chico FWHC, however, hung on. Still, knowing they couldn't fight the battle for reproductive rights alone, the FWHC directors joined forces with the local Planned Parenthood clinic (opened in 1981) to combat the antiabortion onslaught.

On the surface, this coalition appeared fitting, even congenial. For all their history, however, the Feminist Women's Health Centers actively contrasted their mission with that of Planned Parenthood, insisting that FWHCs wanted to give women control and Planned Parenthood wanted to control women. Planned Parenthood also threatened independent abortion clinics' survival. At least one FWHC closed as a direct result of competition from Planned Parenthood.[104]

Planned Parenthood opened a clinic in Chico in December 1981 and began offering abortions in March 1983. Their initial relations with the FWHC
were cool but not hostile. When Planned Parenthood announced its intention
to begin offering abortions, Eileen Schnitger of the Chico FWHC suggested
that it was "unusual" for Planned Parenthood to offer abortions in an area
"where [abortion] services already exist," and she worried about how "responsive" Planned Parenthood might be to women's needs. Chico FWHC director
Shauna Heckert put her reservations more bluntly: "Why didn't they go where
there are no providers?" For her part, Linda Galloway, director of the Chico
Planned Parenthood, saw no need for "ill will" between the two clinics, although she admitted that they would be competing for clients. Still, she noted,
"We [Planned Parenthood] are offering women another choice."[105] After the
clinic opened, the FWHC remained the favored locale for most women—it
provided three times as many abortions as Planned Parenthood—but the
FWHC did lose clients.[106] In addition to drawing clients away from the Chico
FWHC, the Planned Parenthood clinic also siphoned off state family plan-
ning money. According to Heckert, "The State would rather fund Planned
Parenthood because Planned Parenthood, like the State, is interested in con-
trolling population rather than empowering women." As a result, the entry of
Planned Parenthood into the Chico market "devastated" the Chico FWHC.
"They didn't close us down but they did hurt us."[107] For the next few years, the
FWHC continued their general critique of population control and Planned
Parenthood while maintaining cordial relations with the local clinic.

Nevertheless, the antiabortion threat required that the two organizations
overlook their philosophical differences for the sake of presenting a unified
front. Chico FWHC directors declared a de facto truce with Planned Parenthood and joined forces with them to combat the antiabortion onslaught. As a
result, the Chico clinic and its offshoots abandoned, at least temporarily, their
larger critique of population control policies.[108] This decision indicates that
the directors privileged the continuation of direct services even if that decision reinforced the power of an institution that allegedly worked to decrease
women's control over their own bodies. Although the decision was painful,
the women of the Chico FWHC agreed that securing access to abortion and
other reproductive services for women was a necessary, if not ultimately sufficient, means of securing women's bodily autonomy.[109] The truce with Planned
Parenthood acknowledged the shifting terrain in the battle for reproductive
freedom. Maintaining services despite terrorist attacks marked a victory for
individual women and for the larger struggle to secure and support reproductive rights for women.

Managed Care

Perhaps the biggest challenge to the survival of the California Feminist Women's Health Centers was the rise of managed care. In the late 1980s, California began experimenting with mandatory Medi-Cal managed care.[110] Before these experiments, most Medi-Cal clients and the uninsured were cared for through a network of safety-net providers such as federally funded community and migrant health centers, Indian Health Center sites, county-run clinics, and independent centers such as the FWHCs. All these centers depended on Medi-Cal funding.[111]

Before Medi-Cal was folded into managed care, the patient population reliant on public funding was seen as undesirable, allegedly costing more to treat than the providers earned in state reimbursement. As a result, when the Chico health center opened, they were the only provider in town that took Medi-Cal patients. With the rise of Medi-Cal managed care, however, Medi-Cal patients became desirable because the state paid the health maintenance organization (HMO) for every Medi-Cal patient it enrolled. Thus mainstream providers began competing for Medi-Cal contracts. For the population served by Medi-Cal, this new approach theoretically gave them more options for securing care. The safety-net clinics, however, were forced to contract with an HMO or lose the client base that sustained them. Many of the safety-net sites worried that a managed-care contract would not be enough as clients left the clinics for more mainstream providers.[112]

Echoing the concerns of safety-net clinics, feminist activists at FWHCs feared for their survival in the wake of the takeover by managed care. They worried that their client base would disappear, and they were unsure whether they could secure a managed care contract even if they wanted to.[113] The Feminist Women's Health Centers also faced philosophical and political dilemmas that made them wonder whether survival under managed care was worth pursuing. They worried that by giving in to managed care they were becoming more fully integrated into the medical model they had once challenged. As one woman from the Chico FWHC worried, "In setting ourselves up as gatekeepers, and building alliances with the state and primary providers, we're helping construct a health care model we don't even believe in." If FWHCs built those alliances effectively, she asked, "will we still be feminist women's health centers?"[114] This concern may have been exacerbated because the centers had never prioritized their role as providers of health care services. They continued to see their mission as creating "a world where women controlled their own bodies, reproduction, and sexuality,"[115] and they regarded their ability to remain woman controlled—indeed, laywoman controlled—as central to their goals and identity. Would managed care destroy the central mission of the clinics while keeping them alive? Dido Hasper wondered in 1994 if, by giving into managed care, women were "hammering nails in our own coffin, with doctors running our show[.] We'd turn our woman-controlled clinics into gynecological offices." Still, Hasper recognized that the clinics had been changing since the beginning, becoming increasingly less "theirs" over the years. She suggested that rejecting managed care meant certain closure, while some managed-care arrangement might be palatable. If not, she noted practically, "at least the clinics will bring a higher price."[116]

In 1996, the Chico center and its Redding satellite clinic secured managed-care contracts; however, they had to restructure their clinics, "upgrade their image," and change their name to the generic and apolitical Women's Health Specialists. Although it allowed the center to provide continued access to abortion and other reproductive services, the changeover nearly destroyed the center financially.[117] Still, at the beginning of the twenty-first century, the center recovered economically, enabling it to expand its services into even more rural areas and rededicate itself to providing health and wellness information to women outside medical settings.

The Chico FWHC began in 1975 to meet the reproductive health needs of its community and to secure the political goals of women's liberation. The center offered abortions and other health services in a context that stressed women's choice, medical demystification, and knowledge sharing. It strove to normalize abortion as a medical procedure and legitimate form of fertility control. Still, the women of the center never saw their mission as exclusively focused on health care. They promoted self-help, condemned population control, and denounced the medical exploitation of women.

The history of the Chico FWHC illustrates the kinds of accommodations that grassroots organizations often make if they survive beyond the political moment that created them. The leaders of the Chico center adjusted their practices and goals in response to often hostile outside pressures. They changed, however, by weighing those compromises against the political and social importance of their continued survival for the women they served, both in their clinics and through their broader educational and political efforts. While they worried whether each compromise eroded the mission, they understood that their mission had always included health care and politics. Further, the women involved with the center realized that the promise and potential of an institution depended on its social and cultural context. As a result, the political understanding of their mission and services changed in response to changing circumstances. Certainly, providing reproductive health services and fighting the antiabortion forces on many fronts displaced many of the hallmarks of the earlier center's work. Self-help gynecology did not disappear from the center's work, but its role was greatly diminished. Similarly, lay health workers were not shut out of the clinics entirely, but they stepped aside, begrudgingly, to let medical professionals and other licensed health care workers perform the hands-on care. Still, the women involved with the center always believed that they continued to promote a political mission.

Although the changes described in this chapter likely came at great personal cost to the women involved, they do not necessarily mark the demise of a feminist approach to abortion provision and reproductive health care. The women of the center continued to fight for women's empowerment at every turn; their tools changed, but so did the weapons of their opponents. Their compromises represented transformed strategies in a changed political landscape of possibility. Clearly, offering abortion services to women in the face of varied assaults for more than forty years was a political act. And yet, the women who directed the clinic still hoped for a broader and deeper impact. In 2007, director Shauna Heckert acknowledged that Chico health activists once "thought the revolution was coming sooner than we think now," but she insisted that the center was still "in the business of confronting the power structure."[118] After battling into the twenty-first century, they revived their challenge to population control policies, even if they rarely denigrated Planned Parenthood by name. They insisted that women have the right to and the need for information about their bodies that is not created by or passed through the medical profession. They still believed that a speculum and a flashlight could reveal personal truths and unmask medical myths. In sum, they still saw long-term social change as their priority, as well as their challenge.

5

Lesbian Health Matters!
Lesbians and the
Women's Health Movement

In the early 1970s, Francie Hornstein was living in Iowa City. A recent graduate of the University of Iowa, she was active in the Women's Liberation Front, and she hoped to transform her particular interest in women's health issues into feminist action. Her first efforts, bringing her feminist sensibilities into "a local free clinic," were frustrated by the pervasive sexism even in this "alternative" setting. Still, she vowed to serve the health needs of women. When Carol Downer and Lorraine Rothman came to Iowa to demonstrate the "Self-Help Clinic," Hornstein witnessed "the most revolutionary concept in the area of women's health care." As she gained information and watched women learning from each other, she "saw very clearly just how we were going to create women's medicine!" In the aftermath of this demonstration, Hornstein and two of her Iowa City compatriots packed up and moved to Los Angeles to work with Downer and Rothman at the Feminist Women's Health Center.[1]

After arriving in LA, however, they began to hear grumblings from some lesbians, who asked, in effect, "Why would three nice lesbians like you want to work so hard for straight women?" Hornstein was shocked to hear the movement framed in such heterosexist terms; she understood women's health as a movement "for all of us." To challenge what she believed was a misguided political position, in 1973 she wrote what became a foundational document in the women's health movement, *Lesbian Health Care*. In it she made the case for how the women's health movement met the needs of lesbians and all women.

Hornstein declared that she wanted "all of my lesbian sisters to have competent, sensitive, woman-administered health care. And I want no less for heterosexual women or women who are not having sexual relationships at all." She condemned the lesbian critique of the movement as "foggy, irrational thinking." She countered: "The whole idea that we, as lesbians, were being used by heterosexual women to do the work that would benefit only straight women was very narrow thinking . . . both in an immediate practical sense as well as in a wider political sense." Most important, however, she noted that abortion and contraception—the ability to control fertility—were "vital to all of us who are Feminists in light of the use of women's bodies by men for their purposes—from rape to population control—two issues that affect every one of us, regardless of our sexuality." Finally, she denied that reproductive health affected only straight women. Hornstein reminded her readers that many lesbians had children and many others hoped to. Consequently, she claimed: "We need women's medicine as much as any other women." In sum, she insisted, "the myth that the women's health movement is for heterosexual women must be destroyed" because the movement's efforts to wrest control of women's bodies away from men benefited straight and lesbian women equally. For Hornstein, then, lesbian health was rightly and unambiguously a subset of women's health and thus best addressed through the women's health movement.[2]

Hornstein clearly believed that the significance of the women's health movement extended well beyond the provision of health services. By promoting self-help, by highlighting the benefits of returning women's health to women's hands, she described a movement to secure women's liberation. She insisted that lesbian-identified women and straight women alike needed the tools offered by the feminist health movement.

Hornstein's story was not unique—many lesbians worked in the women's health movement, seeing it as key to all women's liberation, even as the reproductive needs of heterosexual women seemed to dominate the work. But some lesbians strove to bring lesbian health demands more centrally into the movement. While this effort yielded some success, it was not enough for lesbian health activists who dreamed of health care free from homophobia and heterosexism, who desired a movement dedicated to the health needs of lesbians. As lesbians took on this work, several questions vexed their efforts. What were lesbians' most pressing health issues? What might lesbian-centered health provision include? Who counted as a lesbian? Between 1970 and 2000, lesbian health activists working within the feminist health movement and beyond it struggled with these questions.

This chapter traces the history of "lesbian health." It argues that lesbian health began as an area of feminist health neglect and a simultaneous demand for more lesbian-centered research and services. In the 1970s and '80s, feminist health activists scrambled to redress the neglect and meet the demand by offering lesbian health services, spearheading lesbian health research, and promoting a lesbian health agenda. Despite these efforts, the boundaries and content of an imagined lesbian health agenda remained elusive. Reproductive issues attracted significant attention in the late '70s and early '80s, and HIV/AIDS, perhaps surprisingly, galvanized some lesbian health activists in the '80s and '90s. But beyond a demand for health care free from homophobia and heterosexism, health workers, researchers, and activists remained unsure how to define and deliver lesbian health.

Two interconnected issues plagued the efforts to define and meet lesbian health care needs. First, lesbian identity—as a political and social marker of sexual desire, affectional preference, and political allegiance—fit uncomfortably as a category of health research and health provision. It was unclear who counted as a lesbian. Second, the category of lesbian health stymied efforts to pin it down, complicated both by the ambiguity of the category of "lesbian" and by the difficulties of framing the relationship between lesbian identity and lesbian health needs, either at the individual or group level. Were lesbians essentially women who rejected patriarchy at every level? Or did lesbian identity connote a particular life experience with distinct health needs? It was clear that lesbian health, as a category of health provision and health research, required an end to homophobia and heterosexism. But after this conceptual foundation, the boundaries defining lesbian health remained fuzzy throughout this period. Would lesbian health include issues unique to lesbians or more common in lesbians than in non-lesbians? Did all health issues in lesbians benefit from a lesbian health approach? Did lesbian health focus primarily on the health concerns and needs directly related to lesbian identity? These questions arose repeatedly as conceptual pitfalls impeding the progress of lesbian health research, health, and organizing. Indeed, they challenged the very foundation of a lesbian health movement. One lesbian health activist put it in 1989: "Nobody really knows what lesbian health is, or what it could be."[3]

Gay Liberation

As Francie Hornstein's example shows, lesbian health as an activist project incubated in and emerged from the feminist health movement. It was made imaginable, however, by the rise of a larger movement dedicated to securing rights and liberation for gay men and lesbians.

Although organized efforts to improve the social status of homosexuals began in the 1930s, they became increasingly more active and visible in the 1950s within what was then known as the homophile movement. This movement was largely, albeit not exclusively, segregated by sex. The Mattachine Society, founded by Harry Hay in New York City in 1950, catered to the social

LESBIAN HEALTH MATTERS!   151

and political needs of homosexual men, and the Daughters of Bilitis, founded by Del Martin and Phyllis Lyon in San Francisco in 1955, focused on lesbian issues. Both provided influential models for later organizing. These homophile groups and others that followed focused primarily on civil rights issues, including employment discrimination.[4]

In the late 1960s, a new but overlapping social movement began, framing the demands of homosexual men and women around a distinctly different axis—one that rejected the politics of respectability and instead demanded recognition of and respect for sexual and gendered behaviors outside the norms of the middle-class, white mainstream. The gay liberation movement did not dismiss the homophile movement's focus on securing individual rights; it also created an in-your-face demand for cultural recognition and acceptance. Gay liberation celebrated sexual freedom, encouraged "gay pride," and demanded respect for gender nonconformity. In gay pride parades, openly gay community establishments, and artistic creations, gay and lesbian people fought for their rights by living out loud.[5]

Gay Politics Meet Gender Politics

Some lesbians found their political community within gay organizations and identified primarily with efforts to challenge oppression born of homophobia. They were less interested in taking on sexism as their issue. The pathbreaking activist Barbara Gittings, for example, began her work in the San Francisco Daughters of Bilitis, taking responsibility for its newsletter, the *Ladder*. She frequently collaborated with Frank Kameny of the DC Mattachine Society in an effort to secure civil rights for gay men and women. Gittings had no particular affinity for issues she associated with feminism—access to childcare and abortion, for example—and she ultimately found her community among gay men. As she put it, she identified as a lesbian and not a feminist: "As long as prejudice continues to exist against my people, my primary identification will be with them."[6]

Other lesbians, though eager to call out homophobia and heterosexism, were also concerned about the damaging effects of sexism. These lesbians also identified as feminists and frequently bristled against the sexism they encountered within homophile and gay liberation organizations. This sexism materialized as neglect of lesbian issues, enforcement of gendered organizational roles, blindness to race and class privilege, and outright misogyny. Del Martin, who tried to bring lesbian issues into feminism, eventually found homophile organizations inhospitable to women. In 1971, she famously described her reasons for leaving the male-dominated homophile movement after fifteen years of "working for coalition and unity." In language filled with rage and betrayal, she described why, like Robin Morgan before her, she said "goodbye to all that":

> Goodbye to the wasteful, meaningless verbiage of empty resolutions made by hollow men of self-proclaimed privilege. They neither speak for us nor to us. . . . Goodbye to the male chauvinists of the homophile movement who are so wrapped up in the "cause" they espouse that they have lost sight of the people for whom the movement came into being. . . . Goodbye, too, . . . to my sisters who demean themselves by accepting "women's status" in these groups—making and serving coffee, doing the secretarial work, soothing the brows of the policy makers who tell them, "We're doing it all for you, too."[7]

Martin's complaints echo the complaints of women involved in earlier organizations of the Left who eventually refused to ignore their own interests for the sake of a "larger cause."[8]

In Martin's proclamation we can also see her discomfort with some of the sexual liberation and gender flexibility goals of gay liberation. She denounced, for example, the gay bars that served only to "dispens[e] . . . drinks and sex partners," the homophile publications that doubled as pornography, and the "defense of wash room sex."[9] She clearly did not champion a sexual freedom that pushed against public norms of propriety.

Lesbians with feminist priorities also found that their interests as lesbians were often dismissed by the women's movement. Some leaders of the National Organization for Women (NOW), for example, feared that any attention to lesbian concerns—or any visibility of lesbians—would taint the feminist movement and make it less palatable for "mainstream" America. Consequently, when Del Martin and Phyllis Lyon, founders of the Daughters of Bilitis, the nation's first lesbian civil rights organization, reached out to NOW to work together for a common cause, their overtures were rebuffed. Similarly, officers within New York City NOW fired the lesbian author Rita Mae Brown from her job as the editor of the group's newsletter. Most infamously, in 1970, Betty Friedan, then president of NOW, described the threat to feminism posed by the "lavender menace." This pronouncement and the continued dismissal of lesbian concerns from the feminist agenda led to the demonstration at the Second Congress to Unite Women where a group of radical lesbian feminists, including Brown, donned "Lavender Menace" T-shirts and circulated a "Woman-Identified Woman" manifesto. This manifesto began with the oft-quoted claim that "a lesbian is the rage of all women condensed to the point of explosion."[10]

Born in rage at the intersection of these two movements, *lesbian feminism—*

an umbrella term that covered a variety of social positions and cultural allegiances—provided organizational and political homes to lesbian refugees from feminist and gay organizations. Developed in the late 1960s and early '70s, it emerged when lesbians working with gay organizations and feminist groups believed that the needs of lesbians were not being met through either movement. Although lesbian feminism encompassed a variety of politics, at least two conceptual beliefs undergirded its organizing. First, it offered a critique of heterosexuality as "natural," framing it instead as an institution that oppressed women. Second, because heterosexuality was no more natural than homosexuality, lesbian feminists urged all feminists to choose women as their primary emotional and sexual partners, thus refusing to contribute to the patriarchy. Within this framework, partnering with women, as lesbians or woman-identified women, became a political act of feminism.[11]

Lesbian feminists frequently espoused the value of a separate women's (or occasionally womyn's) culture and women's institutions. Although few lesbians packed up their VW vans and decamped to womyn's land to lead lives beyond the reach of patriarchy and capitalism, lesbian feminists frequently created women-only gathering spaces, including restaurants, music festivals, and co-ops.[12] These efforts reflected a belief that building a community and a shared culture provided a bulwark against male domination.[13]

This position—that all women could and should be lesbians—rankled lesbians and straight women alike. Many lesbians believed that they had no choice in who they desired, and they viewed woman-identified women as inauthentically lesbian. Straight women (sometimes dismissively referred to as male-identified women) were often similarly offended that their relationships with men were interpreted as cavorting with the enemy.

The lesbian feminist project, then, revealed and stoked significant ambiguity at the center of lesbian identity. According to the sociologist Arlene Stein, lesbian feminists "found themselves caught between two projects: fixing lesbians as a stable group and 'liberating' the lesbian in every woman."[14] The ambiguity was not merely theoretical. It mattered significantly as lesbians constructed a health politics. The porous borders of lesbian identity and the politics at the center of some of its projects compounded the difficulties of conceiving and enacting a lesbian health agenda.

Lesbians, feminists and otherwise, imagined, demanded, and developed "lesbian health." In a variety of ways, they led efforts to put the health needs of lesbians at the center of social activism. Lesbians' health needs overlapped with women's health needs, and lesbians surely benefited from and participated in the efforts to combat sexism in medicine. Lesbians also contributed to and benefited from efforts to combat homophobia in the health professions and to provide health care to gay men and lesbians. Neither of these movements, however, put the health needs of lesbians first; lingering heterosexism and sexism in these movements helped foment a more targeted focus on lesbian health both within these movements and independent of them.

Gay Health Activism

Influenced by other grassroots health efforts of the 1960s and '70s, some gay activists from homophile and gay liberation groups organized around health. They hoped to both improve the quality of care for gay and lesbian patients and improve the climate for gay and lesbian health care workers. This effort acknowledged and condemned physicians' frequent disdain for their gay patients, noting that men seeking treatment for sexually transmitted infections (STIs), known at the time as venereal diseases (VD), experienced particular disrespect.[15] But medicine, because it constructed a model of homosexuality as an outward expression of an inner pathology, shaped the understanding of homosexuals as a group.[16] Much of the nineteenth- and early twentieth-century medical, psychological, and "sexological" literature focused on ascertaining the cause of the "disorder" or "perversion" and considered ideas for its treatment. This morally repugnant position justified the widespread discrimination of gay men and lesbians. As Gittings put it in 1967, "The charge of sickness is perhaps our greatest problem. We can't really progress in other directions until the unsubstantiated assumption of sickness . . . is demolished."[17]

Perhaps the first high-profile action of this movement was the effort to remove homosexuality as a category of illness from the *Diagnostic and Statistical Manual of Mental Disorders* (*DSM*) in the early 1970s. Using a combination of actions—protesting and heckling at the American Psychological Association's (APA) annual meeting, performing staid academic presentations of psychological research, and strategizing in backrooms—activists finally saw victory in December 1973 when the Trustees of the APA voted to remove homosexuality as a category of psychiatric disorder from its upcoming revision of the *DSM*. This decision was affirmed in a second vote, this time by all the voting members of the association in 1974. The win was not absolute, however. In a move meant to appease those individuals who believed that homosexuality was both pathological and treatable, the new *DSM* included "Sexual Orientation Disturbance" as a classification of patients who were distressed by their homosexuality.[18] Although clearly a milestone in the history of gay activism, it is unclear how this declassification might have changed the treatment gay men and lesbians received from their physicians, when and if they could access medical care.

Gay and lesbian health care providers launched a more sustained effort to shape health care by creating a series of professional organizations to increase gay visibility and combat homophobia. The Gay Nurses Alliance, cofounded by librarian Gittings, paved the way in 1973 for other health professionals, including public health workers and pharmacists, to follow suit.[19] Physicians proved harder to organize. Four medical students in Michigan founded the American Lesbian Medical Association in the fall of 1973, but the organization likely folded in 1976.[20] By 1980, the American Medical Student Association had formed a task force on Lesbian and Gay People in Medicine,[21] but it wasn't until 1981 that the American Association of Physicians for Human Rights formed. It was later rebranded under various, more explicit names. In 1976, activists created the National Gay Health Coalition (later renamed the National Coalition for LGBTQ Health) as an umbrella group that became the "nexus of gay health activism." Men and women worked within these organizations and others focused on eliminating the homophobia directed toward gay and lesbian colleagues and patients.[22]

When activists tried to identify the specific health needs of the gay community, it proved difficult to find issues shared by gay men and lesbians. The prevalence of STIs among gay and bisexual men made agenda setting for gay male health activists clear. The alleged epidemic of sexually transmitted infections posed a clear health danger to gay men. By the mid-1950s, public health workers in New York blamed gay and bisexual men for the city's high rates of gonorrhea and syphilis. By the 1970s, health statistics clearly backed up the claim. The Centers for Disease Control and Prevention (CDC) attributed more than 45 percent of all cases of early syphilis to gay men, and in Denver, 60 percent of all early syphilis cases were found in gay or bisexual men. Further, gay men at the greatest risk for STIs frequently skipped disease screening, likely being "reluctant to trust their health to medical authorities who might discriminate against them." As a result, gay health activists established "VD" testing clinics in several major cities, including Los Angeles, New York, Seattle, Boston, and Chicago.[23]

Lesbians, by contrast, had no clearly identified health needs. And yet, lesbians occasionally sought services at clinics promoted to and for the "gay community." They were not generally welcome. For example, lesbians seeking health care at the Howard Brown Memorial Clinic in Chicago, founded in 1974 as a gay VD clinic, were turned away. In response, they protested that the clinic discriminated against women.[24]

As the HIV/AIDS crisis began in 1981, even more of the energy and funding from a gay and lesbian health movement focused on the critical health needs of gay men. New clinics emerged in direct response to the AIDS epi-

demic, and others that had tried to provide balanced services to lesbians and
gay men found that the demands of HIV/AIDS required all their economic
and emotional resources. For example, the Community Health Project of
New York City, founded in 1983 by a merger of the Gay Men's Health Project
and St. Marks Community Clinic with the goal of providing for the gay and
lesbian community, had, by 1988, devoted all its resources to people with
AIDS or at risk for AIDS because of HIV infection.[25]

In some ways, HIV/AIDS deflected health research and resources away
from lesbians and their health needs. And yet, as this chapter will show, HIV/
AIDS organizing became a focus of lesbian health activism in the 1980s and
'90s. HIV/AIDS organizing involved lesbians working on behalf of gay men
and, eventually, other marginalized groups. It was simultaneously an effort to
fight for the health of lesbians themselves.

Creating Lesbian Health

Let us return to Francie Hornstein's description of the place of lesbians within
the women's health movement. As she saw it, lesbians were integral to the
movement from the beginning, often providing leadership in a variety of
feminist health efforts, from the fight for abortion rights to the promotion of
self-help to the establishment of feminist health clinics. According to some
accounts, lesbians dominated the movement.[26] The women's movement also
frequently provided support for women exploring their sexual desires. For
example, according to one health activist at the Gainesville Women's Health
Center, "Every one of us became a lesbian while working at the clinic."[27] But
not all feminist health groups welcomed lesbians, and others discouraged
public declarations of sexual identity. Many women at the Tallahassee Feminist Women's Health Center, for example, identified as lesbian, but because
the leaders feared a homophobic community response, lesbians were discouraged from being "out." As one activist put it, directors of the center didn't
want "people's homophobia and heterosexism [to] keep them away" from
health services.[28]

Sometimes tensions over sexuality created irreparable rifts. According
to a few straight women involved in the Emma Goldman clinic in Chicago,
some of the founders of the clinic "became lesbian separatists" after becoming
involved with the clinic. The lesbians—at least, from the perspective of the
straight women—came to believe that the clinic was dominated by "straight
women who fuck over lesbians." The specific issues of disagreement included
the place of men in the building, the possibility of heterosexual feminists,
and the extent of heterosexism and homophobia within the organization. On

the latter front, lesbians allegedly believed that the "straight women couldn't deal with the lesbians because they were afraid of the latent lesbianism in themselves and afraid of projecting a lesbian image." The straight women who narrated this story denied the widespread presence of "queer fear" within the group, suggesting instead that power differentials among the group and soured personal relationships encouraged the lesbians to leave the clinic to pursue projects with "lesbianism" at their center.[29] The precise nature of the tensions within this organization and their connection to the politics of sexuality cannot be known from this one account. And yet, it demonstrates how issues around sexuality and separatist politics proved useful to explain difficult internal dynamics within the organization.

Despite the internal skirmishes over sexual identity experienced by some feminist health groups, gynecological self-help affected many lesbians powerfully. It clearly inspired Hornstein. Barbara Hoke, a teacher, "faculty-wife," and emerging lesbian feminist in Tallahassee, also saw in self-help the promise of women controlling their lives and breaking the isolation between each other. After representatives from the Oakland Feminist Women's Health Center demonstrated self-help as part of a radical feminism conference, Hoke sold her house, divorced her husband, and joined the Oakland group.[30] As one advocate put it, "For lesbians, the gynecological self-help movement is much like a course in self-defense. For as lesbians, we are the most likely to be intimidated, patronized, and literally ostracized by a male-dominated medical establishment which knows nothing—and cares even less—about the kinds of health care lesbians need and want."[31] For these lesbians, the feminist health movement—even if it appeared to focus on the reproductive needs of straight women—offered a necessary alternative to male-dominated medicine.

By 1975, however, some lesbians grew increasingly frustrated with a movement theoretically committed to empowering all women while practically focused on the reproductive needs of ostensibly straight women. Some wondered what was in it for them. In "Is There Life after Abortions?," Freddy Brass, a lesbian from Iowa City, lamented the time lesbians spent securing the reproductive health needs of straight women. "Do we have any energy left for ourselves after spending the day as a patient advocate for women getting abortions (or birth control or babies)? Do we even know what there is to be done for ourselves?" She understood the importance of securing reproductive services for all women, but she wanted to turn her attention to issues of "personal relevance." "What I want to work on now . . . is lesbian health care, lesbian health research, and how to acquire the technology to care for ourselves and do that research." This desire to focus on lesbian health encouraged Brass to leave the women's health movement.[32]

Brass left the movement, but many other lesbians stayed, committed to meeting the health needs of women as a step toward women's liberation, and vowing to make the movement responsive to the needs of lesbians. The effort to include lesbians explicitly on the agenda was evident at the 1975 Conference on Women and Health, held on the Harvard Medical School campus. This major conference, attended by roughly 2,500 women, relied on separate working groups for much of its content, including a Third World Women's Caucus and a Lesbian Working Group. In addition to sponsoring eight panels addressing lesbian health issues, the Lesbian Health Working Group presented three major goals for the future: to promote lesbian visibility and decry heterosexism within the women's health movement; to develop a lesbian health agenda; and to organize a lesbian-authored resource focused on lesbian health issues.[33] During these sessions, lesbians expressed their frustrations ("and boredom") about spending so much of their time focused on the reproductive needs of straight women. One woman suggested that the reproductive health focus left no time to concentrate on other topics, including sexuality. Although participants acknowledged the commonalities between lesbians and straight women, they also insisted that "space should be made for lesbians in women-controlled clinics."[34]

While affirming the benefits of the women's health movement for all women, feminist health clinics tried a variety of methods to create lesbian-welcoming spaces. Self-help groups provided an early vehicle for lesbian inclusion, and feminist health centers across the country formed lesbian self-help groups.[35] According to one activist, these emerged in response to the alienation and exclusion many lesbians experienced in "mixed groups." These self-help groups avoided the emphasis on birth control so common in self-help and explored lesbian-specific needs.[36]

Many feminist health clinics also instituted "lesbian nights"—a few clinic hours each week or month that catered to lesbians. Sometimes these initiatives responded to lesbian demand; sometimes they were generated by health activists from within the clinic itself. Lesbian nights rarely survived long, perhaps because demand frequently underwhelmed supply.[37] The Emma Goldman Clinic for Women in Iowa City, for example, began offering monthly gynecological clinics to lesbians in early January 1976 to overcome the perception that the clinic had a heterosexual bias. By April, discouraged and frustrated because lesbians had failed to show up, clinic leaders abandoned the effort.[38]

This example suggests that feminist health activists had trouble attracting lesbians to their clinics. Only after their lesbian nights project floundered

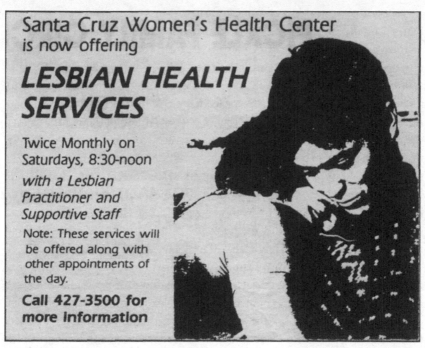

Santa Cruz Women's Health Center
is now offering

LESBIAN HEALTH SERVICES

Twice Monthly on
Saturdays, 8:30-noon

with a Lesbian
Practitioner and
Supportive Staff

Note: These services will
be offered along with
other appointments of
the day.

**Call 427-3500 for
more information**

FIGURE 5.1. Lesbian-focused services lasted at least until 1986 at the Santa Cruz Women's Health Center. *Matrix*, June 1986. Herstory Archive: Feminist Newspapers, Lesbian Herstory Archives. Courtesy of the Archives of Sexuality and Gender.

did the women from Emma Goldman, some of them lesbians themselves, ask lesbians in the community about their current health care practices and their attitudes toward Emma Goldman. The survey yielded important findings. First, lesbians who responded to the survey indicated that they regularly sought health care and were generally pleased with the services they received. This challenged the widespread assumption that "lesbians . . . are totally alienated from seeking health care." Second, the clinic discovered that many lesbians avoided it because of its "heterosexual bias." Although the authors of the study protested this point, they conceded that "many lesbians have become alienated from feminist health care because they feel as invisible within its purview as they do in the traditional structures." Third, survey respondents couldn't imagine how Emma Goldman might usefully serve them because the respondents couldn't identify any specific lesbian health needs.[39] This document suggests that feminist health centers' efforts to provide lesbian health services had both failed to overcome their reputations as heterosexually focused institutions and overestimated the demand for lesbian health, especially as it was ambiguously conceived.

By contrast, a health center in Cambridge, Massachusetts, knew what lesbians wanted, but its workers proved unwilling to meet their request. The Women's Community Health Center tried from the beginning to incorporate lesbian health concerns into their self-help programs and their health services.[40] But when some lesbians in the community demanded access to lesbian-identified health workers, the leadership of the clinic balked. In a 1976 statement, clinic leaders explained their position. Although their aim was that the clinic would "create an environment in which women feel free to express their sexuality-related health needs and questions," they rejected a suggestion that it should provide lesbian health workers on request. They feared that such a policy would "perpetuate divisions between heterosexual and lesbian women," provide lesbians with privileges not available to other groups of women, and force health workers at the center to identify ("label") their sexuality. As clinic leaders reported, "Many of us are not able or willing."[41]

The workers at the clinic eventually changed their thinking. While acknowledging their earlier "refusal to perpetuate divisions between ourselves," they had by 1979 come to recognize that women experience different forms of oppression, based in part on the very differences the women had once hoped to overcome. Their acknowledgment of difference allowed them to "unite and support each other." Consequently, they developed a lesbian fertility consciousness group and planned to offer a participatory clinic with lesbian health care workers.[42]

The Boston Women's Health Book Collective, creators of the foundational compendium of woman-generated knowledge about women's bodies and health, had their own difficulties including lesbian perspectives. Lesbian's health and sexuality received only a brief mention in the original 1970 newsprint edition of *Women and Their Bodies*, and the 1971 New England Free Press edition, *Our Bodies, Ourselves*, replicated the original content.[43] For the 1973 Simon & Schuster edition, the collective recruited women involved in the gay liberation movement to write a chapter by and for lesbians. The product, "In Amerika They Call Us Dykes," suggests an unhappy collaboration. The lesbian authors distanced themselves from the larger project: "We had no connection with the group that was writing the rest of the book . . . and in fact we disagreed, and still do, with many of their opinions."[44]

The content of this chapter generally failed to identify a lesbian health agenda. Sandwiched between chapters on relationships and nutrition, "In Amerika" focused mostly on the lesbian experience in the United States, describing lesbian relationships, the perils of coming out, class divisions within lesbian communities, and the importance of bars as social spaces. A brief section, "The-Rapist: Lesbians and Psychiatry," which denounced the psychoanalytic framework that declared lesbians sick or maladjusted, provided the closest engagement with straightforward health issues.[45]

That the flagship women's health publication had to farm out its lesbian content to a separate organization, and that this organization failed to articulate specific lesbian health concerns, suggests that lesbians had yet to develop a clear health agenda. Over time, Our Bodies, Ourselves developed more lesbian-specific content and a critique of homophobia; but as of 1982, a lesbian reader still complained, "Only about 1/3 of the book applies to me."[46]

Although feminist health activists frequently argued that their fight against medical sexism would ultimately benefit all women, gay and straight, lesbian feminists working outside feminist health organizations insisted that a movement to benefit all women must include a critique of heterosexism and homophobia. Members of the Radicalesbians Health Collective, a New York City group, for example, wrote their own position paper on "lesbians and the health care system." In this 1971 text, the collective condemned the medical profession in general and psychology in particular. The collective's critique of medicine partially reflected that of the larger women's health movement. They denounced, for example, the paternalistic nature of the medical encounter, encouraging instead the widespread use of laywoman health educators, especially at neighborhood clinics. They also demanded that more women become gynecologists: "Why must we ask men questions about ourselves?" In these examples, the health goals of lesbians clearly overlapped with the goals of the larger women's health movement.[47]

The Radicalesbians Health Collective's focus on heterosexism and homophobia, however, was unmatched by the larger movement. Collective members testified to the mistreatment of lesbians, especially by the psychological professions. J, for example, described her experience with a psychiatrist when she was nineteen and eager to talk about the recent death of her mother. The psychiatrist suggested that her problems would be solved "if I found the right man, got married, and started a family of my own." More outrageously, P's psychiatrist recommended that she have sex with men; he volunteered his services. "So we had sex about 5 or 6 times during therapy sessions which I paid for."[48] In general, the collective members charged that psychologists saw lesbians as sick and recommended heterosexuality as treatment. The collective members demanded that the medical and psychological professions stop regarding lesbianism as a problem. Clearly, the collective identified medical sexism as a significant problem for all women, but their critique also highlighted the devastating effects of homophobia and heterosexism. Unless the women's health movement addressed these issues, this document implied, it would never meet the needs of lesbians.[49]

By the mid-1970s, the lesbian feminist movement also identified alcoholism as a particular problem in the lesbian community. In 1975, for example, the *Lesbian Connection*, based in East Lansing, Michigan, published a three-part series on "Lesbians and Alcoholism." These articles identified the "modern tragedy of lesbian alcoholism," claiming that one in seven lesbians was an alcoholic. "Kristi," the author of the articles, blamed homophobia, for condemning lesbians as "queers and perverts," as well as the gay bar scene, the "only place where lesbians can be lesbians." In these articles, the author explained why lesbians might suffer disproportionately from alcoholism: "Not only are we oppressed by strait [*sic*] society, but we are also trapped by a subculture that condones drinking, and further ensnared by an institution that definitely encourages it."[50] These statements from the lesbian feminist movement highlighted the possible health consequences of homophobia and demonstrated the inadequacy of a feminist critique of medical sexism without a similar critique of homophobia.

The women's health movement helped create and define the category of lesbian health. Emerging as a critique of the women's health movement, lesbian health was first identified as an absence, as a category of neglect, a symbol of the heterosexist assumptions of the women's health movement. In response, representatives of the women's health movement, both gay and straight, insisted that lesbians, because they were women, benefited from the movement's efforts to wrest control of women's bodies from men, constructing lesbian health as the beneficiary of the broader improvements in women's health created by the feminist health movement. Finally, health activists understood that lesbians might want to explore their bodies, sexuality, and health needs with other lesbians, so they established lesbian-centered programming and clinics. In this way, the health movement constructed lesbian health as a category of service offered to lesbians. The larger movement, however, did not place homophobia at the center of its critique of medicine. For the most part, that critique came from activists aligned with lesbian feminism outside the parameters of the women's health movement.

Establishing Lesbian Health Institutions

Although some feminist health clinics offered "lesbian nights" and sponsored lesbian self-help clinics, these gestures were not enough to meet the health needs of many lesbians. Uncomfortable with the homophobia of mainstream medicine and the heterosexism of some feminist alternatives, lesbians were more likely than heterosexual women to skip routine health exams and to feel uncomfortable during health visits.[51] In order to bring health care to underserved lesbian communities, a few lesbian feminists founded lesbian health clinics. These institutions provided an alternative to the women's health clinics that focused on the needs of straight women and the gay clinics that frequently treated lesbian health as an afterthought if at all.

Lesbians in Seattle founded one of the first independent lesbian health clinics in 1974. These women, calling themselves the Lesbian Health Collective (LHC), had worked in a variety of health clinics around the city and had identified the need for a health care space by and for lesbians. They noted that many lesbians could not "stomach" male gynecologists or the heterosexist assumptions of most women's clinics and therefore frequently declined to access recommended gynecological health screenings. The founders also noted that lesbian-identified health care providers deserved work spaces that validated their lesbianism rather than forcing them to be "hidden lesbians in the predominantly heterosexual women's clinics." These women also found contraceptive counseling "depressing" and happily left it to their "straight sisters." They reached an agreement with the Fremont Women's Clinic to provide lesbian-specific programming once a week and lesbian-centered health screening and care once a month.[52]

In describing their mission, the women of the LHC insisted that they did not provide "a service for lesbians." Instead, they imagined they were meeting their own needs by serving their community.[53] Nevertheless, they admitted that the community who sought health care at the clinic was quite "narrow" and that they were "anxious to serve more people."[54] Although this clinic seems to have survived longer than the "lesbian nights" offered by several feminist health clinics, it probably folded after slightly more than two years.[55]

On the other coast, lesbian activists in New York City also opened a lesbian-centered health clinic in 1974. St. Marks Community Clinic began in 1970 as a free clinic to meet the health needs of the "street kids" and other medically underserved populations in Manhattan's East Village.[56] In the 1970s, the neighborhood—always in flux—provided a home to countercultural hippies, Ukrainian and Puerto Rican immigrants, ramshackle squats, and purportedly the world's largest gay bathhouse. Homelessness, drug dealing, and crime were common.[57] By 1973, lesbian volunteers at the clinic began to see lesbians as an underserved population—discouraged from seeking medical care by the homophobia and heterosexism of medical clinics and private practice alike. They particularly resented that straight women might receive free medical screening from clinics supported by federal family planning funds. These women, who eventually called themselves the Women's Health Collective, sometimes the Lesbian Health Collective, of St. Marks Clinic, began offering a women's clinic one night a week in March 1974.[58]

Women's nights at St. Marks Clinic were staffed by lesbian volunteers and promoted to the lesbian community. Still, the collective refrained from calling its facility a lesbian clinic, at least in its early years. Collective members insisted that no woman would be turned away unless they were only seeking birth control or other reproductive services. Although the collective highlighted the need for the clinic by insisting that "no illness should place us in the hands of professionals who have contempt for lesbianism and for our rights as health care consumers," they explicitly welcomed "older women" to the clinic as women without reproductive health needs.[59]

The Women's Health Collective gradually came to control St. Marks Community Clinic by taking over the board and setting a quota for the number of men and physicians who could govern. St. Marks continued to offer general medical clinics two nights a week, and it also developed a gay men's night staffed by gay men. For a few years, St. Marks was the rare clinic that catered to women's nonreproductive health needs, the needs of gay men, and medically underserved people, often youths, in the neighborhood.

The disinclination of the St. Marks Women's Health Collective to provide reproductive health services set them apart from other feminist health clinics of the era. In other aspects, however, they were clearly part of the same activist impulse. In particular, they depicted themselves as a challenge to medicine as usual, "an alternative to the hierarchical, male medical model."[60] As founder Barbara Herbert framed it, the clinic provided "technicians to serve people, not professionals to give answers."[61]

Collective members came to rethink their relationship to health care as a goal in itself. According to Herbert, in the beginning, the collective members "were people who believed in liberation, in destroying hierarchy and smashing the patriarchy. And then we came up against bad diseases."[62] In the face of significant illness and scarce resources, access to care emerged as the most crucial service the clinic could provide. To its founders' surprise, the collective that once pursued liberation focused increasingly on health care—providing health services and securing treatment for those needing specialized attention. Health care became the end in itself.

By the end of the decade, the clinic's internal relationships began to fray, primarily over sexual politics and the place of alternative health care. Men— male physicians particularly—staffing men's nights resented their weak representation on the governing board. Physicians, including some of those associated with the women's collective, also grew increasingly uncomfortable with the alternative healing methods offered on women's nights. Tensions over these and other issues grew intolerable, and in 1980, the clinic split into two

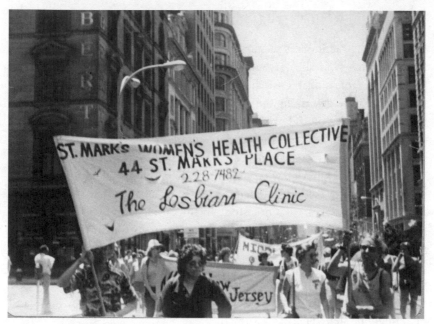

FIGURE 5.2. St. Marks Women's Health Collective only occasionally promoted itself as a lesbian clinic, as it did at the New York City Pride March pictured here. Copyright Lesbian Herstory Archives.

factions. One St. Marks, governed by the Women's Health Collective, continued to offer health care to lesbians and older women until 1995; another St. Marks initially offered health care to three discreet populations—the general public, gay men, and lesbians. This latter St. Marks turned to the health needs of gay men as the AIDS epidemic struck. In 1983, it merged with the Gay Men's Health Project to form the Community Health Project. By 1988, the Community Health Project had devoted itself to AIDS testing and care, and by 1989, only 10 percent of its clients were women.[63] The Community Health Project rebranded itself as Callen-Lorde Community Health Center in 1998.

When the Seattle Lesbian Health Collective and St. Marks Women's Health Collective offered lesbian-centered health services in the 1970s, they challenged the heterosexism and homophobia within mainstream medicine, free clinics, and feminist health movement. Their survival, however, was always tenuous, threatened by internal schisms, financial instability, and inconsistent demand. Moreover, the scope of their practice remained murky. St. Marks, for example, defined its focus outside of women's reproductive concerns. They could not claim special expertise in lesbian health issues, however, beyond their own sensitivity and the experience they gained over time. When these clinics opened, lesbian health research barely existed.[64]

Lesbian Health Research

In the 1970s, practitioners seeking guidance in the medical literature on the health problems of lesbians would have learned very little. Through the end of the decade, professional research on lesbian health virtually did not exist, save for the literature describing the pathology of homosexuality and "inversion" and a few articles on the psychological characteristics of lesbians.[65] Clearly lesbian health had not yet garnered much interest among health professionals.

Responding to this absence and consistent with the feminist project of woman-centered knowledge production, lesbians launched their own grass-roots, community-based research. Frances (Francie) Hornstein's 1973 *Lesbian Health Care* stands out as a milestone in the development of lesbian health research. *Lesbian Health Care* focused on how sexually transmitted infections (STIs) could be passed between women. Based on two years of feminist research, combining information gained at self-help clinics and conversations with trusted medical professionals, this publication claimed that STIs were rare among lesbians but noted that some genital infections (e.g., warts and lice) might be shared between women.[66]

This focus on STIs, widely presumed to be rare in lesbians, might be a surprising starting point for lesbian-centered health research. Still, it highlights an aspect of lesbian health that was most central to lesbian identity and most different from the experience of heterosexual women. It also reflects the health concerns of gay men and young, sexually active women. Finally, while STIs were presumed rare among lesbians, research documenting their prevalence did not exist until 1978.[67]

Hornstein's work on STIs also acknowledged that not all women who identified as lesbians "relate[d] sexually exclusively with women." She noted that some lesbians occasionally had sex with men, and that these women were at risk from the "serious health hazard[s]" of heterosexuality. This discussion highlights the slipperiness of the category of lesbian and how difficult it was to isolate lesbian health needs. Lesbians suffered from STIs even if their identity as lesbians might theoretically protect them from the "perils" of heterosexual sex. The lived experience of lesbians often included heterosexual practices.[68] That some of these women might have identified as bisexual was not mentioned, suggesting either the rare employment of the category or its political dismissal in lesbian feminist circles.

Other groups of health activists quickly followed with their own efforts to investigate and publicize the health needs of lesbians.[69] Spearheaded by Judi Stein, the Women's Community Health Center in Cambridge, Massachusetts, resolved to create a lesbian health pamphlet in 1975, and they solicited input in the lesbian and feminist press. As far as I can tell, this pamphlet never materialized.[70] In 1979, however, the Santa Cruz Women's Health Collective published the pathbreaking *Lesbian Health Matters! Lesbian Health Matters!* sought to consolidate health information specific to lesbians, provide information without heterosexist bias on a variety of health topics (menopause, alcoholism, self-care, "gynecological health"), educate health care providers about the health needs of lesbians, and build "strength and solidarity among lesbians."[71] The pamphlet engaged with issues of particular concern to lesbians, such as alternative fertilization, and it addressed issues shared by straight and gay women (e.g., vaginitis) from a lesbian perspective. The book mixed the practical (avoid coffee while battling a bladder infection) with the political (lesbians often turn to alcohol to escape the stresses of homophobia). In the end, the book identified the need for more research about lesbian health. The authors "suspect[ed]," for example, that certain health conditions were more common (breast cancer, alcoholism) or less common (syphilis, cervical cancer) in lesbians than in straight women, but they called for more research to provide "more accurate answers."[72]

At roughly the same time, lesbian health activists on the East Coast hatched a plan to ask lesbians (finally!) about their health and their relationship with the medical system. Conceived in 1978 by Caitlin Ryan, the project remained fallow for several years while Ryan pursued other projects. In 1982, while enrolled as a graduate student in social work at Smith College, she relaunched the project, collaborating with the New York City social worker and psychotherapist Bernice Goodman. After securing sponsorship from the newly created National Gay Health Education Foundation and funding from the Ms. Foundation, Ryan and Goodman recruited graduate student Judith Bradford. Pursuing a PhD in social policy and social work at Virginia Commonwealth University, Bradford brought her institutional affiliation and her emerging skill with survey design and data analysis to the project.[73]

Ryan and Bradford set three main goals for the survey. First, it aimed to provide a baseline inventory of the health status and concerns of lesbians. Without this baseline, Ryan and Bradford understood it was impossible to generalize about lesbian health care needs, identify gaps in current health services, and develop appropriate interventions.[74] Until activists identified central lesbian health needs, Ryan and Bradford feared lesbians "would continue to be discriminated against, underserved, [and] invisible" to mainstream medicine.[75] Second, the survey hoped to steer future research in lesbian health. By mapping areas of concern and neglect, the authors of the survey sought to set the research agenda. Third, the survey authors understood that "lesbian health" remained an amorphous concept. The survey thus attempted to "think through what lesbian health might mean," simultaneously "defining and exploring" the boundaries of lesbian health.[76]

In the fall of 1984, Ryan and Bradford sent out nearly four thousand questionnaires to women's centers, gay and lesbian organizations, gay newspapers, feminist bookstores, and personal contacts in prisons and the military. Participants returned nearly 50 percent of the surveys, a strong response rate, but their efforts to collect demographic diversity largely failed. Eighty percent of the participants were between the ages of 25 and 44, 61 percent had at least some college education, and 88 percent identified as white. (Six percent identified as Black and 4 percent as Latina.) Overall, then, this survey primarily provided a snapshot of the health status of an educationally and professionally elite segment of the lesbian-identified population—those whose access to health care and economic pathways to health were greatest.

The National Lesbian Health Care Survey (NLHCS) gathered and analyzed data from 1,925 lesbians from every US state and several territories. Not published until 1988, the NLHCS was the "most extensive study of lesbians" published in the twentieth century.[77] The survey documented several things: depression or sadness was the most common health problem reported; lesbians and straight women shared many health problems (e.g., arthritis, menstrual cramps, allergies); nearly one-third of the lesbians surveyed had been pregnant, and another third hoped to be; financial barriers kept many lesbians from getting needed health care; and many lesbians resented the heterosexist attitude of their health care providers. Nevertheless, 80 percent of the respondents reported that the health care they received was good or very good. In addition to these findings, the published report argued that lesbians' health would improve only through broader social acceptance of lesbianism. Ryan and Bradford concluded: "Unless service providers are able to view lesbianism as an acceptable lifestyle and not a symptom of mental illness or deviance, they risk delivering services that will be harmful rather than helpful or will prevent lesbians from accessing them."[78] This conclusion reinforced the claims of lesbian feminists in the early 1970s who insisted that heterosexism and homophobia endangered lesbians' health.

Despite the significance of the NLHCS as the first widespread effort to gauge the health of lesbians, its results failed to settle the boundaries of lesbian health, in part because the survey failed to capture a definitive sample of lesbians. It could describe the health only of the fairly homogeneous group of lesbians the survey had reached.[79] As a result, informal interpretations of the data suggesting, for example, that lesbians used alcohol in excess more than non-lesbians could not be definitively sustained. Further, it remained unclear whether lesbian health must be defined as a category of need in contrast to that of non-lesbians; or whether lesbian health could be understood as the sum total of health experiences of lesbians. In other words, should lesbian health focus on issues unique to lesbians, disproportionately afflicting lesbians, or common among lesbians?

By the beginning of the 1980s, lesbian-identified health professionals joined community-based efforts to create a body of research on lesbian health. These included a handful of lesbian physicians, psychologists, and medical students who were at least "somewhat out" at work and willing to assume the uncertain professional consequences of studying lesbians.[80] As the physician and early lesbian health researcher Susan Johnson described it, "I suppose it crossed my mind that it might be risky, but I guess I just didn't care."[81] These early researchers were simultaneously activists and professionals; they addressed an unmet need of the lesbian community by framing lesbian health issues for a professional audience.

In the 1980s, the medical literature on lesbian health, based almost exclusively on survey data, converged on several general claims: that lesbians frequently avoided medical professionals; that lesbians frequently withheld their lesbian identity from their health care providers; that many lesbians reported mistreatment from their physicians after revealing their identity; that particular health risks or lifestyle advantages of lesbians remained largely unstudied; and that the rates of alcoholism among lesbians appeared to be significantly higher (five to seven times higher) than in heterosexual women. These overarching findings demonstrated the need for further research into the health status of lesbians and the health consequences of homophobia.[82]

In the 1970s and '80s, research on lesbian health reflected activist passion and significant foundational problems. Throughout this period, the definition of lesbian remained generally unanalyzed. For the most part, lesbians qualified as lesbians for research purposes if they said they were. (Bisexuals, however they were defined, were sometimes considered in the same category as lesbians, sometimes in the category of straight women.) The researchers circulated surveys through friend networks or at various lesbian cultural sites including bars, musical festivals, and bookstores. The "lesbian" documented through this method of data collection was overwhelmingly white, middle class, well educated, and young.[83] It captured those who embraced a cultural identity; it did not attempt to locate and survey those who participated in particular behaviors. Further, because cultural factors including race, ethnicity, and religion all influenced the acceptance of the label, relying on lesbian identity to recruit subjects may have undersampled the very women who might have felt the effects of homophobia most intensely: working-class women, poor women, and women of color.

The research also highlighted the ambiguity of the project itself. These early researchers struggled with the boundaries of their efforts, realizing that they were "defining and exploring simultaneously."[84] The research failed to clearly identify what health issues concerned lesbians qua lesbians and how (and whether) their experiences of health and illness differed from other women. Pat Maher, the director of lesbian health projects in the New York City Office of Gay and Lesbian Health Concerns, said in 1984, "Trying to delineate what lesbian health issues are is like groping in the dark."[85]

Reproducing Lesbians

The heart of the lesbian-centered critique of the feminist health movement was its alleged focus on women's reproductive health needs. Lesbians, or so the argument went, did not need abortion or other forms of birth control. Further, there was a widespread belief among some elements of the community that lesbians didn't have children.[86] Barbara Butcher, for example, a volunteer at St. Marks, recalled, "No lesbians had babies back then. . . . You just never heard of that." She claimed that it wasn't until the 1980s that "gay women" said, "Oh, I want a baby. I'm going to have one."[87]

Many lesbians did have children, of course, most frequently from heterosexual relationships dating from before they identified as lesbian and from sexual encounters contemporary with their lesbian identity. For some of these women, motherhood created significant conflict in their lives. Lesbians in the 1960s and '70s, for example, frequently lost their children in the aftermath of divorce, and the fights over the status of male children in "womyn's space" affected both straight women and lesbians.[88] In the early 1970s, lesbian mothers began meeting in rap groups to discuss their shared concerns, including maintaining custody, raising sons, and coming out to their children.[89]

While lesbian mothers discussed their shared struggles, lesbians who wanted children also gathered to consider their options in community. In the 1970s, women's centers and clinics began to sponsor workshops for lesbians seeking motherhood.[90] Because adoption was generally unavailable for out lesbians, ideas for conception dominated these early conversations.[91]

Many lesbians, then as now, conceived children through sexual intercourse with men. Sometimes these encounters produced accidental conceptions; at other times, lesbians pursued sex with men to become pregnant. Sometimes the men in these encounters were willing participants in the effort to make a baby; sometimes they were "unsuspecting."[92] But many lesbians hoped for alternatives to conception through sexual intercourse.

For some women, these dreams hinged on technological developments far removed from the immediately possible. As early as 1975, lesbians, especially lesbian separatists, began to imagine cloning and parthenogenesis as woman-centered forms of reproduction and called for more research into these methods, especially the latter. In parthenogenesis, an egg cell, without fertilization by sperm, divides spontaneously, giving rise to embryos and eventually offspring, described in some circles as "virgin births." This form of reproduction occurred in some relatively simple species like sea urchins, and its wild possibilities captured the imagination of scientists and science fiction writers alike. Lesbian separatists found parthenogenesis attractive because it completely bypassed the need for sperm (and men), and it conceived only female children.[93] Many lesbians were skeptical. Frances Chapman, in her 1975 description of a "radical lesbian biology workshop," concluded that it was "misdirected [to] technologiz[e] what is essentially a natural function."[94] Chapman needn't have worried—human parthenogenesis remains a fantasy.

In the early 1970s, lesbians who wanted to avoid intercourse with men had few options for acquiring sperm. A woman could ask a friend or a friend of a friend for a donation. Even when donors agreed, however, known donors occasionally created thorny quandaries about paternal involvement and family structure. Even more worrisome, known donors created potential custody issues downstream.[95]

Women found it difficult to secure anonymous sperm through the 1970s. Reproductive physicians had access to anonymous donors through networks or, less frequently, through fledgling sperm banks. These physicians, however, generally refused to inseminate lesbians or single women.[96] As a result, lesbians created alternatives. Some used their networks of friends and families to secure willing-but-anonymous donors. "A friend could ask another friend unknown to you, to secure a donor unknown to the first friend." In this accounting, preserving anonymity was framed as security.[97] The historian Katie Batza described the efforts of "sperm runners"—women who drove across town with containers of donated sperm tucked between their legs or inside their bras for warmth, sometimes handing off vials to another sperm runner in an effort to maintain donor anonymity.[98] One woman noted in a lesbian comic strip: "I feel like an urban sperm-guerilla."[99] Other women apparently ran independent insemination services. "Lily," for example, ran a sperm selection, donation, and insemination service out of her home in the San Francisco Bay Area. She screened the mostly gay donors for sexually transmitted infections, weeded out donors with genetic diseases or addictions, and shared information about appearance and aptitudes with prospective mothers so that they could choose the donor.[100]

Although Lily provided sperm and performed the insemination to some, other lesbians had to make do on their own. Publications in the feminist and gay press provided guidance on calculating a fertile period, choosing insertion methods (syringe or diaphragm), and warning about dangerous procedures. Some even suggested methods to improve chances of conceiving a child of a particular sex. These instructions highlighted the power of these do-it-yourself methods while acknowledging the homophobia that limited lesbians' reproductive choices.[101]

While lesbians could and did conceive babies outside an organized movement, feminist health clinics—frequently prompted by their lesbian staff—brought lesbian reproduction into the women's health movement. In the mid-1970s, lesbians at the Los Angeles Feminist Women's Health Center, including Francie Hornstein, began discussing and researching donor insemination; by 1975, they considered offering artificial insemination (more commonly described as assisted reproduction or alternative fertilization) services to their clients.[102] In 1977, Hornstein, with the help of several Los Angeles FWHC colleagues, became pregnant through donor insemination.[103] It wasn't until 1978, however, that the Los Angeles FWHC officially offered conception services to their lesbian clients. Initially, the clinic only helped clients find donor sperm and performed the insemination. Other feminist health centers also offered this service.[104] By 1979, physicians at the Los Angeles FWHC and other some feminist health clinics agreed to secure sperm from sperm banks on behalf of their clinic patients.[105] This allowed the centers to formally expand their conception services.

As lesbians across the nation devised creative ways to get sperm into bodies, they also turned to a new institution, the cryobank, known colloquially as the sperm bank. Banking sperm—storing frozen sperm for later use—was developed first in cattle production in the 1950s and took off quickly, producing more than one hundred million calves from frozen sperm by 1972. Human sperm, however, proved more delicate than bovine sperm. Although two reproductive physicians reported the birth of children conceived with frozen sperm as early as 1953, worries about the procedure's safety, reliability, and integrity remained. The first commercial sperm bank opened in 1972, but by 1977, only one thousand children had been born after conception with frozen sperm. In the 1980s, the emergence of HIV made the use of fresh sperm increasingly risky, as the virus could be transmitted to women through insemination. It was safer to store the sperm "on ice" until the donor could be tested six months after the donation. This fear of HIV/AIDS—along with technological refinements—encouraged the use of frozen sperm stored in sperm banks.[106]

Throughout the 1970s, sperm banks "denied services to unmarried women."[107] Physicians, however, could acquire banked sperm without divulging the marital "qualifications" of their clients. By 1979, some physicians agreed to secure sperm from cryobanks to serve their lesbian and single clients, bypassing the gatekeeping strategies women faced. Frustrated by the practicalities and the politics of this workaround, in the early 1980s, a few lesbians working in feminist health clinics and in gay and lesbian clinics created lesbian-friendly alternatives. In 1982, the Oakland Feminist Women's Health Center opened the Sperm Bank of Northern California (SBNC) as the first nonprofit sperm bank in the country. It refused to interfere with women's reproductive decision-making; the SBNC did not ask clients to divulge "any sort of social criteria," including marital status, and it allowed women—as opposed to medical providers—to choose the donor.[108] According to Batza, SBNC broke "the stranglehold of physicians and the sperm banking industry on access to sperm."[109] Other health feminists followed their lead. In 1984, the lesbian nurse practitioner Sherron Mills founded Pacific Reproductive Services, a sperm bank for "women planning alternative families" regardless of marital status. Mills, one of the founders of Lyon-Martin Women's Health Services, San Francisco's lesbian health clinic, understood that while the reproductive health needs of married heterosexual women were met in traditional medical settings or feminist health clinics, the needs of lesbians and single women hoping to become parents were not.

Feminist sperm banks enabled more feminist health clinics to offer reproductive services, including insemination, to their lesbian clients.[110] These initiatives integrated lesbians more fully within the larger effort to secure reproductive control for all women. Lesbian reproductive health projects clearly placed women's health in women's hands.

By the end of the 1980s, increased visibility of alternative vehicles for conception and increased availability of reproductive services for lesbian conception led to a lesbian baby boom, or "gayby" boom. By 1989, the lesbian baby boom had even caught the attention of the New York Times.[111] Nevertheless, the extent of the lesbian baby boom was likely exaggerated. A study published in 1987, for example, suggested that while nearly 60 percent of the 1,900 lesbians surveyed considered having a child after they assumed their lesbian identities, only 3 percent of those women actually "obtained" a child through pregnancy or adoption. The women who pursued pregnancy or adoption faced significant obstacles. Of the forty lesbians who sought to adopt, only four succeeded. Of the twenty-six who tried donor insemination, only eleven succeeded. Lesbians were most successful when they followed the path with the least medical, governmental, or organizational gatekeeping: intercourse with "cooperative" or unsuspecting men.[112]

Many lesbians had critiqued the women's health movement for its focus on women's reproductive needs, arguing that this reflected the heterosexist bias of the movement. But lesbians had reproductive needs as well, and in the mid- to late 1970s, lesbians working with the feminist health movement and independent of it developed pathbreaking methods and supportive networks to enable lesbian parenthood. This flurry of activity—researching parthenogenesis, teaching insemination methods, procuring sperm, and providing insemination services—testifies to the integration of lesbian reproductive needs into the feminist health movement.

AIDS Activism

In the 1970s, lesbian health activists struggled to establish a lesbian health agenda. In the 1980s, however, HIV/AIDS—a disease often associated with gay men—became an urgent, if contested, lesbian health concern. Lesbians assumed a variety of positions within AIDS work, but their efforts engendered many questions and inspired heated debates. On whose behalf did lesbians perform AIDS work? Should lesbians dedicate their time and effort to the AIDS crisis when a lesbian health agenda remained unclear? Were lesbians at risk for HIV infection? Should lesbians devote time and energy to the HIV/AIDS movement when other health issues took a greater toll on the community? In the 1980s and '90s, HIV/AIDS was clearly a health crisis that animated many lesbian activists. It occupied a central place on the only vaguely defined lesbian health agenda, and it allegedly diverted attention from discovering and addressing more pressing lesbian health issues. Into the 1990s, however, lesbians argued about the place of AIDS in a lesbian health agenda. Debates flared over who benefited from AIDS activism.

In the early 1980s, as AIDS began to ravage gay male communities in several major cities and beyond, the fledgling gay and lesbian health movement focused its limited resources on the epidemic. By 1982, men and women in cities across the nation were creating organizational responses to what was quickly looking like a crisis. In New York, San Francisco, Houston, Los Angeles, and elsewhere, activists launched educational, philanthropic, and social service organizations to meet the diverse needs created by the epidemic. New York City's Gay Men's Health Crisis (GMHC), San Francisco's Kaposi Sarcoma Research and Education Foundation (later the San Francisco AIDS Foundation), and the AIDS Foundation Houston were some of the major organizations launched in the epidemic's earliest months. By 1987, however, many people involved in HIV/AIDS work had grown frustrated by the slow pace of progress, a pace that left individuals dead and communities ravaged.

In response, Larry Kramer, one of the founders of the GMHC, urged the creation of a new organization focused on political action. The AIDS Coalition to Unleash Power, better known as ACT UP, arose to agitate for change.

From the beginning, many lesbians turned their attention and their effort to the crisis. Lesbians delivered food to AIDS patients, used their bodies to protest FDA rules, led AIDS social service organizations, and demanded more HIV/AIDS research. They were caregivers, educators, theorists, agitators, health providers, researchers, and case managers. According to some accounts, "Lesbians . . . emerged as such important caretakers of gay men with AIDS and as the community's new leaders."[113]

Lesbians joined the effort for a variety of reasons. For some, their motivation was personal, forged in the grief of watching friends and family die. Many of these women worked on behalf of their gay "brothers." As one activist explained, AIDS was "not a direct lesbian problem," but many lesbians devoted themselves to the cause "for our gay brothers [and as] a political issue for the community." Another activist acted out of her love for gay men. She refused to watch passively as the people she loved died. So "yes," she declared unapologetically, "I am giving my energy to gay men."[114]

Other lesbians saw their AIDS work as a battle for gay and lesbian rights and against homophobia and shared oppression. The ACT UP New York activist Maxine Wolfe, for example, insisted that she was "in this movement for myself." Her "queer consciousness" led her to AIDS work because she was frustrated by the sexism and homophobia of the male-dominated Left, the homophobia of feminism, and "the inability of lesbians to organize around or even figure out what their issues were."[115] Marion Banzhaf, who had once worked at the Tallahassee FWHC and who cofounded the short-lived Washington, DC, Abortion Rights Movement (ARM) of Women's Liberation, joined ACT UP in July 1987. Although a veteran of feminist and anti-imperialist causes, Banzhaf had not worked much with gay men; indeed, she had "sort of dismissed them as being narcissistic and just party hogs." But with the emergence of AIDS and the rise of increasingly virulent homophobia, she understood that "the discrimination that was happening against gay men in particular was going to bleed over to the lesbian community." When she heard that William F. Buckley had called for tattooing AIDS sufferers, she realized the gravity of the situation. "So we had to organize together to fight that kind of stuff."[116]

Many lesbians active in AIDS work brought a feminist political analysis to their activism.[117] Zoe Leonard, a New York City activist with ACT UP (and later one of the most prominent artists of her generation), for example, regarded AIDS work as a "movement for social change with a feminist agenda."

This framework encouraged Leonard to see AIDS as a lesbian issue.[118] In particular, lesbian feminists brought a politics of inclusion into the movement, pressuring AIDS organizations, researchers, and service providers to take seriously the threat AIDS posed to women, especially women of color, trans women, and lesbians.[119] According to the ACT UP member Anne-christine d'Adesky, lesbians and straight women, both cis and trans, deployed a feminist perspective to force attention to "the needs of lesbians around HIV/AIDS; to women drug users; to sex workers." D'Adesky insisted that "women and lesbians [had] always worked intersectionally—who made the connections, demanded the outreach, connected across social justice movements."[120] These lesbians viewed their AIDS work as both an obligation born of their political commitments and an opportunity for social change and political development.[121]

This commitment to feminism among many lesbian AIDS activists created some challenges as they discovered that their priorities did not always match those of the mostly white, mostly middle-class, gay men who dominated the movement. Indeed, lesbians realized that their male AIDS compatriots were frequently indifferent to women's struggles.[122] Some lesbian activists worried that the political analysis forged in feminist and lesbian-feminist spaces would be ignored or diluted in AIDS work dominated by middle-class white men. Karla Jay, for example, understood that taking on "a political, medical, and social battle that center[ed] on gay men" after a decade of largely separate struggles posed significant risks for a lesbian-centered politics, but she also saw the opportunities.[123] Lesbian involvement in ACT UP highlighted these tensions. According to the writer and activist Sarah Schulman, working in ACT UP meant working with men who had never supported women's struggles for autonomy, "men who had never fought rape [or] marched for abortion rights."[124]

Others worried about reciprocity, convinced that gay men would not work for lesbians like lesbians were organizing for gay men.[125] The anger that gay men had not—and the fear that gay men would not—organize around lesbian needs animated significant controversy about lesbian AIDS activism.[126] But other activists denounced the framework that conceived of lesbian AIDS work as activism for the benefit of gay men. In the provocatively titled "Has AIDS Finally Bonded Lesbians and Gay Men?," Deborah Bergman dismissed as misguided an understanding of AIDS work as coalitional, where diverse groups horse-traded their efforts under the agreement that "I'll support your issue if you'll support mine." She encouraged the use of a community framework "to recognize that we share the same values. . . . We share with gay men the need to secure the freedom to love in our own way . . . and to live our lives unbattered by violence and bigotry."[127]

Despite widespread lesbian involvement in AIDS activism and service projects, some lesbians worried that this work prioritized gay men's health at the expense of lesbian lives. Skeptics pointed to the relative rarity of HIV/ AIDS in lesbians. As late as 1985, there were no reported cases of lesbians with AIDS.[128] In September 1989, the CDC reported only seventy-nine lesbians with AIDS among the roughly 9,717 adult women diagnosed.[129] When compared with the thousands of lesbians with cancer, for example, the significance of AIDS for lesbians seemed negligible.[130] Jackie Winnow, a San Francisco AIDS activist turned cancer activist, acknowledged in 1989 the importance of lesbians in the AIDS movement. She understood why lesbians joined in the fight against AIDS, because it allowed them to feel generous and "heroic" and because it served the community "where our hearts lie." She conceded that AIDS work was necessary and important. But when Winnow turned to her communities for support after her breast cancer diagnosis and found none, her perspective changed. With bitterness and frustration, she noted: "No one takes care of women or lesbians except women or lesbians." Still stinging with disappointment, she wondered why the lesbian and gay community didn't "mobilize around the urgent needs of women and lesbians[.] Why don't we even consider our needs urgent?" After her diagnosis, she founded the Women's Cancer Resource Center in Berkeley. Her experience with the center only increased her frustration as she believed that women spent their energy on AIDS work, leaving nothing left over to address the life-threatening health issues common among lesbians.[131] Other critiques suggested that the focus on AIDS had delayed the development of a lesbian health movement. The editors of the *Sourcebook on Lesbian/Gay Health Care*, for example, blamed AIDS mobilization for the dearth of a lesbian health agenda: "One of the most glaring casualties of being overlooked as a result of mobilizing around AIDS is lesbian health concerns. Once again, women's concerns have become overshadowed by male issues."[132] The lesbian feminist Beth Elliott saw in lesbian attention to AIDS a deeper misogynist agenda. The identification of lesbians with the cause of AIDS, she noted, threatened to "replace lesbian feminism with a forcibly-integrated community in which lesbians play the female role."[133]

But most lesbian AIDS activists refused to frame AIDS activism as a zero-sum game that benefited gay men to the detriment of lesbians. They insisted that AIDS activism and service provision challenged homophobia and heterosexism and therefore aided lesbians as well as gay men. As the activist Laura

Giges put it, "Homophobia does not discriminate by sex." Consequently, she insisted, "in view of the historical survival of lesbians and gay men through unified efforts, AIDS is by necessity a lesbian issue."[134]

The published statistics clearly underestimated the number of lesbians with AIDS. Many HIV-positive women in the early years of the epidemic were dying of opportunistic infections without ever receiving an AIDS diagnosis because the progression of the disease in women had yet to be established.[135] Indeed, the CDC only widened its definitions of AIDS to include invasive cervical cancer and other conditions common to HIV-positive women in October 1992.[136] Further complicating the interpretation of health statistics, the CDC criteria for "lesbian" required exclusive sex with women since 1977. Women who reported no sex since 1977 or sex with men *and* women were not considered "lesbian" in these studies, regardless of their self-identity.[137] In addition, lesbians were frequently hidden in these statistics, as patients were categorized by risk category rather than sexual identity. This approach to data gathering and interpretation rendered lesbians living with HIV nearly invisible.[138]

The statistical rarity of lesbians in official counts of HIV/AIDS infections encouraged some lesbians to deny AIDS as a concern in their community. That the allegedly few HIV-positive lesbians likely became infected through IV drug use or sex with men reinforced some lesbians' belief that lesbianism kept them safe. According to this way of thinking, lesbians rarely acquired HIV through sex with women, and thus HIV-positive lesbians became infected via pathways incidental to or in conflict with their sexual identity. This position suggests that some lesbians overlooked or ignored the sex workers, IV drug users, and women who had occasional sex with men when they imagined the lesbian community.

But was sex between women free from risk? Debates about woman-to-woman sexual transmission became "a political battle" that that played out in the feminist and lesbian press in the late 1980s and early '90s.[139] Even lesbians who believed lesbians could and did transmit HIV through woman-to-woman sexual contact admitted that it was rare. Indeed, it was officially undocumented. Although the lesbian press frequently reported that woman-to-woman transmission of HIV had been confirmed, epidemiologists repeatedly challenged these claims.[140] In 1992, the HIV Surveillance Branch of the CDC claimed that all the HIV-positive women who reported sexual contact exclusively with women since 1977 (then 164 such cases) were IV drug users or had received blood transfusions. (Two women who had initially denied it later admitted to having had sex with men.) As a result, Susan Y. Chu and colleagues noted that while "female to female transmission of AIDS" could not be excluded, "it appears to be extremely rare."[141] The relative safety of sex play between women encouraged AIDS researchers, public health workers, and many lesbians themselves to frame lesbians as low risk, sometimes as "the group at least risk," for HIV infection, especially when they acted sexually "as lesbians."[142] The boundaries of lesbian sex were, of course, heatedly contested.[143]

Nevertheless, transmission of HIV through woman-to-woman sexual contact seemed theoretically possible, so some lesbians demanded more research into the question, claiming that the absence of this research proved that lesbians were being neglected by the AIDS community.[144] Indeed, in January 1990, some AIDS activists "demanded that the CDC proclaim lesbian sex to be a transmission route for HIV."[145]

The argument that lesbians might transmit HIV sexually encouraged some activists to develop AIDS prevention guidelines for lesbians. In 1985, for example, the Women's AIDS Network (WAN) in San Francisco joined forces with the San Francisco AIDS Foundation to create a series of brochures focused on AIDS and women. When WAN created a brochure targeting lesbians, however, the director of the foundation balked, insisting, "Lesbians are not at risk for AIDS." In the end, the foundation agreed to publish the brochure—not to meet a public health need, but allegedly to reward lesbians who were "working so hard in AIDS services, they deserve[d] a brochure."[146] Lesbian safer-sex literature, then, reflected the political effort to construct lesbians as a population at risk for HIV infection and the condescension of those in the movement who denied it.

The safer-sex guidelines published for lesbians focused on the possible transmission of HIV through bodily secretions including saliva, blood (including menstrual blood), vaginal fluids, and feces. Like other targeted HIV/AIDS education campaigns, safer sex for lesbians focused on the use of latex (or plastic wrap) barriers to prevent the exchange of bodily fluids between partners. Safer sex required dental dams for oral sex, latex gloves for internal manual stimulation, and condoms for sex toys.[147]

While some lesbians welcomed these guidelines as evidence that lesbians' risk for HIV/AIDS was finally taken seriously, others regarded them as unnecessary and possibly dangerous. Cindy Patton, a leading writer about AIDS and women, noted that the first safe-sex guidelines for lesbians reflected the sexual behaviors and protective needs of men rather than considering the "subject position of women."[148] Barbara Herbert, a lay health activist turned physician health activist, expressed her extreme frustration with the guidelines in 1989:

They are a classic example of the worst in medical education, which is to say, there's a device, so let's use it. There's no evidence that they work, and I have questions about whether a square of latex the size of a piece of toilet paper could provide any protection. They may in fact present a cruel joke for those who really are at risk and think they're getting protection. Saran wrap leaves me particularly terrified because my experience is that many lesbians might use alcohol or a drug before making love and it would be possible to suffocate on the saran wrap. It seems unacceptable that someone could potentially die trying to protect themselves from a risk that is not clearly defined.[149]

As a result of the widespread dissatisfaction, some activists argued that the lesbian safer-sex recommendations needed to be tossed out and re-created "from scratch."[150]

The political meanings of safer-sex guidelines for lesbians aside, evidence suggests that lesbians—even HIV-positive women—generally ignored much of this advice. According to Lena Einhorn, for example, lesbians' assumptions about the safety of their sexual practices supported their dismissal of safer-sex advice.[151] While it made intuitive sense to some lesbians to avoid sharing sex toys, dental dams and latex gloves proved to be hard sells. Even safer-sex educators reportedly "rarely pull[ed] latex out of their nightstands."[152]

In a 1997 roundtable discussion, five HIV-positive lesbians rejected the "safe sex" approaches they learned from formal channels. Instead, they practiced safe sex by considering and enacting what they were "okay with." These women made choices based on their experiences, desires, and comfort with risk. While they tried to "play it safe," they generally avoided barrier methods, rejecting gloves and latex dams. They refused to replace conversations about desire and pleasure with logistical exchanges about illness and disease. One HIV-positive woman described her encounter with a partner who didn't feel safe being sexual with her without latex gloves. As a result, she "felt unattractive and diseased. . . . I felt like a germ." Another woman noted that she wouldn't feel comfortable if someone said, "'I can't stick my fingers in your pussy without a glove on.' I would feel like shit." A few of the discussants— some of whom were AIDS educators—tried to follow stricter guidelines, to play by the book, but they found it inconvenient, unsatisfying, and stigmatizing. For the most part, they felt comfortable with their decisions because they were skeptical that women could transmit HIV through most of the sexual practices they enjoyed. According to the AIDS activist Frenchie Laugier, "Everyone should be a lesbian [because] lesbians are so safe."[153]

When this conversation was first published in the "Lesbian and AIDS" issue of *Newsline*, a few outraged readers accused the editor of "spreading death in our community."[154] This suggests the depth of division over safer sex within the lesbian and the AIDS communities. These women's choices were nevertheless supported by epidemiological data. They were also supported by lesbians who dismissed woman-to-woman transmission as "hysterical," anti-sex, and an example of "AIDS envy." Beth Elliott, for example, compared woman-to-woman transmission of HIV to the "urban legend . . . about a poodle in a microwave."[155]

According to some lesbian AIDS activists, the ruckus about woman-to-woman transmission left lesbians confused and misinformed about their actual risk of acquiring the disease. As Amber Hollibaugh, a longtime lesbian activist and eventual director of the Lesbian AIDS Project at New York City's GMHC, put it, "Lesbianism is not a condom." Lesbians could and did acquire HIV through a variety of familiar, well-known channels including sex with HIV-positive men and IV drug use.[156] Indeed, Hollibaugh argued, "[lesbians] are a specific population of women with high numbers of HIV-positive members, but no official recognition or accounting."[157]

Hollibaugh also insisted that the focus on female-to-female transmission supported a "circumscribed lesbian sexual border" that imagined narrowly who counted as lesbians and what lesbians did sexually and otherwise.[158] The activist Abby Tallmar described this as the "Myth of Homogeneity," a belief among privileged lesbians that "most lesbians are like themselves: white, middle-class, politically active and sexually traditional," while ignoring the lives and practices of lesbians outside this imagined community.[159] According to Hollibaugh, designating lesbians as low risk for HIV infection "led to many erroneous and tragic conclusions and confusions" for individual lesbians.[160] She demanded that lesbian AIDS activists and lesbian feminists adopt an expansive notion of lesbian community—one that included

> working-class women, women in prisons, reform schools, and juvie halls, women locked down in mental institutions for being too queer, women of color, women in the military and in the bars, women surviving in "straight" marriages and dead-end jobs who longed each day to touch another woman, women who were peep-show girls, sex workers, carnival strippers, women who shot drugs and women in recovery from those drug and the streets, women in trailers, small towns, and cities across America, women who filled the floors of the factories, fast-food restaurants, and auto plants of this country, women whose lives were situated in PTAS [sic], shopping malls, and Teamsters' unions.[161]

For Hollibaugh, these women, who might not even call themselves lesbians, were precisely the women most at risk for AIDS and were rendered invisible because they lived outside the bounds of "sisterhood."[162]

In summary, in the 1980s and '90s, many lesbians devoted their health activism toward the AIDS crisis. For some, this was primarily an effort to combat the dire health consequences of homophobia, misogyny, racism, and class privilege—an effort, in other words, that relied on a feminist and queer politics. For others, it reflected the political work of lesbian inclusion, bringing lesbians into the conversation about the HIV-infected and broadening the conception of who a lesbian was and what lesbians did. Both efforts placed AIDS on the lesbian health agenda. Indeed, the larger discussion of AIDS within lesbian communities helped broaden the conception of the boundaries of the lesbian community and identified a health issue that demanded a lesbian-specific response.

Professionalizing the Lesbian Health Movement

The late 1980s and early '90s saw a flurry of activity on lesbian health matters at a number of levels, in part in reaction to the quite visible organization focused on HIV/AIDS. Grassroots lesbians demanded more attention for their particular needs at gay community health centers.[163] Gay civil rights groups included lesbian health as one of their concerns.[164] Books on lesbian health reached out to both medical and popular audiences.[165] Individual lesbians touched by illness created organizations and foundations to address lesbian health needs.[166]

In the 1980s, a few municipalities, including New York and San Francisco, developed lesbian health programming, inspired by the health crisis created by the AIDS epidemic.[167] It wasn't until the 1990s, however, that lesbian health attracted the attention—and the funding—of the federal government. In 1993, lesbian health activists met with Secretary of the Department of Health and Human Services Donna Shalala to request more federal attention to the health needs of LGBT individuals. In February 1994, lesbian and bisexual activists met in a Lesbian Roundtable to formalize recommendations to Health and Human Services and to establish a lesbian health agenda.[168] These recommendations included the expansion of federally funded research on lesbian health issues. The Institute of Medicine (IOM) took up this challenge, and in July 1997, it convened the Committee on Lesbian Health Research Priorities. This nine-person group, staffed primarily with health care academics, had little experience with the issues. Only Judith Bradford, one of the directors of the 1988 National Lesbian Health Care Survey, had any obvious experience with lesbian health. Cynthia A. Gómez, a PhD psychologist and HIV/AIDS policy researcher, was likely the only person of color. The committee was charged with assessing the extant research on the physical and mental health issues of lesbians, reviewing the methodological challenges involved in the research, and proposing a research agenda for the future. *Lesbian Health: Current Assessment and Directions for the Future*, published in 1999 by the IOM, was the pathbreaking product of this workshop.[169]

The IOM report highlighted the problems with the then current research on lesbian health. The report, for example, cited research that demonstrated that lesbians had higher rates of some high-risk behaviors (e.g., smoking, problem drinking) and lower rates of some protective conditions and behaviors (e.g., pregnancy and oral contraceptive use) than women in general. As a result, researchers long claimed that lesbians were at increased risk of certain conditions, including breast cancer and heart disease. The report cautioned, however, that no epidemiological evidence verified that lesbians truly suffered disproportionately from either breast cancer or heart disease.[170] (The report conceded that lesbians, by virtue of having less heterosexual intercourse, were "probably" at decreased risk for cervical cancer.[171])

The report noted that most of the research on lesbian health had relied on small convenience samples (e.g., surveys distributed to women's music festivals and lesbian organizations) that did not represent lesbians as a whole. This methodology created an ascertainment bias and thus contributed to the current uncertainty about the true health profile of lesbians. The report also pointed to the ambiguity of the category of lesbian itself. To illustrate the problem, the report cited a study that broke "lesbian" into three possible characteristics: current same-sex desire, current identity as lesbian or bisexual, and same-sex behavior since age eighteen. The study showed that less than 16 percent of "lesbians" claimed all three aspects. This study highlighted the methodological incoherence plaguing the category and called into question the legitimacy of comparing the extant literature on lesbian health.[172]

The IOM report fueled the visibility of the lesbian health movement and gained professional legitimacy for lesbian health research and other projects. In 1999, for example, the American Public Health Association called for more research on sexual orientation and gender identity.[173] In June 2001, the *American Journal of Public Health* devoted an issue to LGBT public health.[174] Most, but not all, of the articles in this issue, however, lumped all the constituent populations of this acronym together, masking the unique aspects of lesbian health. Still, more researchers felt emboldened and inspired to undertake lesbian health research.

Some of this new research provided the population-based perspective called for in the IOM report. For example, a 2000 article published in the *Archives of Family Medicine* claimed to be the first study of lesbian health based on population data. It drew on data collected from the 1997 Los Angeles

County Health Survey, where all phone numbers in Los Angeles County had an equal chance of being included in the sample. The study confirmed earlier work that showed that lesbian and bisexual women were more likely than heterosexual women to have poor health behaviors—especially smoking and problem drinking—worse access to health care, and lower rates of satisfaction with their health care providers.[175]

Because this study did not rely on targeted outreach to lesbian communities, it presumably sidestepped some of the pitfalls of convenience-sampling studies by avoiding the overselection of particular lesbian communities. Nevertheless, population-based studies still generally relied on lesbian self-identity as a category of analysis, even as "lesbian" became increasingly ambiguous as a meaningful public health analytic.[176] To provide a more clearly defined object of study, some epidemiologists began to research the health of "women who have sex with women" (WSW). The category of WSW emerged in 1995, shortly after "men who have sex with men" (MSM) was introduced in 1994.[177] Both MSM and WSW began as categories in HIV/AIDS literature. Within this context, these terms indicated an attempt to center behaviors rather than identities as risk factors for HIV infection and to acknowledge the social constructedness and cultural embeddedness of gay and lesbian identities.

This new vocabulary and approach significantly expanded the breadth of the women who might be served by a lesbian health agenda. It did not, however, clarify the scope of the category of "lesbian health." A review of the literature between 2000 and 2006 found that "sexual orientation was measured in more than 100 different ways" and that the results of the different classification schemes resulted in different understandings of the health consequences at play.[178] Further, some health scholars argued that the categories MSM and WSW were problematic "on theoretic, political, ethical, and epidemiological grounds" because they undermined the personal value of self-identity, severed sexual behaviors from their social contexts, deflected attention from the social dimensions of sexuality, and "obscure[d] elements of sexual behavior that are important for public health research and intervention."[179] Consequently, although the research on lesbian health increased, the category's contested boundaries remained unresolved.

In the 1970s, lesbians inside and outside the feminist women's health movement fought to have their health care needs addressed. They demanded lesbian health. In response, health activists offered lesbian self-help groups and lesbian health clinics, developed lesbian reproductive services, and launched lesbian health research. Lesbians also took on HIV/AIDS as a community health crisis, even if the relationship of the lesbian community (itself a disputed construct) to AIDS was contested and uncertain. Nevertheless, this flurry of activity, while meeting both political and medical needs, failed to satisfactorily define a comprehensive lesbian health agenda or develop an understanding of how lesbian identity or same-sex sexual behaviors interacted with health care needs or promoted a conception of "lesbian" that sufficiently captured an identity that hinged on some combination of feminist politics, social marginalization, affectional preferences, and sexual behaviors. As the next chapter shows, disputes over the boundaries of lesbian identity and its relationship to community animated the history of one of the only lesbian health clinics in the United States.

A Clinic of Our Own:
Lyon-Martin Women's Health Services

On January 25, 2011, the board of directors of Lyon-Martin Health Services announced that the San Francisco clinic would suspend operations after more than thirty years of providing health care to the LBT community. The board blamed a desperate financial crisis, including significant debt.[1] This declaration was premature, however. Within two weeks of the original announcement, the local community—including former and current patients—raised more than $250,000, much of it earned through gay karaoke, "Homo Hoedowns," drag shows, and other queer-identified fundraisers.[2] In the aftermath of tremendous grassroots community support and administrative maneuvers, the clinic regrouped and survived this crisis, one of many throughout a history of struggle, crisis, accomplishment, and pride.

This chapter explores the instantiation of "lesbian health" within the institutional setting of a feminist—in this case, lesbian feminist—health clinic. While the parameters and the significance of the label "lesbian" had long been a sticking point in the evolving lesbian health framework, identity-based demands became an even more vexing concern in the provision of lesbian health care. By tracing the history of this health clinic from its founding as a lesbian clinic in 1979, this chapter highlights the sexual, racial, and gender politics at the center of its history. It demonstrates the instability of the clinic's identity, requiring the clinic, its board, its staff, and its community supporters to continuously reaffirm, redefine, and reenact its lesbian focus. Ultimately, it shows how identity politics kept the struggling institution afloat while simultaneously threatening its future.

Identity politics describes a political strategy based on organizing around group identity and focusing on group-specific problems. It marked a shift away from a struggle to secure general rights (access to education, employment, the vote) to focus on group-specific problems (racism, patriarchy, homophobia). Although elements of this strategy were clearly in play in the nineteenth century, identity politics emerged as a powerful strategy for social change in the 1960s and '70s, in part as a response to a class-based critique of the civil rights movements and a gender-based critique of the New Left.[3] Although already a visible and potent organizing tool, it was first described as "identity politics" in 1977 by the Combahee River Collective, a group of African American feminists in Boston: "This focusing upon our own oppression is embodied in the concept of identity politics. We believe that the most profound and potentially the most radical politics comes directly out of our own identity, as opposed to working to end somebody else's oppression."[4]

Identity politics characterizes many of the most visible and significant social movements of the 1960s and 1970s. These movements began with a belief that a shared social identity—be it race, sex, or sexuality, among others—created common experiences, including a shared experience of oppression. By organizing as members of marginalized groups to build community, create visibility, and challenge oppression, social movements based on identity politics mobilized hundreds of thousands of people to work for a more just and equitable world.

Identity politics movements were both cultural and political projects. They depended on at least three central tenets: an "affirmative conception" of self to combat the toxic forces of denigration and oppression (e.g., black is beautiful, sisterhood is powerful, gay pride); the development of a collective identity that created bonds of kinship beyond other community networks and family ties; and a sense of loyalty to other community members—a willingness to look after and fight for other members of the group.[5] The political communities based on identity politics have provided a potent political force to demand and effect social change. They have also knit together imagined communities, providing a source of affirmation and a buffer of protection against an often hostile society. Identity politics created schools and stores, established shelters and clinics, founded magazines and presses, and sponsored marches and parades. They have increased the visibility of previously marginalized communities, changed the tactics and goals of political organizing, and recast the political landscape.

But for all their power, identity politics have also been criticized, sometimes denounced. Scholars have challenged the deployment of identity politics on a number of grounds: that they have generally ignored "intragroup difference," at times demanding that group members deny or suppress aspects of their identity;[6] that they have failed to challenge systemic economic oppression;[7] that they frequently have relied on essentialist categories of identity;

that they have required constant surveillance of the boundaries of the identity category;[8] that they have failed to secure "political acceptance;"[9] and that they have abandoned a commitment to coalition across identities, creating instead "a fragmented mosaic of political groups."[10]

The history of Lyon-Martin highlights the promise and the pitfalls of identity-based politics and institutions. The clinic was created because a group of middle-class, white lesbians wanted to provide safe and accessible health care to the lesbian community. At its founding, the clinic sought to meet the health care needs of middle-class lesbians as well as poor lesbians with few resources. But as the clinic's patient base diversified, by accident and by choice, the lesbian community who supported the clinic with their money and their time confronted many of the weaknesses of a politics based on identity. Who constituted the lesbian community? To whom did the lesbian community owe its loyalty? How did the community accommodate difference? How did lesbians know when a space was theirs?

"A Lesbian-Born Idea"

The seeds of Lyon-Martin Women's Health Services were planted in 1977 when Patricia Robertson, a white lesbian and second-year obstetrics and gynecology resident at the University of California, San Francisco, overheard a comment by a colleague. "Lesbians can't get PID [pelvic inflammatory disease]," he said when encountering a lesbian whose symptoms resembled PID. Robertson was aghast at the assumptions this statement reflected. Surely lesbians could get PID, and this patient, in Robertson's view, obviously had. When she sought confirmation in the medical literature, she found almost no research on lesbian health at all. (Indeed, before 1980 almost all the medical literature on lesbians focused on the cause of homosexuality in women or on the approach to a "cure."[11]) Consequently, she began to consider the widespread ignorance and uninformed assumptions concerning lesbian health needs, and she resolved to use her position to improve the situation. She initiated a research project with the support of San Francisco General Hospital to investigate the incidence of sexually transmitted infections (STIs) among lesbians. To gather her evidence, she, her partner Lesley Anderson, an orthopedic surgery resident, and some of her medical colleagues created and then voluntarily staffed a weekly evening clinic for lesbians.[12]

Although Robertson and her colleagues saw their efforts primarily as a research study, an act of knowledge production, they also believed that it benefited an imagined community of lesbians.[13] According to Alana Schilling, an early project volunteer, they thought that the research and the health care screening it provided "could also serve our public."[14] Schilling's language is important here. She laid claim to a lesbian community ("our public") that would benefit from health care outreach by being identified as people who deserved medical attention. To recruit subjects for the study, volunteers blanketed with posters known lesbian haunts, including women's music festivals, a lesbian-owned café, and the Women's Building in San Francisco. These cultural sites suggested the geographic, racial, and cultural borders of that community. More than two hundred women attended the lesbian clinic during its short life (September through December 1978), and 148 of these women were considered suitable for the study.[15] Not surprisingly given the targets of the publicity, 92 percent of the participants were white and 96 percent of them were employed.[16]

And yet, even at this very early moment, it was unclear which women who showed up at the clinic were sufficiently lesbian for the purposes of the study. Robertson decided on an admittedly "arbitrary" definition: her study included only women who had been "sexually active only with women in the past six months." Nevertheless, the vast majority (89 percent) had had "coital experience with men." Although for research purposes Robertson and her team needed a clear, even if arbitrary, definition of lesbian, they nevertheless were happy to provide STI screening for all women who sought care at the makeshift lesbian health clinic.[17]

The study found no active cases of sexually transmitted diseases among the lesbian sample. Robertson and her coauthor, Julius Schachter, a microbiologist specializing in sexually transmitted infections, concluded that the absence of STIs was likely because of the small number of sexual partners the subjects reported (a mean of 2.3 the previous year) or because "woman-to-woman contact is a less efficient means of transmitting infection" than heterosexual intercourse. The study also reported that the average interval between Pap smears for this group of lesbians was more than twice as long than for other women treated at San Francisco General (twenty-one months versus eight months).[18] Although this speculation was not reflected in the published article, Robertson and her coworkers believed that this longer interval was likely the result of homophobia; lesbians were less likely to seek routine medical care for fear of encountering ignorance, discrimination, and intimidation.

The belief that medical homophobia discouraged lesbians from seeking regular contact with health care providers was more than a hunch. Indeed, a survey created and circulated by the Bay Area Physicians for Human Rights, an organization of gay physicians founded in 1978, discovered that heterosexual women were 66 percent more likely to have a regular physician than lesbian-identified women, and that 60 percent of lesbians found their health care inadequate. The survey also found that more than 40 percent of lesbians reported having trouble securing respectful, ethical, and competent health care "because of their orientation."[19]

In the face of what they saw as an intense need for affordable health care sensitive to lesbian needs, Robertson and two other white women who had volunteered in the study project—Sherron Mills, a nurse practitioner, and Alana Schilling, a medical administrator—founded Women's Alternative Health Services Inc., a nonprofit company dedicated to meeting the health needs of lesbians. The goals of the organization were ambitious. It sought to improve the health of lesbians by providing medical care in a setting free from homophobia and heterosexism. It also sought to address the dearth of research on lesbians by sponsoring lesbian-specific studies. Further, it hoped to develop and disseminate health education materials to the lesbian community. Finally, it planned to create an educational venue to train nonhomophobic health practitioners.[20] Lyon-Martin Women's Health Services, named after the lesbian pioneers Del Martin and Phyllis Lyon, was the vehicle to achieve these ambitious goals.[21]

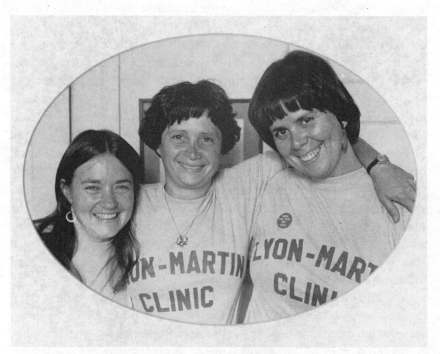

FIGURE 6.1. Lyon-Martin founders Sherron Mills, Patricia Robertson, and Alana Schilling. Permission by Alana Schilling.

By naming their clinic after Martin and Lyon, the founders signaled both their feminist and their lesbian bona fides.[22] In 1955, Martin and Lyon founded the Daughters of Bilitis in San Francisco, one of the earliest and most important lesbian organizations in the US. Focused initially on providing a social network for lesbians, it became a potent force in the political fight for lesbian rights. Although Martin and Lyon were initially identified with the gay rights movement, they became increasingly focused on feminist issues as well. When they applied to join the National Organization for Women (NOW), for example, they forced the issue of lesbian rights onto the agenda of the resistant organization. Martin also wrote *Battered Wives* (1976), a classic text in the burgeoning domestic violence movement.[23]

In building a clinic to meet the health needs of lesbians, the founders understood that the category included professional women as well as downwardly mobile and working-class women. They also hoped that the clinic would meet the health care needs of the young lesbians who flocked to San Francisco seeking the promise of a gay mecca or escaping the often violent homophobia of their natal homes and families.[24] Like most community clinics of the moment, Lyon-Martin wanted to provide care for the economically needy. As Schilling put it, "We had to . . . serve those women who had nothing. And that those lesbians who were coming here, who were homeless and all of that, to keep them safe. . . . Our intention was to keep serving people who had nothing."[25] Consequently, the clinic charged on a sliding scale, providing free health care to those who could not pay.

Founders of this clinic saw their work as part of at least two social movements centered on health. The founders identified as feminists and saw their efforts as part of the larger women's health movement. Indeed, giving women practitioners a feminist workplace dedicated to helping other women was part of their goal.[26] They also understood their work as part of the gay and lesbian health movement, aimed at increasing knowledge about the health needs of gay men and lesbians and providing health services without the corrosive effects of homophobia. As lesbian feminists, they sought to provide a counterweight to a system plagued both by sexism and homophobia.[27]

By creating Lyon-Martin, the founders identified firmly with the community it was designed to serve. As Robertson described it, Lyon-Martin "was a Lesbian-born idea, it was nurtured by Lesbians. . . . Everyone shared in finding out about ourselves as Lesbians. Everyone got together to help each other." Here Robertson put her community—"ourselves as Lesbians"—at the center of the need for and the creation of Lyon-Martin. Schilling similarly believed in the project because it "could also serve our public."[28] This belief that the clinic was built to benefit "ourselves as Lesbians" and "our public" served as a guiding principle for the future of the clinic, giving it an imagined community of stakeholders and clients. It also created a recurrent and vexing problem, perhaps a political liability, as some members of the "community" benefited from expanding lesbian-friendly health care options and thus needed Lyon-Martin less, while some potential patients who clearly needed Lyon-Martin's services challenged the boundaries of the community.

By some measures, Lyon-Martin could be viewed as a latecomer to the feminist health care scene. As early as 1970, women working in the free clinic movement began offering "women's nights" or other forms of women's clinics to meet the health care needs of women and to provide care free from the sexism so pervasive in the free clinic movement. Some of these women's clinics became relatively independent units within a larger free clinic institution (e.g., the Berkeley Women's Health Collective of the Berkeley Free Clinic); others began as part of a free or community clinic and eventually separated completely (e.g., Arcata's Northcountry Clinic for Women and Children); while others grew from feminist roots outside of extant health care institutions (e.g., Los Angeles Feminist Women's Health Center). After the 1973 *Roe v. Wade* decision, the growth of these clinics and health centers accelerated. The scope and impact of these clinics and centers varied greatly. Some failed to launch in any significant way, others lasted less than a year, and still others continued to provide health care with feminist roots, if not feminist care, well into the twenty-first century.

Although many lesbians participated in the women's health movement, created lesbian self-help groups, and organized lesbian nights at some health centers, clinics that focused primarily on the health needs of lesbians were rare. St. Marks Clinic in New York City opened a women's clinic in March 1974 that served women who ostensibly did not require reproductive health care. It therefore catered to lesbians, postmenopausal women, and celibate women. It also targeted its publicity to the lesbian community.[29] In Seattle, lesbian feminists created a lesbian health collective in 1974, which offered a medical clinic and an educational lesbian health care forum, each once a month. This effort seems to have lasted at least two years.[30] The Emma Goldman Clinic in Iowa City established lesbian nights in 1976 but promptly canceled them when the expected lesbians failed to appear.[31] These efforts suggest that lesbian-centered health care was an aspirational goal of many health feminists in the 1970s, but that in most locales it did not remain a priority.

Feminist health care clinics mushroomed in the 1970s, but gay health centers arose much more slowly. Over the course of the 1970s, more than twenty gay community health clinics emerged, but as the historian Katie Batza has shown, these clinics generally provided little more than testing for STIs. In the vernacular of the time, these were known as VD (venereal disease) clinics. Three with staying power—the Gay Community Services Center in Los Angeles (1972), Howard Brown in Chicago (1975), and the Gay Health Collective of the Fenway Community Health Center in Boston (1974)—were founded with the health needs of the gay male community in mind.[32]

San Francisco was not a trailblazer in either the feminist health movement or the gay and lesbian health movement. The city had a women's health clinic, but its visibility was overshadowed by health centers in Oakland, Santa Cruz, and Berkeley. Further, according to the sociologist Elizabeth Armstrong, most lesbian organizing in the San Francisco Bay Area occurred outside of San Francisco proper.[33] Gay men's health efforts were no better. Although Berkeley was home to the Berkeley Gay Men's Health Collective, offering VD testing two nights a month as well as a VD clinic at one of the city's bathhouses, gay men in San Francisco had to rely on the city's San Francisco City Clinic, the city- and county-supported sexual health clinic.[34] At its founding, then, Lyon-Martin was one of the few health clinics in the Bay Area devoted to any segment of the gay community.

When Lyon-Martin Women's Health Services first opened in 1979, it was a small, makeshift production, operating two nights a week out of borrowed space with an all-volunteer staff, financed with the $500 proceeds from a women's music concert. Every night the staff would cart in the patient charts, medical supplies, and educational materials to the clinic and carry them away again at the end of the shift. The tenuous nature of the clinic, however, did not discourage clients. In 1980, working at full capacity, it served more than five hundred patients.[35] Demand for service quickly outgrew the clinic's space, so in 1981, it moved into the private practice space of a lesbian podiatrist, Arlene Hoffman, in the upscale Pacific Heights neighborhood. At this point, the clinic provided health care five days a week, doubling its caseload. Most of these patients identified as lesbian; some were middle-class women who were willing to pay out of pocket for health care without homophobic hassles; many others were young, unemployed, recent San Francisco arrivals.[36]

By 1983, the clinic needed still more space, so it moved to a larger facility in San Francisco's Mission District. The relocation to the Los Portales Medical Center, both because of its increased capacity for patient care and because of its geographic and cultural location in San Francisco, changed the clinic in many ways. First, the all-volunteer staff was no longer sufficient to meet the needs of a full-time health center. Consequently, the clinic hired medical practitioners and an administrator. Second, the increased costs of running the clinic could no longer be met by patient fees. Before the move to the Mission District, the clinic, unable to bill insurance companies directly, asked its patients to pay up front for medical services. As the clinic expanded, it needed to find sources of revenue beyond the pockets of its patients. Lyon-Martin sought and received city and county funding and began accepting patients insured by Medicare and Medi-Cal, California's Medicaid program. Third, the geographic placement of the clinic in the Mission District brought unforeseen results. Although well placed to attract patients familiar with the lesbian-friendly Valencia Street, the larger Mission neighborhood was home to many Chicano families and recent immigrants from Central and South America. Because Lyon-Martin was a neighborhood health center and because it was the only medical facility in the neighborhood that accepted Medi-Cal patients, by 1986, roughly 40 percent of the clientele of this "lesbian" clinic consisted of women who considered themselves straight. A significant percentage of these heterosexual clients were monolingual, Spanish-speaking women, often elderly. So what began in 1979 as a clinic serving mostly white, mostly employed lesbians had become by 1986 a clinic with a substantial percentage of straight women, many poor, and increasingly nonwhite.[37]

By 1987, the clientele of the clinic was clearly bifurcated. On the one hand, the clinic saw white lesbians with insurance who were willing to pay up front for services and negotiate for reimbursement on their own; on the other hand, it served straight, white and nonwhite, women with Medi-Cal.[38] This division in the patient base led many staff and board members to wonder whether Lyon-Martin was fulfilling its mission to meet the health needs of lesbians in San Francisco. They also wondered whether the mission of the clinic should be changed to legitimize the health services the clinic was providing to poor women, including poor women of color. This tension surrounding the possible mismatch between clinic goals and clinic services influenced the clinic's identity forever after.[39]

To gauge the health needs of San Francisco lesbians, Lyon-Martin administered a survey in 1987 to women involved in the Bay Area Career Women (BACW), a social and networking organization for Bay Area lesbians in professional or business careers. Among the white (89 percent) and largely middle-class respondents, the vast majority did not go to Lyon-Martin, citing its location in the down-at-the-heels Mission District, its lack of direct insurance billing, and its status as a community clinic without a full-time doctor.[40] For most lesbians with health care options, Lyon-Martin was unappealing.

The choice of BACW as its referent was significant.[41] By reaching out to professionally identified women as the imagined clientele, the survey failed to connect with lesbians who had the fewest health care choices and helped shape the aspirations of the clinic in directions that could never be met. Financial expediency was likely an important motivator for reaching out to middle-class or aspiring middle-class lesbians to attract both cash-paying clients and donors with deep pockets. Without more patient dollars or other means of support, the clinic was financially unsustainable.

These results discouraged the women most committed to keeping Lyon-Martin a lesbian health center, as they suggested that most lesbians—at least, most middle-class lesbians—were uninterested in the services Lyon-Martin offered. And yet, lesbians with options *did* seek health care at Lyon-Martin, both as a way to support the clinic and to obtain lesbian-centered care without the usual heterosexism and homophobia. Because Lyon-Martin still attracted lesbian patients, the board and community stakeholders opposed transforming Lyon-Martin into yet another community clinic. Ironically, the dedication to lesbians limited the clinic's options. Because roughly half of the clients were insured and more than half of the clients were white, the clinic was not eligible for funding sources targeting ethnic minorities or the economically disadvantaged.[42] In other words, the clinic did not see enough middle-class, lesbian patients to sustain itself, but it served too many for it to qualify for funds to serve its other patients.

How could Lyon-Martin reconcile its commitment to lesbian health care with a clinic waiting room peopled with poor, straight-identified women? In January 1988, the board and staff created a new mission statement that solidified rather than resolved the clinic's ambiguous agenda:

> Our goal is to provide comprehensive quality health care for women by women with special attention to lesbian health care needs. We would like to serve women of all ages, ethnic backgrounds, sexual orientations and disabilities in a safe, personal, supportive, non-judgmental environment. . . . We would like to offer these services to women of all different economic levels while maintaining the clinic's financial self-sufficiency.[43]

This mission statement captured the clinic's ambivalence. It wanted to give lesbians special attention, but it also wanted to treat all sexual orientations. It hoped to serve poor women, but it needed to stay financially self-sufficient. Perhaps most important, this mission statement acknowledged the needs and identities of the women the clinic actually served while reinforcing its ties to the lesbian community. This compromise allowed the clinic to move forward, but its identity and its agenda remained fuzzy.

At the end of the 1980s, Lyon-Martin was forced to reconsider its identity and its mission because many self-identified lesbians had more desirable health care options in terms of location, physical setting, and continuity of care. By 1988, the gay and lesbian community in San Francisco had enough political, economic, and social clout that "gay-friendly" medical settings

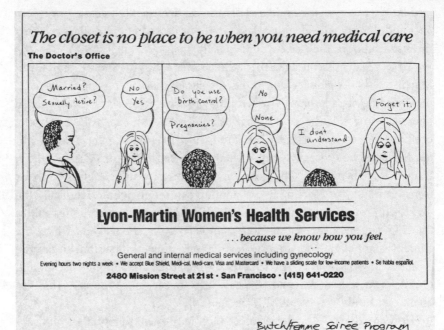

FIGURE 6.2. This Lyon-Martin advertisement captured the heterosexism typical of medical encounters. It also suggested that lesbians would not need contraception to avoid pregnancy—a suggestion at odds with the sexual history of many lesbians. Permission by J. M. Jaffe of Lyon-Martin Community Health Services. From the San Francisco LGBT Groups Ephemera Collection. Courtesy of Gay, Lesbian, Bisexual, Transgender Historical Society.

became increasingly available.[44] And yet, while middle-class lesbians had options, poor women had markedly fewer. The heterogeneous client population was an unintended and unforeseen consequence of timing, location, and unmet health care needs.

Expanding the Clinic, 1989–1993

Into this ambiguity came a new executive director, Marj Plumb, in 1989. Plumb, a white, lesbian woman, had just finished a stint as administrative director of the Berkeley Women's Health Clinic. At the time, Lyon-Martin was a minor player in the health care landscape, with a small staff of four or five who saw about two hundred patients a month. Plumb's mandate from the board (and the desire of the staff) was to increase the capacity of the clinic and to stabilize its financial base. When Plumb arrived, she vowed to "grow the clinic," but she was also determined to "grow the clinic in a multicultural way."[45] Under her guidance, Lyon-Martin continued to move in several directions, but it did so with intention.

Plumb instituted a strategic planning exercise to help the Lyon-Martin staff and board set the agenda for the next few years. The exercise revealed that opinions were strongly held and clearly divergent. At a planning retreat, one participant wondered whether Lyon-Martin was a lesbian institution or a lesbian welfare project.[46] Participants struggled to determine what made a lesbian clinic "lesbian" and whether Lyon-Martin could remain lesbian-identified when most clients did not identify as lesbian. They wondered how they could serve any clients at all with the current financial model. The resulting strategic plan, finalized in May 1990, was a hybrid document, with priorities that suggested an attempt to retain the original vision while moving in new directions. It included a new mission statement that reiterated its core commitment to lesbians while also announcing a simultaneous commitment to "all women" and promising a "special outreach to women of color, low-income women, older women, and differently abled women."[47] As a result, this plan attempted to guide the clinic in two distinct ways—firmly back to its lesbian base, and just as firmly to other women who had a difficult time securing compassionate, capable health care.

To become more fully a lesbian clinic, Lyon-Martin determined to become more insurance friendly by gaining preferred provider organization (PPO) status with more local insurance plans, and they vowed to arrange for hospital privileges with at least one San Francisco hospital, thus providing more continuity of care. Also, acknowledging that the Mission District was unlikely to attract middle- and upper-class lesbian women, the plan committed the clinic to a move by September 1990. This proposed move fulfilled two perceived needs: the need for more space (which would allow the clinic to double its client base in five years) and the need to be in a more lesbian-friendly part of town.[48] At the same time, as the plan recommitted the clinic to lesbian health care, it also pushed the clinic in directions it was already moving toward, providing health care to the community's most needy women—poor women, disabled women, and women of color, regardless of sexual orientation. Making lesbians, including middle-class, white lesbians, and the city's neediest women both feel comfortable at Lyon-Martin was complicated, especially because the clinic had a reputation in the city as a "white women's clinic."[49] To address this perception, Plumb, with the support of the board and the staff, worked to diversify the board, the staff, and the clientele.

Under Plumb's leadership, the clinic sponsored a variety of programs that increased the clinic's visibility in and outreach to lesbian communities while also reaching out to marginalized communities of color and other elements of the gay community. These programs included the Last Drag, a smoking cessation program for lesbians, gay men, and bisexuals; Lambda Youth and Family Empowerment, a multicultural youth substance abuse and self-esteem program for lesbian, gay, bisexual, and questioning young people; and a substance abuse prevention program for mothers. Plumb also expanded the lesbian parenting program sponsored by the clinic to include support services to gay, bisexual, and lesbian parents and parents-to-be.[50] These programs reflected a refusal to see lesbians and their needs in isolation.

Plumb's most lasting influence on Lyon-Martin was her decision to seek federal and local funding for HIV and AIDS services. San Francisco, where the gay male community had been devastated in the early years of the AIDS epidemic, became a pioneer in the treatment of people with AIDS, developing what came to be known as the San Francisco model of care. This model acknowledged that HIV-positive people needed care from a variety of medical disciplines and help navigating a host of extramedical concerns. San Francisco General Hospital developed the first outpatient AIDS clinic in the world, Ward 86. At these facilities, patients received services to meet a variety of medical, social, and psychological needs. Social workers connected patients with a vast array of community organizations for counseling, housing, and food delivery. Ward staff encouraged friends, lovers, and families of patients to participate in the caregiving.[51] Community members provided entertainment, hand-holding, and sometimes marijuana-enhanced treats at a time when marijuana was illegal.[52]

Although the vast majority of early AIDS cases were diagnosed in men, the number of women diagnosed rose steadily in the 1980s. By 1988, women composed about 9 percent of all AIDS cases, and they were increasingly reported among new AIDS cases. More than half the women diagnosed with AIDS were Black.[53] The situation in San Francisco, however, differed significantly. Throughout the 1980s, while the absolute number of women diagnosed with AIDS generally rose slightly, women never accounted for more than 3 percent of those newly infected. Likewise, compared to the nation as a whole, Black women represented a much smaller percentage of the total women diagnosed with AIDS in San Francisco in the late 1980s, usually hovering around 30 percent.[54]

Although San Francisco had been a national leader in creating health and social services for gay men with HIV/AIDS, women with AIDS in San Francisco and elsewhere were significantly underserved. There was some women-focused programming. The AIDS Foundation sponsored the Women's AIDS Network, and the Lesbian AIDS Project formed in July of 1987 to locate lesbian IV drug users for education and testing.[55] But there was no integrated home for HIV-positive women in San Francisco to receive health care and social services. Women with AIDS or AIDS-related complex (ARC) were welcome at Ward 86, but some women complained that the ward and some of the social services focused on men's needs. For example, J. H. noted that Ward 86 initially "didn't have any sanitary napkins."[56] Another women noted that gay men received more resources than straight folks or women with kids, a situation that was particularly vexing in AIDS housing.[57] Both of these women worried about their ability to care for their children and what might happen to them after they died. As J. H. put it, HIV-positive women needed women-specific assistance: "I need a real support group—someplace where we can sit around and plan for our kids, our family needs, to help us with our sickness."[58]

Plumb's dream to fill this gap was made possible by increased federal attention to HIV/AIDS. In August 1990, the United States Congress enacted the Ryan White Comprehensive AIDS Resources Emergency (CARE) Act, created to fund programs for low-income, uninsured, and underinsured victims of AIDS and their families. Plumb saw this as an opportunity for Lyon-Martin to reach beyond its lesbian focus while still meeting the health needs of marginalized women. In 1990, Lyon-Martin secured federal CARE Act funding to address the needs of women with AIDS and became the only place in San Francisco dedicated to serving women with AIDS.[59]

Lyon-Martin did not entirely ignore HIV/AIDS before Plumb. Beginning in the mid-1980s, the clinic held occasional forums on women and safe sex and developed and distributed safe-sex kits. Then-executive director Francine (Fran) Miller claimed that these kits were the "first to contain guidelines for lesbians as well as heterosexual women."[60] But in a July 1987 interview, when Miller was asked about lesbians and safe sex, she stumbled, unable to discuss safe-sex guidelines with confidence because "I don't feel very articulate about them." She noted that rough sex and sex during menstruation weren't "safe," and she agreed that "those little dams" should be available to lesbians who wanted them. But her description of how the dental dams performed in practice—"it's hard to breathe, but it's not the worst thing in the world"—and her claim that few lesbians had been diagnosed with HIV signaled her skepticism that HIV/AIDS was a pressing concern for lesbians or Lyon-Martin.[61]

As Lyon-Martin launched its new programs under Plumb's direction, the leaders of the clinic framed HIV/AIDS as a neglected lesbian health threat. For example, in 1992, Rita Shimmin, the HIV services coordinator, argued that lesbians were at risk for HIV infection and underserved by HIV/AIDS organizations. As she framed the problem, "Invisibility will not shield us from

HIV. It can only increase our risk." Although Shimmin acknowledged that lesbians and bisexual women frequently became infected through sex with infected men and using infected needles to shoot drugs, she also condemned the neglect of "sexual activity between women" as a risk factor for HIV transmission.[62] Shimmin thus demonstrated why a lesbian health clinic should invest in HIV/AIDS outreach and care.

Lyon-Martin also sponsored a support group for HIV-positive lesbians. Despite the effort, these groups failed to attract many women; in the early years of the program, only two regularly showed up. Dorothy Bartolomucci, a white woman, and Yolanda Jones, an African American woman, frequently appeared in press coverage of Lyon-Martin's HIV/AIDS programs. Jones and Bartolomucci attributed lesbians' absence from the support group to "denial," and they described the significance of "show[ing] up for each other" for their continued well-being and survival. They also hoped to dispel the myth that lesbians were safe from HIV/AIDS. Bartolomucci offered her own story as a cautionary tale: "So many lesbians were so sure we couldn't get this disease ... and I believed them."[63]

In 1992, Lyon-Martin strengthened its efforts to connect its HIV/AIDS programming to its lesbian-centered mission. Funded by a major grant from the American Foundation for AIDS Research (amfAR), it developed HIV prevention efforts focused on lesbian and bisexual women. Lani Ka'ahumanu, a bisexual rights pioneer, created programs to reach three groups of women believed to be at particular risk: lesbians and bisexual women who had sex with high-risk men to get pregnant; female sexual partners of HIV-positive women; and lesbians and bisexual women who frequented women's dance and sex clubs. According to Ka'ahumanu, the program directed to the latter—called Safe Sex Sluts and "dedicated to demolishing denial"—was the most visible and successful.[64] Ka'ahumanu trained a team of lesbian and bisexual peer educators (the Peer Safe Sex Sluts Team, or PSSST) who performed safe-sex skits at clubs and other community spaces. PSSST was apparently so popular that when the grant expired after two years, Ka'ahumanu kept the group going with an expanded array of genders.

Despite these efforts to link lesbians with HIV/AIDS, the HIV/AIDS programs moved the clientele of Lyon-Martin even further from the lesbian-identified community. Although the HIV/AIDS *testing* services saw a predominantly lesbian clientele, the HIV/AIDS *prevention* programs that targeted the lesbian community were short lived. While the Safe Sex Sluts were popular performers, it is unclear how significant their prevention efforts were.[65] Moreover, most HIV-positive women clients were heterosexual; only a handful identified as lesbian or bisexual. In the wake of these new programs, the clinic

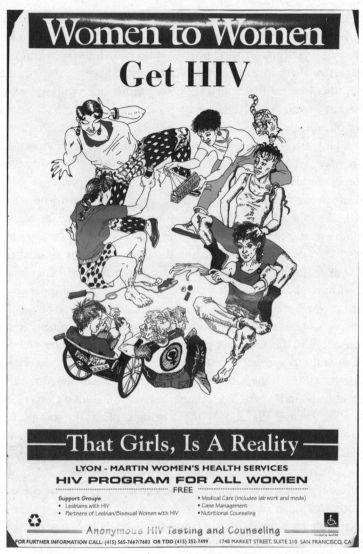

FIGURE 6.3. An HIV awareness poster targeting lesbians, created by the Lesbian and Bisexual HIV Prevention Project, ca. 1992. Despite this attempt to normalize safer-sex practices among lesbians, it proved to be a hard sell. Image by Zanne deJanvier. Courtesy of Lani Ka'ahumanu.

saw a smaller percentage of lesbian-identified clients, an increased percentage of women of color, and a much-increased percentage of poor women.[66]

Plumb refused to interpret the clinic's changing demographics as a betrayal of its lesbian-centered mission. She justified her new programming on many levels. First, she insisted that white, middle-class lesbians were not seeking care at Lyon-Martin because they did not need Lyon-Martin. As she put it, when even the health care giant Kaiser Permanente was promoting itself as "a gay-friendly health organization . . . when you couldn't throw a stone in San Francisco and not hit a gay doc," middle-class lesbians with insurance had attractive alternatives to a community clinic. Second, she insisted that "lesbian" was an identity that had the greatest resonance with white women. In contrast, Plumb believed that many women of color had sex with other women but did not necessarily see themselves as lesbians. Consequently, Plumb maintained that to reach more women who had sex with women, the clinic needed to target its services to women of color instead of just lesbians of color. Finally, Plumb argued that by engaging in AIDS work, Lyon-Martin would encounter and assist many desperately needy women who were often stigmatized by their sexual choices—a stigma shared by lesbians.[67]

Plumb's reference to women who have sex with women (WSW) deserves analysis. WSW became a public health designation in 1995 as an attempt to move away from the use of identity categories in favor of behavioral categories within public health research. Plumb's use of this designation can be read as her attempt to categorize these women as possible lesbians, closeted lesbians, or sometime lesbians and therefore appropriate clients of lesbian health services. In this sense, her gesture to women who have sex with women was an attempt to appease board and community members determined to maintain the clinic's lesbian identity. At the same time, she urged stakeholders to redraw the boundaries of their community, focusing not on lesbian identity but on sexual marginalization. Without being explicit, she was asking for a move away from identity politics to an embrace of queer politics, a politics that rejected allegedly self-evident categories of identity as the basis for movement organizing.[68] This double reading allowed stakeholders with considerably different politics to continue to work with and for the same clinic even if they were working toward different ends.

For Plumb, then, Lyon-Martin could survive as a lesbian clinic only if it abandoned the idea of remaining a "lesbian-only clinic." As she put it, there had been no way to remain lesbian-only after it expanded beyond "seeing thirty people a month at San Francisco General." The staff and the board agreed, for the time being, and supported building Lyon-Martin as a lesbian clinic that served women who had the fewest health care options. They vowed to "keep it as a community clinic, keep it lesbian-focused, but see that as a much broader frame."[69]

Reaching out to women of color proved easier than reaching out with women of color. Plumb, the staff, and the board knew that they had to diversify to better understand the communities they served. Adding more women of color to the board proved rocky, however. The board diversified, but as a result, several board members, both new and old, reported feeling "unsafe" at meetings. Some of the new board members complained that the board was more interested in bringing women of color into the clinic and onto the board than facing their own racism. For at least one woman, the situation was untenable. L. Dymond Austin, a self-proclaimed "Black; Lesbian; Womanist; Parent," resigned from the board in January 1992, insisting, "I do not feel a part of the Board of Lyon-Martin. I do not feel listened to. I do not feel like I am taken seriously. I do not feel safe." She recounted her initial enthusiasm for the changes the clinic and board were trying to enact and expressed her gratitude that she was asked to be part of it. In the end, she concluded that the board had been unwilling to "reach out and interact with people of color on a level of which would truly move the agency toward multiculturalism."[70]

Diversifying the staff apparently proceeded more smoothly; by 1992, more than 50 percent (five of nine) of the clinic's staff were women of color.[71] Still, some at the clinic insisted that Plumb had not done enough. For example, Plumb had hired a Black woman, Rita Shimmin, to head up the HIV services for the clinic. Shimmin applauded Plumb's efforts to bring women of color into the agency, but Plumb recalls Shimmin urging her to push harder, insisting that "you've done a pretty good job of diversifying the clinic, but, you know, you keep hiring safe women of color. . . . You keep hiring women that are essentially like you, just dark-skinned. And if you really want to have a diverse agency, you need to actually take risks."[72]

To close the distance between the clinic's clientele and its staff, and perhaps to take more staffing risks, Plumb hired an African American woman who lived in public housing to run peer-led HIV prevention programs in the projects. This program highlighted the difficulty of running a truly multicultural, multiclass organization. In the end, the project failed, as Lyon-Martin allegedly proved unable or unwilling to engage with the lived experiences and the financial needs of the women they were attempting to recruit, train, and serve.[73]

Under Plumb's guidance, the clinic expanded and transformed. In 1989, when Plumb arrived, the operating budget was roughly $325,000; the budget for 1992 was $820,000. The expansion was fueled and funded primarily by the HIV/AIDS programs. In addition to reaching more women, some of whom probably had sex with women, the HIV programs also allowed Lyon-Martin to hire a full-time doctor for the first time—a doctor who could then see patients, lesbians included, who had non-HIV-related conditions.[74]

Plumb provided leadership, vision, and resourcefulness that allowed the clinic to grow financially, spatially, and programmatically. Although there were moments of dissension and distrust, often over the efforts to diversify the board and the staff, the changes she instituted were largely supported. Nevertheless, by the end, according to her own assessment, Plumb was in over her head: "I had built this thing way over my capacity to lead it."[75] She left, rather abruptly, a thriving but conflicted institution. Without Plumb's confidence (or bravado, perhaps) that Lyon-Martin's services were consistent with its mission, the clinic gradually lost its footing and much of its funding. Without Plumb's leadership, the consistency she saw between Lyon-Martin's commitment to lesbians while serving the poor became increasingly invisible to the clinic's board, staff, and community supporters.

Losing Its Direction, 1993–2000

Plumb's departure in 1993 left a gap at the top of the organization that took almost a decade to fill. Between March 1993 and May 2001, seven different women served as executive director or interim executive director.[76] At times, the clinic operated (or not) without even an interim director. When Plumb left in 1993, the staff and the board were firmly behind the broadened vision of the clinic. Without her leadership, however, the resolve behind the clinic's expanded scope grew shaky. Without a spokesperson who could explain how Lyon-Martin was still a lesbian clinic even as lesbians composed less than half of its client base, the clinic found it increasingly difficult to attract private funding, dedicated leadership, appropriate health care workers, and committed board members.

Many community members who had once supported the clinic were distressed to see the clinic limping along. They often identified the turn to HIV/AIDS services as the moment when the clinic lost its way by neglecting its own. In the mid- and late 1990s, the number of lesbian-identified clients at Lyon-Martin hovered around 35–45 percent of the larger client load.[77] In the HIV/AIDS programs, however, lesbian-identified clients never represented more than 10 percent.[78] As a result, when Lyon-Martin stakeholders wondered how the clinic had strayed from its lesbian-centered mission, they focused on the HIV services—and Plumb's pursuit of these funding streams—as the source of the problem. Founders, board members, and past donors condemned Plumb's decision to chase the money rather than stay the lesbian-specific course.

Clearly, many women who worked at Lyon-Martin, lesbian and straight, white and Black, were thrilled to provide care to some of San Francisco's neediest residents. Some of them were especially delighted that the lesbian community was looking beyond its own self-interest by supporting a clinic that did not exclusively serve its own. For some of the women who worked at Lyon-Martin, the diversity of the clientele was key to their affection for it. When the nurse practitioner Tamara Ooms was asked what made Lyon-Martin worthwhile to her, she replied: "It was the most amazingly diverse group of women . . . in one place. . . . I mean, you know, from your . . . wealthy lesbian in Marin County who just wants to come there because . . . she has insurance but she still does want to come to Lyon-Martin, to your . . . crack alcoholic, transgender, HIV-positive, homeless . . . woman on the corner. . . . It was just a really fascinating, diverse group of folks."[79] Naomi Prochovnick, an HIV caseworker and longtime employee, agreed: "Imagine the waiting room. You've got someone who hasn't bathed in weeks and may or may not be talking to themselves and belligerent, and you've got someone who's sitting there waiting for their Pap. It was fantastic."[80]

But for others, the imagined and actual waiting room symbolized the cultural struggle at play. The physician assistant Rose Quinones told how Lyon-Martin went from "this very kind of groovy, fuzzy, dyke-couches-and-women's-posters and . . . advocacy energy to a poor African American woman with HIV and mental illness screaming and yelling, poor dentition, demanding to be seen right away. . . . [A] very different energy to sit in a waiting room with a different population. So it went from [a] kind of middle-class, downwardly mobile group of people to truly poor, disenfranchised, undereducated, underinsured people. [It was a] struggle to share that space."[81] Beth Rittenhouse, an HIV case services manager, also described the face-off: "Our patients . . . are all sitting there together. Some of them have shopping carts, and . . . they are very mentally ill or have active substance use problems—maybe talking to themselves—with a completely different population of people who might be working, who are sort of looking at each other on the couch like, 'Hmm,' . . . in the waiting room. 'What is really going on here, and who is the clinic serving?'"[82]

While some of the staff relished the broad-based clientele, the diversity of the waiting room marked the distance between the clinic's clientele and the lesbian community that founded and supported the clinic over the years. It was not that the lesbian community opposed health care for poor, multiply marginalized women. They just did not embrace HIV/AIDS treatment as their own cause or responsibility.[83] Indeed, women who had thought they had built a clinic for their own community found twelve years later a waiting room full of, as Prochovnick put it, "icky, stinky, smelly, noisy homeless women."[84] While some of these women might have identified as lesbians and others might have had sex with women, they did not fit within the imagined lesbian community. As a result, many of the women who had once seen the clinic as "theirs," even if they never sought services there, no longer felt connected to it.

The distance between the clinic's donors and its clientele presented a dilemma for fundraising. One of the first major fundraisers for the clinic was an annual Lesbian Mixed Doubles Tennis Tournament (butch-femme versus butch-femme).[85] In the early years, it was relatively easy to attract well-heeled lesbians to a tennis match to support the health care of other lesbians. But eventually this became a hard sell. Shimmin, the HIV services director, noted that the women who once supported the clinic were challenged by the changing client base. She asked, "Did the women who supported the clinic . . . know how to change? Did they sign on to support really poor women, . . . women of color, and women who are, you know, doing all the bad things in life?"[86] Apparently, many were not.

By early 1999, the many problems of Lyon-Martin had escalated to a crisis, and the board reached back to a time when the clinic seemed to have a trusted leader. One of the board members called, in desperation, Marj Plumb, who remembered: "We're down to three board members. Our executive director just left and she's suing us. We have four other active employee lawsuits. We've lost medical staff. I just wanted to let you know, we're having a meeting next week, and we're probably going to close the clinic." She eventually convinced Plumb, who had just started a doctoral program in public health at Berkeley, to return to the clinic as interim executive director "until they could figure out what to do."[87]

When Plumb returned, things were grim indeed. The clinic had no executive director, no clinic director, and no development director. It had a deficit of more than $100,000, and the number of donors had gone from 1,500 in 1990 to 150 in 1998.[88] Desperate staff reported to the board that the phone lines were cut, contract deadlines were missed, and funds were mismanaged.[89] Although many of the people watching the clinic decline blamed the AIDS programs, regarding them as a detour from the original charge of serving lesbians, Plumb would have none of it. She placed the blame on the ineffective agency leadership and the breakdown in fundraising.[90] When asked what killed the clinic at this particular juncture, she claimed that it was because "they didn't ask people for money. That's what killed the clinic!"[91] They had stopped sending newsletters and direct-mail appeals for donations. Not only had fundraising stopped, but Medi-Cal billing (and thus reimbursements) was four years behind, in part because of inadequate accounting software and in part because of staff shortages. Under Plumb's guidance, the clinic's board, experiencing its own crisis, created a ninety-day "Stability and Recovery

Plan." To address the personnel and financial crises, the plan set several goals: hire a qualified executive director, develop a budget, update financial systems, negotiate loan repayment plans, and improve organizational structure were some of the items on the urgent to-do list.[92] She also urged the board to consult with staff and other stakeholders to solidify the clinic's mission.[93] Without articulating clear goals for the clinic, the path forward would remain unclear.

Plumb was quite clear about how she saw the mission of the clinic. She directed the board and the staff to "serve poor people. Lesbians with health insurance will never come here. Besides, there are plenty of poor lesbians who would use the clinic if they only knew about it. Community clinics serve poor people. You are the keeper of that sacred trust. Don't break it."[94]

While Plumb's position was clear, many of the supporters of the clinic were unconvinced. In 1999 and 2000, the clinic held a series of meetings with the staff, the board, and community stakeholders to identify the shortcomings of Lyon-Martin and articulate how they wanted to see the clinic move into the twenty-first century. By 1999, the staff was committed to serving poor women regardless of sexual orientation, but they were concerned how the clinic's actual practices fit with the clinic's official mission and public presentation.[95]

Plumb and the board also sought input from community members, sending a solicitation letter in June 1999 inviting "stakeholders" to a series of meetings focused on discussing the future of the clinic. The solicitation acknowledged the dual roles of the clinic: "The agency is actually many things, it is a local health care provider with a special focus on lesbians, a national leader in lesbian health care, and a community clinic serving low-income women and women of color." The letter noted that the clinic was at a crossroads and needed help deciding whether it could continue to fill all these roles or whether the clinic should continue at all.[96]

In deciding who were included in the category of stakeholders, Plumb and the board shaped the final outcome of the negotiations. By turning to the founders, early funders, and wealthy and visible lesbians, the solicitation itself turned the clinic's future back toward its past. These community stakeholders strongly endorsed a recommitment to rebuilding Lyon-Martin as a medical facility for the lesbian community.

The outcome of these solicitations and meetings essentially pitted the health needs of poor, multiply marginalized women who depended on the medical and psychosocial services offered by Lyon-Martin against the health needs of lesbians who did not yet seek health care at the clinic but who might be recruited. The staff sided with the current patients; the board, persuaded by the views of community stakeholders, embraced a recommitment to a lesbian clinic. In February 2000, the board unanimously agreed that Lyon-

Martin Women's Health Services would refocus on "its original charter—services to lesbians." As a result, the board committed to a gradual expansion of services to lesbians and a withdrawal of services from non-lesbians. Although the board insisted that "no one in need of services [would] be turned away," it did plan, for example, to "transition" HIV services to non-lesbians somewhere else. The board insisted that it had not been a mistake to provide "HIV care when we did, but the need [was . . .] to move on . . . and to identify our next 'cutting edge' lesbian issue."[97]

In the following months, the clinic did in fact increase its outreach to lesbians and its presence in shaping the local and national lesbian health agenda.[98] Nevertheless, Lyon-Martin never abandoned its HIV/AIDS services, perhaps because it could not afford to. In 2000, roughly 50 percent of its $1.2 million budget came from funds earmarked for HIV/AIDS or homeless health care programs. Without these funds, the clinic could not stay afloat.[99] Still, economics does not entirely explain why Lyon-Martin retained its HIV and homeless services. While many of the board members and stakeholders believed in the value of a lesbian-centered clinic, many of the staff members were unconvinced of its need and of its practicality. As Naomi Prochovnick put it, a lesbian health clinic made sense in the 1970s when lesbians could not find sensitive and competent medical providers. Prochovnick insisted that by the 1990s, however, in San Francisco at least, "the need for a specialized clinic for lesbians was not that dramatic." Besides, she claimed, the majority of the white, middle-class lesbians "for whom this clinic was designed" had a form of insurance never accepted by Lyon-Martin. Consequently, it made no sense to Prochovnick and many of the other staff members to turn away from the women who needed Lyon-Martin to court women who did not.[100]

The clinic weathered the crisis of 1999 and 2000. Nevertheless, because it renewed its emphasis on lesbian health while maintaining its HIV/AIDS services, the clinic did not resolve its internal divisions. Recurrent crises continued to plague the clinic. From November 2004 through January 2005, for example, the clinic closed because of a staff walkout.[101] Indeed, conflicts over who should be allowed to seek care at Lyon-Martin were already brewing along a different axis.

Trans Patients at a Lesbian Clinic

During the same time Lyon-Martin struggled to accommodate all the women who sought medical care at the clinic, they also debated whether a women's health facility should provide care to trans people, both trans women and trans men. Just as the HIV prevention, support, and treatment programs brought significant funds and many multiply marginalized, straight-identifying women to Lyon-Martin Women's Health Services, they also unexpectedly brought transgender individuals into the women's clinic. Many of the women who used medical and psychosocial services offered by Lyon-Martin were trans women (known at the time as MTF). Trans women, especially trans women of color, had high rates of HIV infection.[102] According to Prochovnick, the risk factors for transgender people were "through the roof. Lots of substance abuse, lot of unsafe sex, lot of sex for drugs, . . . just all the factors that put people at risk."[103] In addition to the use of injection drugs and participation in sex work, trans women had other risk factors, including sex with men who frequently had sex with men and densely connected sexual networks.[104]

Before 1993, there had been little research on the health care needs of trans people beyond transition care. Even more alarming, there were few studies of HIV prevention efforts among trans people, despite high rates of HIV infection, especially among trans women sex workers.[105] In addition, there were no health facilities in the nation specifically designed to meet the primary needs of trans people, and facilities established to serve gay men or HIV-positive people often failed to attract trans patients. When trans people sought health care, they frequently encountered ignorance and transphobia. Sometimes they were denied care outright. As a result, trans men and trans women frequently put off seeking health care until they were quite ill.[106]

In San Francisco, staff at an HIV clinic in the Tenderloin—an impoverished neighborhood well known for sex work and drug use, and one ravaged by AIDS—noticed a dearth of trans-identified patients. They knew that many transgender people in the neighborhood were HIV-positive but weren't coming to the clinic. In response, the clinic opened a nighttime trans clinic in 1993 under the name Transgender Tuesdays. Over time, this clinic became the first primary care facility for transgender people in the nation.[107] Despite this pathbreaking clinic, it did not nearly meet all the health care needs of the San Francisco trans community, and Lyon-Martin, with a city contract to serve HIV-positive women, became a mostly welcoming alternative.

The staff seemed to take this new client population in stride. As case manager Prochovnick put it, "We served anyone who needed women's health care."[108] Some members of the board, however, were less accepting. For them, as a lesbian clinic first and a women's health clinic second, treating patients they considered anatomically male did not fit with their sense of the mission. They also worried that an acceptance of trans women might lead to the treatment of trans men. How could they remain Lyon-Martin Women's Health Services if they served men? The issue remained unresolved for years; most of the staff welcomed transgender patients, and the majority of the board did not. A tacit policy apparently emerged as a compromise: the staff treated trans patients while keeping the board in the dark.

In the mid-1990s, the city of San Francisco stepped in to resolve the issue. In the spring of 1993, the Lesbian, Gay, Bisexual, Transgender Advisory Committee of the San Francisco Human Rights Commission (HRC) created a Transgender Committee. The committee, chaired by the transgender activist Kiki Whitlock, educated the HRC about the diversity of the trans community and the widespread discrimination its members experienced. In September 1994, the HRC issued a report detailing the human rights abuses against the transgender community. This report, written by the transgender activist Jamison Green, prompted the city to create an ordinance adding gender identity to its antidiscrimination clause along with race, age, weight, disability, and other social axes of inequality.[109] As a result, the law in San Francisco prohibited discrimination based on gender identity in public accommodations, including health clinics. Presumably to inform the clinic of its obligations under the new law, the HRC reached out to Lyon-Martin to apprise the clinic of its legal obligations to treat trans clients. In July 1995, the board of Lyon-Martin responded. It agreed to serve "pre-op FTM's and post-op MTF's"—that is, people who might need gynecological care based upon their so-called female anatomy—and it recommended that the clinic "develop protocols for FTM hormonal therapy." The board refused to sanction, however, the treatment of individuals it considered to be men: "As a clinic specializing in women's health care, we can only serve those clients that are anatomically and physiologically female and therefore have female medical issues. While we recognize the importance of identity in medical care, serving clients that are anatomically and physiologically male is currently outside the scope of our medical practice."[110] The HRC let this policy stand for a while, perhaps because they believed, and rightly, that the clinic did indeed treat trans women regardless of whether they intended a medical or surgical transition, despite the policy outlined above. But, probably in response to a complaint, in June 1996 the HRC warned Lyon-Martin that if its "current policy [was] to deny services to pre-operative MTF women," it was in violation of the law. The HRC maintained that preoperative trans women were in fact women and denied Lyon-Martin's position that "female medical issues are confined only to people who are anatomically and physiologically female." The letter concluded by insisting that trans women "should have the opportunity to be served in a high quality women's clinic."[111]

Perhaps feeling like they had no choice, or perhaps because they were ready to embrace transgender medicine, in July 1996, the executive director of Lyon-Martin informed the Human Rights Commission that the Lyon-Martin

Board of Directors had voted "to offer our scope of services to all persons seeking women's health care. This includes pre-op MTF. . . . Any transgender person seeking women's health care is welcome to come here to access our services."[112] As part of its now official commitment to transgender medicine, the clinic also applied for and received permission from insurance underwriters to provide hormone treatments "as part of gender re-assignment therapy."[113] These expanded services were not reflected, however, in a revised mission statement until five years later. In 2001, the board agreed to the following: "Lyon-Martin partners with women to enhance their well-being by providing access to high quality health and social services, with a focus on the current and emerging needs of lesbian, bisexual, and queer women, transgender people, and women who have sex with women." Still, the mission statement also ended with the declaration: "We are leaders, advocates, educators, and activists on behalf of women's health."[114] Efforts to add "and transgendered people" to this last sentence failed.[115]

Just as it had highlighted the tensions between middle-class, lesbian patients and poor, straight, HIV-positive women, the waiting room also captured the cultural clash between some of the cis women patients and the trans patients. Quinones described the resistance to trans women, who, Quinones claimed, often looked like men. Although many lesbians welcomed other cisgender, female-identified, non-lesbians at the clinic, especially if they "enabled us to keep the doors open," they often rejected the presence of people they regarded as men. Quinones noted that some lesbians framed their rejection in terms of safety: "You know, a lot of women had been victimized . . . physical and sexual abuse, and they felt unsafe around men." Another staff member merely attributed it to discomfort.[116]

Trans men, who started to attend Lyon-Martin in significant numbers after the turn of the twenty-first century, also raised concerns. Quinones described the scene: "Some of our patients were taking testosterone, and they would get big beards, big buff muscles, smell like guys, sweat, have BO, boy BO, and some of them had chest surgery so they would have their breasts removed. . . . They looked like men. Their energy was like a man. And here were all these women sitting in a women's clinic next to a man . . . and it was like, who is this? When is this not ours anymore?"[117] These tensions— among patients, and between the staff and the board—prevented the clinic from wholeheartedly welcoming trans-identified patients, although the clinic served them.

The board's resistance to transgender patients must be understood in a larger political context. Although second-wave feminism has been frequently characterized as "trans-exclusionary," recent scholarship by Finn Enke, Cristan Williams, and others has shown that trans women have frequently been "integral to" some of the "most iconic feminisms" of the 1970s. Nevertheless, when Lyon-Martin began, there was no clear consensus that transgender people belonged in the same social or activist space as feminists or lesbians.[118] Janice Raymond's 1979 manifesto, *Transsexual Empire*, for example, made the case that transsexuals sought "to colonize feminist identification, culture, politics and sexuality," raping women's bodies in the process.[119] The Michigan Womyn's Music Festival was wracked for years over the issue of whether to admit women who were not "woman-born-women."[120] These larger political issues were only magnified in a health clinic with expertise in women's health care.

The 1990s marked an increase in transgender activism, forged by new theoretical discussions of gender and sexuality coming out of the academy (eventually known as queer theory) and the devastation caused by the HIV/AIDS epidemic. Because AIDS ravaged many different communities, including gay men, sex workers, and IV drug users, it eventually launched a politics of alliance across many traditional identity boundaries. This politics of alliance resonated with the new queer politics of the academy. In 1990, activists in New York City from the HIV/AIDS group ACT UP created Queer Nation, a group committed to eliminating homophobia and increasing queer visibility. Queer politics in general and Queer Nation in particular eschewed identity politics because they allegedly emphasized "identity and personal development rather than liberation, justice and solidarity."[121] Indeed, queer politics resisted identity categories altogether. According to the theorist Steven Seidman, "Under the undifferentiated sign of Queer are united all those heterogeneous desires and interests that are marginalized and excluded in the straight and gay mainstream. Queers are not united by any unitary identity but only by their opposition to disciplining, normalizing, social forces."[122] One of the achievements of queer politics was to create a new community that brought transgender people and bisexuals together with lesbians and gay men under the banner of "queer"; ironically, the word *queer*, rather than retaining its anti-identitarian foundation, increasingly became a new identity category.[123] In San Francisco, Queer Nation was explicitly trans-inclusive, though not all gay men and lesbians embraced trans activists. To fight transphobia, Anne Ogborn created Transgender Nation in 1992, an interest group created under the Queer Nation umbrella. According to the historian Susan Stryker, this short-lived group helped establish and promote common cause between transgender and queer communities.[124]

Although queer politics created opportunities for lesbians and transgender activists to work together in a movement against heteronormativity, the politics of identity did not disappear. Efforts for trans inclusion elicited heated battles throughout the 1990s, often separating factions along roughly generational lines. By the end of the 1990s, many gay and lesbian organizations had included reference to transgender people in their names and missions, adding a *T* to their LGB acronym. Stryker notes, however, that this inclusion often represented a "failure to grasp the ways in which transgender identity differed from sexual orientation as well as a misconception about how they were alike."[125]

By the twenty-first century, it had become clear that trans men and women frequently identified as gay or lesbian before and/or after their social and/or medical transition. While some members of the LGB community, especially the lesbian community, strove to separate themselves from trans men and women, this position declined as more and more lesbians openly identified as trans. At Lyon-Martin as elsewhere, political positions fell largely, though not completely, along generational lines. According to Dawn Harbatkin, who became medical director in 2006, the "old-guard lesbians[,] . . . those for whom lesbianism was a separatist thing," were most opposed to the broadened mission. In Harbatkin's experience, a younger generation of lesbians, who might also or instead refer to themselves as queer, who might partner with trans men, demanded an inclusive vision of the lesbian community.[126]

By 2003, the clinic—board, staff, and larger community—had generally embraced trans people as not just an unintended consequence of the HIV programs that needed to be dealt with but as a pool of marginalized, underserved individuals who could benefit from sensitive and informed medical and psychosocial services. Despite the accidental influx of transgender patients and the initial resistance to them from the board and some community stakeholders, outreach to trans people eventually became central to Lyon-Martin's focus. By May 2003, the board revised its mission statement yet again, frontloading Lyon-Martin's commitment to transgender people: "Lyon-Martin provides personalized healthcare and support services to women and transgender people who lack access to quality care because of their sexual or gender identity regardless of their ability to pay."[127]

As the clinic embraced transgender patients, its visibility rose in trans medical circles. Nick Gorton, a trans emergency medicine physician in Sacramento, began to donate his time to the clinic twice a week in 2005. Harbatkin, lured away from New York City and a job as medical director at Callen-Lorde Community Health, one of the nation's premier LGBT health centers, had been recruited by Lyon-Martin in part because of her experience with trans health. By 2007, about one-third of the clinic's 1,500 patients identified as trans.[128] Perhaps this increased focus on trans health culminated in April

2007 when the board voted to drop *Women's* from its name, becoming Lyon-Martin Health Services.[129] In a statement to the press, Harbatkin stressed that the mission of Lyon-Martin—to serve women, especially lesbian and bisexual women—had not changed, but she noted that serving women was "not all of who we serve anymore."[130]

Lyon-Martin Women's Health Services was built for the lesbian community by the lesbian community. By donating their time and their money to the clinic, lesbians and some gay men believed that they were taking care of their own. Over time, as homophobia in San Francisco declined and cultural sensitivity to gay and lesbian issues in health care increased, the need for a lesbian-specific clinic declined. As AIDS hit, however, a new set of women—poor women, both women of color and white women, who were often doing, as Rita Shimmin put it, "all the bad things in life"—desperately needed affordable and culturally sensitive health care. Many people associated with Lyon-Martin eagerly shifted their focus, willingly giving their time to serve the most needy; others, however, resented and resisted the turn away from lesbian-centered services.

The waiting room of Lyon-Martin became a place where concerns about the clinic's mission took physical form, where politics of inclusion and exclusion were tested, where claims about "our community clinic" became tools to exclude the already most marginal and most needy. For some stakeholders, a waiting room full of poor women of color, men with beards, or women with Adam's apples proved that the lesbian-centered mission of the clinic had been abandoned and that lesbian clients had been literally and figuratively displaced from their own space. The waiting room came to symbolize, at least for a while, the loss of a safe haven for the lesbian community; for some lesbians, "a place for us" required not just the absence of homophobia but also protection from being forced to confront their own privileged social and economic positions and the limits of their inclusive politics. Safe space, at least for some members of the community, required policing the boundaries of that community.

Ironically, the queer bodies of transgender people, once a lightning rod for dissension, eventually served as the conduit that brought the support of the lesbian community back to Lyon-Martin. By the 1990s, middle-class lesbians had many health care choices, but trans men and women still needed informed, compassionate, and affordable health care. Many trans folks needed Lyon-Martin. As the larger lesbian and gay community came to embrace trans people as part of us rather than part of them, so, too, did the San Francisco lesbian community come to accept Lyon-Martin and its outreach to transgender people as an asset to the community.

Coda: A Clinic Worth Fighting For

The financial crisis of 2011 that began this chapter threatened to be Lyon-Martin's last. But the community who refused to let Lyon-Martin fold was gay, lesbian, and queer identified. A largely queer community embraced Lyon-Martin as a community asset—as their clinic—and they organized fundraisers, exerted political pressure, and volunteered to reconceive and rebuild the embattled clinic. As patient-turned-board-member Pike Long put it, Lyon-Martin provided the best medical care she had ever had, "so [it was] worth fighting for."[131] Although the outpouring of cash from local and national sources in the first three months of 2011 was remarkable and unprecedented, it was not nearly enough to dig the clinic out of debt, and certainly not enough to sustain the clinic going forward. The clinic needed to be rebuilt. This required at least another $350,000 in community donations, a reconsideration of the clinic's scope, a reorganization of the clinic's operations, and the redevelopment of the clinic's board.[132]

Because of her history of resuscitating Lyon-Martin, Marj Plumb was asked to return to the clinic and serve as the clinic's first new board member; she was immediately elected board chair. As she had done before, Plumb provided a compelling justification for the clinic's survival at a moment when survival seemed unlikely. In an August 1, 2011, letter, Plumb wrote:

> As you know, Lyon-Martin began as *the only clinic in the world specifically caring for lesbians.* The clinic has evolved to now serve a unique blend of 2500 underserved women, lesbians, and transgender patients. It is a nationally recognized model for serving our communities and . . . true to our historical beginnings, it is a clinic of last resort for patients who don't "fit" anywhere else. This isn't a question of "maybe we don't need the clinic anymore"; it's a question of *"how could we let a unique clinic, with such a significant place in our history, that is addressing such a compelling patient population, be lost." We ask you to consider Lyon-Martin as the embodiment of core feminist values: creating a just and equitable world.* We deliver the highest quality healthcare to the most marginalized within our community.[133]

Plumb dismissed any discussion of whether any imagined community of "we" might need the clinic, and she highlighted its political, personal, and material significance. She reminded lesbians that Lyon-Martin had been built specifically for them. She emphasized the historical significance of Lyon-Martin—the only one of its kind—and highlighted the potential loss to lesbian history. She underscored the clinic's ability to expand its mission to embrace other marginalized people "within our community." And finally, she appealed to "feminist values" of equity and justice to encourage donors to see the continued survival of Lyon-Martin as their issue. Plumb appealed to notions of identity, but mostly as an artifact of history. She appealed as well to a community, but it was a community of place, values, and history. This approach simultaneously argued for the significance of the clinic's history and the value of its future.

Plumb's plea was apparently successful enough. In September 2011, Lyon-Martin began taking new patients, signaling its commitment to survival. The clinic also needed more federally funded patients to increase its cash flow.[134] But survival required significant organizational changes. Fundraising in 2011 stabilized the clinic's operations but did not significantly diminish the clinic's debt. In 2014, Lyon-Martin merged with HealthRIGHT 360, itself a merger of the Haight Ashbury Free Clinics and Walden House, a residential substance-abuse treatment facility.[135] In November 2017, Lyon-Martin moved again, returning to the Mission District to share a facility with two other HealthRIGHT 360 units, the Women's Community Clinic and the Lee Woodward Counseling Center for Women.[136] This merger allowed Lyon-Martin to maintain a presence as a welcoming haven for queer women and trans folks while sharing the operational infrastructure and the community fundraising with other units dedicated to meeting the health care needs of the area's most needy.[137]

This history of Lyon-Martin reveals a great deal about feminist health organizing and institution building. Most critically, this chapter has highlighted both the limits and the power of identity politics. Lyon-Martin emerged as an antidote to the negative health consequences of medical homophobia. Founders in the late 1970s believed correctly that lesbians were less likely to seek routine medical screening and care than their non-lesbian-identified counterparts. Taking their cues from the feminist health movement and the burgeoning gay and lesbian health movement, the founders enacted a form of institutional self-help, building a clinic by lesbians for lesbians. That this clinic had a community who felt connected to it, who felt that the clinic was theirs, was key to its success and survival at a time when other feminist clinics were closing their doors. In its early years, the clinic provided valuable care to lesbians, both middle class and poor, and to other women. As long as the clinic retained an identifiable lesbian clientele, all the stakeholders, founders, staff, and board members seemed willing to extend care to other needy women, even if they were surprised by the influx of presumably straight women. But the problems with an identity-based approach were evident already at the beginning because it encouraged surveillance of the threshold. Consequently, very early in the clinic's history, some of the patients seeking care were understood as central to the clinic's mission while others were welcomed as incidental and accidental patients, benefactors of lesbian largesse. As the number of these accidental clients increased and their demographic changed, the lesbian community—or, at least, the middle-class component of it—became less able see themselves, their own particular experiences of marginalization, reflected in the clientele. The clinic's commitment to an identity-based mission provoked recurrent and divisive discussion about the clinic's goals.

This chapter has also explored what happens to institutions born in one political moment as the politics change around them. Lyon-Martin, a "Lesbian-born idea," was founded by white women who identified as lesbians and as feminists to provide a safe haven from the heterosexism and homophobia prevalent in medicine at the time. But as feminist health clinics closed, replaced by mainstream medicine's women's health centers, as even Kaiser advertised itself as gay and lesbian friendly, as the lesbian community increasingly included trans men, the clinic needed to evaluate its mission in light of the community's evolving needs. The clinic survived only because it was willing to incorporate, in fits and starts, a new queer politics and a more capacious sense of community.

Finally, this chapter has explored the racial dynamics at play at Lyon-Martin. Although its clients, volunteers, and (eventually) staff were never exclusively white, the infusion of straight-identified Latina clients in the 1980s racialized the concern that Lyon-Martin had strayed from its mission to serve lesbians. Marj Plumb's efforts to diversify the clinic similarly worked to destabilize the clinic's lesbian identity. As a result, much of the discussion about Lyon-Martin's possibly derailed mission focused on women of color. Nevertheless, the clinic never abandoned its commitment to diversity. By the early 2000s, people of color occupied roles from receptionist to peer counselor to physician assistant to executive director. Through struggle and reflection, Lyon-Martin became a racially diverse workplace that welcomed a racially diverse clientele.

"Any Sister's Pain":
Forging Black Women's Sisterhood
through Self-Help

In the spring of 1983, Felicia Ward, a San Francisco–born-and-raised Black woman, attended an Erhard Seminars Training (more commonly known as EST) in California. There she sat next to Luz Alvarez Martinez, a Latina who worked at the Berkeley Women's Health Collective.[1] Martinez had heard about an upcoming Black women's health conference at Spelman College, and she and a friend were raising money to send a group from the Bay Area. "Would you like to join us?" Martinez asked Ward. Ward enthusiastically agreed.[2]

When Martinez reached out, Ward was ready. She yearned to be part of something bigger than herself. Thirty years old in 1983, she was searching for home, a community that fed her emotionally and politically and provided the opportunity for her to give back. She had joined a sorority in college and was looking to replicate the culture of support and service. Her sister was a Black Panther, but the Panthers didn't offer what she sought. When her sister invited her to join an ashram in Oakland, Ward moved in. There she embraced meditation and other forms of self-development. She especially appreciated EST, "because it let me separate who I was from all the noise in the world." Still, she wanted more, and she thought feminism might suit her. When Ward attended a demonstration in San Francisco in April 1983, headlined by Gloria Steinem and Alice Walker, it spoke to her, but she didn't see a way in. The conference at Spelman College gave her a path.[3]

The Black Women's Health Conference held in the summer of 1983 was unlike any other event in Ward's life. She appreciated the rich program focused on a variety of health topics, and she was captivated by the presence of so many Black women coming together across their differences. She was initially overwhelmed by the sheer joy and wonder of being surrounded by

Black women, hugging and laughing and crying together. "I had never been embraced by a Black woman in my life," she recalled later. "[I'd] never been hugged ever. Never . . . and suddenly I'm getting these hugs by Black women." She felt "drunk on love for my people." The experience changed her life.[4]

Like many other women at the conference, Ward was especially influenced by a workshop facilitated by Lillie Allen, Black and Female: What Is the Reality? Ward remembers the room bursting with women, chattering, excited, and curious. Allen began the workshop by proclaiming: "It's time we told our stories. It's time we broke the silence." In response, Black women rose and shared their stories, stories of pain, grief, and accomplishment. As Ward described it, "The whole room broke into tears. . . . I was glad I was on the floor because the whole room was sobbing. I mean, loud wracked sobs." Ward felt her own grief and pain merge with the keening of hundreds of other Black women; she also sensed the potential for healing. Amid the emotion around her, Ward felt safe. In that moment, she "felt like this will save us. This is what will save us, . . . [w]e needed to grieve."[5]

In Ward's telling, the sounds of pain and grief she heard at Spelman connected her to the Africans brought to the Americas in shackles and the violent legacy of enslavement. She heard Black women's sobs as echoes of African men and women protesting their captivity from the hold of slave ships.

> It dawned on me that these sounds are *why* we'd survived. Making these sounds is *how* we'd survived. When our chained bodies feared what the physical self knew had to be coming[,] we knew to holler. Death and destruction. Generations that would only know misery. Holler. But we weren't steeped in shame back then. Shame hadn't chained us yet. Standing there in our midst, ringed by our grievous history, Lillie Allen stood in some new light. She helped us remember what we'd forgotten. Breathe, and cry your heart's sorrow. Rest a moment in the cradle of some safe arms, and then go on and truly live.[6]

The Black Women's Health Conference and Allen's Black and Female workshop gave Ward's life a new purpose, one that linked the devastating history of Black Americans with a path toward psychic and physical healing. As she felt the grief of all the women around her, she became one of the many women who decided, "I want to be part of whatever this is."[7]

Ward was one of the roughly 1,700 mostly Black women who attended the first national Black Women's Health Conference at Spelman College in June 1983.[8] This conference, sponsored by the Black Women's Health Project of the National Women's Health Network, marked a milestone in the history of the women's health movement, a moment when Black women—gay and straight, rich and poor, urban and rural—came together to focus on their specific health needs. Organizing under the civil rights activist Fannie Lou Hamer's famous declaration, they were "sick and tired of being sick and tired." Their presence at the conference testified to their intention to heal their physical and mental wounds in the presence of other Black women. In the cradle of each other's arms, Black women would share their collective grief as a step toward health and healing.

Well before the conference, Black women and other women of color influenced the shape of the larger feminist health movement. They joined self-help groups, founded and directed feminist health clinics, denounced reproductive oppression, and demanded an end to homophobic health care.[9] In the early 1980s, however, Black women increasingly organized collectively and nationally around issues concerning their physical, mental, and emotional health.[10] The Black Women's Health Conference, a watershed moment in what became the Black women's health movement, built upon Black women's health organizing and inspired further activism.

This chapter focuses on the efforts of Black women, especially those engaged in self-help, to define and nurture Black women's health. It argues that the Black women's health movement emerged from the larger feminist health movement and extended it to new audiences. These groups differed in their approaches and their goals, but they each created space for Black women to support each other within a culture that demeaned and disregarded them.

This history of Black women's health activism begins with the story of Byllye Avery and her work with the women's health movement in Florida and her leadership in promoting a movement focused on Black women's health. It then explores the history of two self-help groups, one directly influenced by the Black Women's Health Conference and the national organization it sparked, the other an organization more directly influenced by cervical self-exam and feminist self-help practices. Focusing on self-help practices demonstrates the importance of gynecological self-help and cervical self-exam for some Black health activists, but it also highlights how Black women reframed and expanded self-help, deploying it as a form of psychological counseling and emotional healing that recalled a long history of women's self-help projects in the Black community.

A Clinic in Gainesville: Byllye Avery and the Creation of a Health Activist

The story of the National Black Women's Health Project began in Gainesville, Florida, where Byllye Avery and her new husband, Wesley, settled after they graduated from the historically Black Talladega College in Alabama in 1959 and married in 1960. Soon after their marriage, Avery became unexpectedly

pregnant with their first child. Even though the couple tried to prevent another pregnancy, a second child arrived in 1966.[11] As a mother of two small
children, Avery returned to school at the University of Florida, earning a master's degree in special education in 1969. Her training led to a job in the children's mental health unit of the University of Florida's hospital. A few months
later, Wesley suffered a fatal heart attack. He was thirty-three years old.[12]

Wesley's death changed the trajectory of Avery's life. The tragedy taught
her that many people, especially Black people, didn't understand their health
risks; only after Wesley's death did Avery understand that his hypertension
was life-threatening. Knowledge could save lives, she realized. Accurate
knowledge could have also prevented her unplanned pregnancies. These revelations planted the seeds of health activism.[13]

Wesley's death also planted the seeds of feminism. During their marriage, Wesley had occasionally suggested that Avery read Betty Friedan's *The
Feminine Mystique* (1963). Overwhelmed by her multiple roles, Avery refused.
When she finally read the feminist classic after Wesley's death, Avery immediately recognized her unappreciated work caring for her family and her
simmering resentment as part of the "problem that has no name." As Avery recounted, *The Feminine Mystique* "really opened my eyes, and I could
not close them again." Hungry for more feminist ideas, Avery and her white
friends and colleagues Judith Levy and Margaret Parrish threw themselves
into a study of feminism.[14]

They were not alone. Gainesville, a college town of about sixty-five thousand with a significant Black population, already had a reputation for civil
rights organizing and feminism. In 1968, Beverly Jones and Judith Brown
published a pamphlet, *Toward a Female Liberation Movement*, an early articulation of second-wave feminism. Jones, the wife of a University of Florida
professor, and Brown, a law student, had both been active in the civil rights
movement in Gainesville. But like Casey Hayden and Mary King before them,
Jones and Brown protested the sexism that characterized their experiences
in the movement. This pamphlet, shared widely among women's liberation
networks, put Gainesville on the feminist map. With the help of activists from
New York City, Jones and Brown founded the Gainesville Women's Liberation
shortly thereafter, anchoring a network of local feminist organizations and
institutions.[15]

A request at work added to Avery's emerging activist consciousness. Her
boss at the hospital asked Avery, Parrish, and Levy to present an overview
of reproductive health activism. Avery protested that she knew little about
birth control and even less about abortion, but she and her colleagues gained
expertise through their research. After their presentation, Avery and her col-

leagues became community resources for women seeking abortions, eventually working with the Clergy Consultation Service to help women secure abortions in New York City. When a Black woman could not afford the trip to New York and subsequently died of a self-induced abortion, Avery began considering how reproductive health issues affected Black women and white women differently.[16]

Avery's interest in women's health politics intensified when Carol Downer and Lorraine Rothman came to Gainesville promoting self-help. On one of their cross-country tours, Downer and Rothman sought to organize women around reproductive health and to recruit them into self-help activism. As part of their presentation, the Los Angeles women demonstrated self-exam. Avery remembered the moment she saw her cervix as a profound experience. As she described it in 2005, "This is one of the things you will remember where you were. You will remember when you did it. It was of that importance."[17]

After the *Roe* decision in 1973, Avery, Parrish, and Levy, joined by another white activist, Joan Edelson, resolved to enact their commitment to feminism, reproductive equity, and health education by founding an abortion clinic in Gainesville. Protests by the Alachua County Medical Society had blocked an earlier attempt by Planned Parenthood, so they approached their goal quietly. They rented a building, hired a medical director, and acquired the necessary medical equipment all without alerting the Gainesville medical community. When the Gainesville Women's Health Center (GWHC) opened in May 1974, the medical society was caught off guard, and it apparently declined to protest.[18]

The women of the GWHC, like most feminist health activists, promoted health education as a tool for women's empowerment. Avery's experiences with medical ignorance fueled her commitment to education: "We taught the women everything in the world they wanted to know or didn't want to know about their bodies. We were not passing up this opportunity to educate. We did wonderful education. We took care of them exquisitely."[19]

Abortion provision, however, rather than health education, led her to focus on Black women's needs. Before Avery and her colleagues opened the GWHC, she hadn't realized the extent of Black women's demand for abortion. Although her activism had been sparked by the abortion-related death of a Black woman, Avery didn't "really think that many black women got abortions." At the clinic, however, Black women composed more than 50 percent of the abortion clients while composing only 20 percent of the general population. These statistics gave Avery a new perspective on Black women's repro-

ductive health needs. She and her colleagues tried to attract Black women to
the GWHC's well-woman gynecology services by reaching out through Black
churches and other community institutions, but the gynecology clinic never
attracted many Black clients. Black women's intense need for access to abortion and their simultaneous disinclination to seek other reproductive health
services or educational programming stuck with Avery, but she was not able
to change the situation in Gainesville.[20]

After the GWHC became established, white women in the community
approached the founders looking for support for a birthing center staffed by
midwives. The women of the center eagerly took on this new challenge, but
as they began planning, personal rifts within the center eventually forced a
break. Avery, Levy, and Parrish left the GWHC and took their plans for the
Birthplace with them. It opened in November 1978, and by the end of 1979,
thirty or so babies had been born through the Birthplace. By 1980, the Birthplace had reached its capacity; to meet the demand, they needed to hire a
second midwife. Not interested in midwifery as a career and eager to find
work serving the Black community, Avery left the Birthplace for a job with
Santa Fe College in Gainesville, working to identify and address the needs of
its Black female students.[21]

Connecting to a National Movement

Avery's work with the GWHC and the Birthplace brought her into the larger
women's health movement. Initially, she and the other women from the
GWHC were particularly connected to feminist self-help activists, perhaps
influenced by their earlier visit with Downer and Rothman. Women from
the GWHC, for example, explored the larger self-help gynecology movement
by attending the Women-Controlled Women's Health Centers Conference in
November 1974 in Ames, Iowa. There they met women from several Feminist Women's Health Centers as well as other feminist health clinics founded
on a self-help model, including the Santa Cruz Women's Health Center, the
Emma Goldman Clinic for Women in Iowa City, and the Elizabeth Blackwell
Clinic in Minnesota.[22] The GWHC women became especially friendly with
the women from the FWHC down the road in Tallahassee, but the Gainesville
women considered themselves less "hard-nosed feminists" than the women
of the FWHCs, and they created a clinic that reflected their own approach to
feminism and women's health. They rejected menstrual extraction, for example, and strove to teach women how embrace menstruation, or at least
make its physical effects less onerous.[23] In 1975, Avery and four other women

from the GWHC attended the first national conference on women and health in Boston; there she came to understand her efforts in Gainesville within a larger women's health context.[24]

National feminist health conferences expanded Avery's vision for women's health and challenged many of her long-held beliefs. They also increased her visibility as an African American leader of the women's health movement. In the aftermath of the 1975 Boston conference, and likely as a result of it, Avery became part of the board of the National Women's Health Network (NWHN), an organization founded by white women in 1975 as the "policy arm" of the women's health movement. On the board, Avery joined other women of color, including Pamela Freeman, Dolores Huerta, and Helen Rodríguez Trías. The NWHN provided the context and support for Avery's next project.[25]

By 1980, Avery noticed that the NWHN had failed to address the particular health needs of Black women.[26] Her work with young Black women at Santa Fe College introduced her to the everyday hardships they faced. She vowed to devote the next stage of her activist career to Black women's health needs. This path returned Avery to issues that had bothered her for years: the frequency of illness in her own extended family, Black women's high rates of abortion and low usage of well-woman care at the GWHC, and the struggles of young Black women caught between the demands of school and their families. A focus on Black women's health would let her explore and address these concerns full on. Financially and institutionally supported by the NWHN and assisted by board director Belita Cowan, Avery launched the Black Women's Health Project in 1980.[27]

The timing of Avery's decision to create a Black women's health organization was not coincidental. Black women had been building a feminist movement for at least a decade, and health care and reproductive rights were two areas of significant grassroots organizing.[28] It was not until 1982, however, that the Black feminist Barbara Smith noted in her edited collection *Home Girls* that "we have a movement of our own." In fact, Avery's work was part of a "groundswell," to borrow Stephanie Gilmore's phrase, of Black feminist activism in the early 1980s.[29]

Before she could launch an organization for Black women, Avery understood that she needed to expand her professional and personal networks. For most of her professional and political life, Avery had worked primarily with white women, reading *The Feminine Mystique* at Judy Levin's kitchen table, founding the GWHC and the Birthplace. She understood that she needed to build connections with more Black women, so she repeatedly asked the white women in her circles, "Do you know any black women I can meet?"[30]

Finding a Partner: Lillie Allen and "Black and Female"

It was through a white woman on the board of the NWHN that Avery met Lillie Allen.[31] Allen, the daughter of migrant farmworkers, attended college at Bethune-Cookman College, majoring in health and physical education. At this historically Black college, Allen experienced the effects of the skin color-based hierarchy, feeling ostracized because of her dark skin from the very community "I thought was mine."[32] After graduation, she developed her interests in health education further, earning her master's degree in public health from the University of North Carolina at Chapel Hill in 1974.[33]

Allen was a health educator in the Departments of Family Medicine and Community Health at Morehouse School of Medicine when she met Avery. Since her graduation, she had worked variously as a genetic advisor, a sickle cell anemia outreach consultant, and a teenage pregnancy prevention counselor. Her pregnancy prevention work with teenagers convinced Allen that people did not change their behaviors through narrowly targeted campaigns; people changed their behavior only if they could envision a better life, believe they could attain it, and connect changed behaviors (e.g., contraceptive use or healthy eating) to their chances of success.[34] In order to improve their health and their lives, people needed to believe that they deserved better and that they could effect change.

Allen's personal experiences of oppression and her professional work in health education illuminated the serious physical and psychic harms Black women experienced, and they sparked her lifelong efforts to identify and ameliorate Black women's pain. She wanted to heal Black women's wounds, encourage their connections to each other, and empower them to fight for social change and racial justice. In an attempt to heal her own wounds, Allen became involved in reevaluation counseling (RC), an experimental form of therapy developed in the 1950s. RC was founded on the belief that while humans were "naturally" happy creatures, they sometimes experienced pain—physical or emotional—that compromised their ability to respond appropriately to life's demands. Pain led to compulsive behaviors, paralyzing self-doubt, and bad decisions that reinforced deleterious patterns of thought and action. According to RC's founder and champion, Harvey Jackins, "hurt" people required a psychic reset through a "discharge" of negative emotions. Sobbing, trembling, and shouting were among the physical signs of psychic discharge. Jackson insisted that while discharge required the support of others, observers could not console or soothe. He believed that the process needed to culminate, thereby allowing the person to shed their negative pathways and forge responses more appropriate to life's experiences.[35]

As people on the political Left adopted RC in the 1960s and '70s as a therapeutic practice of self-improvement, oppression became a central theoretical
concern of the method. Because oppression—acting through "classist, sexist
and racist institutions"—inflicted constant pain, RC leaders came to believe
that they must encourage "movements to change society."[36] This reformed
version of RC coupled healing introspection and release with a commitment
to political liberation.

RC appealed to Allen because it was affordable, accessible, and committed to liberation. Still, as she noticed that she was frequently the only Black
person in the room, she became skeptical of RC's commitment to Black liberation.[37] She realized that few RC advocates enacted their anti-oppression
commitments, and she concluded that RC had failed to offer a clear pathway
for social action after "discharge." How were people supposed to build a more
healthful and just community? she wondered. How could they effect social
change?

Black and Female, a self-disclosure and healing process grounded in her
own struggles, was Allen's intervention. Black and Female aimed to heal
Black women's personal wounds inflicted by oppression, develop supportive
ties with other Black women, and empower them to become activists. She
argued that a racist and sexist society had convinced Black women that their
desires and needs did not matter. This "internalized oppression" shaped how
they saw themselves and each other and left them feeling powerless to change
their situation. According to the historian Evan Hart, Allen recognized that
Black women needed skills to enable them to "work outside their oppression
to become empowered individuals."[38]

Allen linked Black women's health to community, arguing that their healing required support from other Black women. She believed that internalized
racism led Black women to blame themselves and other Black women for
conditions and circumstances caused by anti-Black racism.[39] As the activist
Beverly Smith put it, "It's real hard when you are a member of a group that
is so despised. When you look at another Black woman you see all this re-
viled stuff—you see all the stuff you embody and have been told is bad about
you."[40] By gathering in community, by sharing their vulnerability and their
pain, Black women could reject society's lies and together build pathways to
wellness.

Allen argued that Black women's alienation from each other supported a
"conspiracy of silence" about their traumas and struggles. She joined Avery
and other Black feminists who insisted that silence trapped women within
their circumstances because it concealed possible alternatives and it strengthened stigma and shame.[41] Black and Female, which Allen referred to as "Self-

Help," provided Black women an opportunity to shed their distrust of each other and share the secrets that kept them isolated and stuck. It gave Black women a process to share their struggles, confront and reject their false beliefs about other Black women, and gain the confidence to transform their lives and improve their communities.[42]

Avery and Allen shared the goal of improving the mental and physical health of Black women. Although their pathways to self-help differed, Avery believed that she and Allen both sought to empower Black women through mutual exploration, shared vulnerability, and emotional support. She invited Allen to join the team she was creating to plan a conference focused on Black women's health as the launching event of a larger project devoted to Black women. Allen agreed. The exact vision for the eventual project was still unclear, but self-help emerged as a foundational process.[43]

In advance of the Black Women's Health Conference, scheduled for June 1983, Allen worked to bring her ideas for Black women's self-help across the country. The BWHP-sponsored efforts shared with gynecological self-help the belief that self-help empowered women, giving them knowledge and confidence to care for their own basic health needs and to translate their needs and concerns to health professionals when necessary. But as envisioned by the BWHP, self-help also encouraged women to become the "primary health resource" for their families and communities.[44]

In the months immediately before the conference, the BWHP recognized twenty-six different local self-help groups working under the BWHP banner.[45] Their goals and activities varied widely. From the perspective of the BWHP, these groups aimed "to raise the consciousness of women about the severity and pervasiveness of Black women's health problems; to provide a comfortable, supportive atmosphere for women to explore health issues affecting them and their families;" and to create awareness of and encourage connection with the BWHP. Within these parameters, local self-help groups determined their own focus and direction.[46] The first self-help group officially aligned with the BWHP began in Monteocha–Gordon, Florida, a rural community just outside the city limits of Gainesville. It started in September 1981, with an effort to decrease hypertension among the group. The group met weekly to exercise.[47] Others focused on attracting "senior citizens" to the movement while still others organized "disadvantaged youth." In these early years, self-help groups also sought to recruit Black women to the Spelman conference.[48]

Cervical self-exam did not play a significant role in most of the Black women's self-help organizing. Still, some Black self-help groups did experiment with gynecological self-help as part of their work. A Chicago group, for example, focused on "learning gynecological self-help skills." This group also encouraged discussion of abortion and "consciousness raising," topics that proved contentious in many Black women's groups. But the gynecological approach was not limited to big cities with histories of feminist activism. The self-help group in Ideal, Georgia, a community of barely more than six hundred people, hosted a women's health weekend that included presentations on birth control and childbirth and demonstrations of gynecological self-help and self-breast exams.[49]

The Black Women's Health Conference: A Movement Launched

Avery, Allen, and other organizers understood the first-ever conference devoted to Black women's health concerns as the launching point for a national movement. They had seeded self-help groups across the country to provide foundational models for the promise of Black women's health activism and to create an appetite for health activists to join a national movement in Atlanta. The conference planners took time and care to create an event that was both culminating and foundational. Committed to attracting Black women from all backgrounds and circumstances, organizers encouraged local and national fundraising to help low-income women attend. Nearly 25 percent of the attendees received some sort of financial support to make the trip possible.[50]

The conference succeeded beyond the organizers' expectations, attracting between seventeen hundred and two thousand participants, representing a cross section of Black womanhood. They came in packed vans, on planes, in cars. Daughters brought their mothers. Aunts brought their nieces.[51] According to one account, the conference attracted old and young women alike, "women in uniforms, [M]uslims, lesbians, political activists, women with straight hair, afros, and dread locks, women from all walks of life."[52] According to Avery, "They came with PhDs, MDs, welfare cards, in Mercedes and on crutches, from seven days old to 80 years old—urban, rural, gay, straight."[53] She believed that the conference likely provided the first opportunity for such diverse Black women to "sit down and talk to each other."[54]

Many women were inspired by the conference. Janice Route Blaylock, a nurse with three children, for example, felt "totally energized by the wonder of the conference." In its aftermath, she remembered the conference as "a catalyst for change in my life. It was the starting point for my on-going personal empowerment." Dázon Dixon Diallo had been a student at Spelman when the conference came to campus. She ditched her job to "hang out with this incredible movement of women." The conference sparked a need for her to be more engaged in her community. In early 1984, this spark led her to the

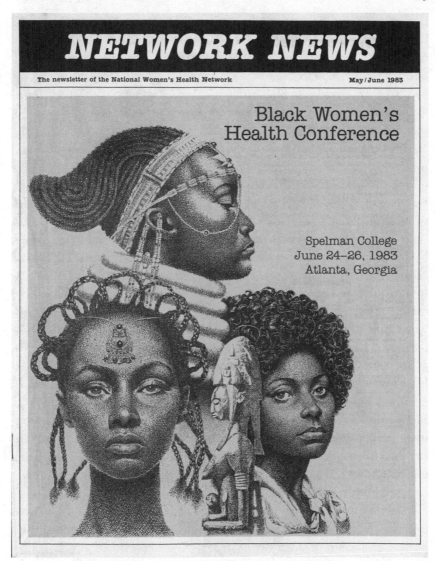

NETWORK NEWS

The newsletter of the National Women's Health Network   May/June 1983

Black Women's Health Conference

Spelman College
June 24–26, 1983
Atlanta, Georgia

FIGURE 7.1. Publicity for the Black Women's Health Conference highlighted Black women's diversity and their common roots in Africa.

Atlanta FWHC, where she worked as a lay health worker for almost six years. She left to found SisterLove Women's AIDS Project in July 1989, an Atlanta organization devoted to HIV education, prevention, advocacy, and research.[55]

According to the participants, much of the conference's power came from the sheer number of Black women in one space. For most of the women, it was the first time that they were in the presence of so many Black women.[56] The size of the conference allowed for women to see themselves reflected in the

230   CHAPTER 7

faces of hundreds of others and meet other Black women. Sharon Gary-Smith traveled to the conference from Seattle, where she directed a community-based health center. She approached the conference with apprehension, "wary of Black women, and the South." She admitted that before the conference, she had "seldom worked with Black women."[57] For Gary-Smith and others, learning about and from other Black women proved the most powerful lesson of the conference.[58]

The program was as diverse as the participants. It highlighted topics common to feminist health conferences, including birth control, sexually transmitted diseases, childbirth, sexuality, mental illness, and domestic abuse. But the program also highlighted issues that resonated strongly with Black women, including workplace hazards, environmental contaminants, conditions for incarcerated women, infant mortality, and lupus. Under the banner of "self-help demonstrations," women could be tested for diabetes and sickle cell disease, learn tips for weight control and smoking cessation, and hear how to measure blood pressure at home. These sessions described how race and racism affected health, offered community strategies for wellness, and provided tools for individuals to improve their health. Gynecological self-help— the core of some feminist self-help practices—barely appeared on the program, being limited to a two-hour demonstration by an activist from the Atlanta FWHC and another from a Black women's self-help group in Chicago.[59]

Despite the variety and relevance of the many panels, Allen's workshop, Black and Female: What Is the Reality?, provided an experience widely remembered as the central moment of the conference. The conference planners had themselves participated in the workshop and were eager to make it available.[60] Not all conference attendees were welcome; Black and Female was reserved for Black women.[61]

Allen began Black and Female by asking the women in attendance what it "really" felt like to be a Black woman. The question hit a nerve. Many audience members responded to this deceptively simple question with tears;[62] in some accounts of this moment, the audience howled and sobbed as they admitted their own experiences of pain.[63] Crucially, they also recognized the pain of other Black women.

Word of the power and significance of this workshop spread. Attendees demanded more access to the workshop, and conference organizers added extra sessions, each subsequent version in a room larger than the last. The activist Loretta Ross described five hundred women squeezing into one room, sitting on the floor, lining the walls, and listening from the hallway through an open door as a "movement moment."[64] Organizers estimated that roughly 1,500 women at the conference attended the Black and Female workshops. In the aftermath, some of them were moved to build space in their own communities for Black women to share their pain and support each other's healing.[65]

The conference highlighted the hunger for a health movement focused on the needs of Black women, and many participants eagerly pledged to organize with women in their communities. But they also encouraged Avery to launch a national organization. Although the conference had been organized as a project of the NWHN, attendees at the conference demanded that the BWHP develop independently. Avery, despite the objections of some members of the NWHN, acquiesced, and the newly independent organization emerged under Avery's directorship in partnership with Allen, incorporating as the *National Black Women's Health Project* (NBWHP) in March 1984.[66]

"Black and Female" remained the name for workshops and training led by Allen; the groups inspired by Black and Female were known as "Self-Help Groups." According to Allen, Black and Female and the Self-Help Groups it sparked provided the "vehicle that kept women together and moving" after the conference while Avery developed the structure and the funding for the national organization.[67] Self-help groups, already seeded across the country before the conference, multiplied in the aftermath, providing the "primary focus" of the NBWHP, bringing Black women across the country into a movement centered on their healing and wellness.[68] Black and Female Self-Help provided a process for Black women's empowerment and healing: clear-eyed introspection, unguarded truth-telling, shared vulnerability, and unconditional support. In April 1984, the NBWHP hired Sharon Gary-Smith as the director of National Self-Help Programs, and she and Allen led trainings for women who hoped to facilitate groups in their own communities. According to Gary-Smith, these groups provided the "glue" that brought women together to improve the health of their communities, families, and themselves.[69] As she described it, the groups aimed to "provide a safe, validating environment . . . to come together to share [our] stories; to be appreciated for the struggles we have all participated in; to review our circumstances; and to make decisions designed to change our lives and our health status." Self-Help, then, was not only a vehicle for Black women to share their struggles—it aimed to empower Black women to change their lives.[70]

In time, the NBWHP developed a manual to clarify the process and goals of Self-Help.[71] The guide described Self-Help as a "strategy for Black women" to pursue wellness by addressing "emotional, spiritual, mental and physical health concerns . . . [and by] helping each other make healthy decisions." It attributed disproportionate rates of illness, especially stress-related illness in Black women, to "the persistent distress" caused by pervasive "racism, sexism, classism and heterosexism" that surrounded them and limited their ability to "exercise control" over their lives. According to the guide, Self-Help Groups aimed to reveal how oppression, stress, and illness converged in the lives of Black women:

> Our commitment to our health includes a commitment to understanding the umbrella of oppression that hovers over us. . . . By better understanding the ways in which these interlocking oppressions affect our health status, we can look at our wellness within the broader social/political/economic context that is our reality. In this way, our efforts to promote our health are clearly political in nature as we take control of our lives and support each other to do the same.[72]

This manual highlighted how Black women's health problems were rooted in oppression rather than the failings of individual women to exercise, "eat right," or access care. Nevertheless, it argued that Self-Help provided a political solution by developing a "conscious activist network" of Black women, empowered, knowledgeable, and committed to individual and community wellness. As activist Ross put it, "The whole process of Self-Help was supposed to lead to social justice work, that you get rid of this baggage, this remembered pain, so that you can free up your mind, your body, your soul, your spirit to do more work and service to your community."[73]

Self-help energized a movement focused on Black women's health. Black women across the country—sometimes in affiliation with the NBWHP and sometimes not—created self-help groups to address their emotional and physical health. While the Black and Female approach was the foundation for NBWHP-sponsored Self-Help, it did not appeal to everyone, especially not in the long term. Indeed, its detractors saw it as a cult.[74] Instead, Black women across the country tailored their self-help methods to meet their own needs. Some of these groups focused on various health education topics, while other groups gathered to promote exercise, healthy eating, or smoking cessation.

Self-Help as envisioned by Allen and the larger NBWHP connected Black women with a long tradition of community response to systemic racism and the egregious health conditions for Black Americans it created. In the presence of state neglect, African American communities frequently organized to establish institutions, organizations, and campaigns to promote health services, increase health access, and disseminate health education. As the historian Susan L. Smith argued in her pathbreaking work, *Sick and Tired of Being Sick and Tired* (1995), women provided much of the grassroots organizing and service provision of these projects throughout the long first half of the twentieth century: "Black women's organizing efforts at the community level sustained a black health movement that targeted health improvement as a means to racial advancement. . . . The cumulative effect of health activism in thousands of rural and urban communities across the country was the creation of a mass movement that turned to the health arena to keep alive the black struggle for equality."[75]

The Black women's self-help movement of the 1980s differed from previous efforts by Black women focused on improving the health of their communities, in that the self-help movement encouraged Black women to put themselves first. The conference coordinator Eleanor Hinton-Hoytt insisted that the conference aimed to "help Black women learn to take care of their bodies and to take charge of their lives."[76] Nevertheless, Black women's obligations to their community remained at play. Self-Help Groups ultimately sought to create a "ripple-effect" that began with individual Black women and eventually empowered them to "address key health problems in [their] communities."[77]

Organizational Transformation

By 1989, the NBWHP had reached a crossroads. At the grassroots level, the organization seemed to thrive. Black women launched self-help groups across the country and local affiliates of the NBWHP in at least twenty-two states.[78] Gary-Smith claimed that there were "more than four hundred emerging, seventy-four developing, and twelve established self-help groups."[79] These groups gained inspiration from the national organization, but they remained largely administratively and economically separate.[80] This independence allowed local groups to shape their programs to meet local needs, but it also left them frequently scrambling for funding. At the same time, Avery led the NBWHP's national programming from the headquarters in Atlanta. Although she had envisioned a decentralized national organization that worked through linked chapters, in the end, the organization primarily worked through the Atlanta office.[81]

By the end of 1989, the NBWHP was in trouble, plagued by financial problems, organizational weakness, divergent visions, and interpersonal strife. Avery won the prestigious MacArthur "genius grant" in 1989 for her work with the NBWHP, and it brought her a new level of attention that distracted her from her administrative duties. Her managerial skills, never her strong suit, became increasingly problematic. She and the board agreed to hire an executive director while she assumed the role of the founding president.[82] This distanced her from the day-to-day management of the NBWHP. At roughly the same time, in the wake of some contentious discussions about the role of self-help—both as a tool to build trust and support within the organization's leadership and as a process for building a grassroots Black women's health movement—Allen left the organization to found Be Present, Inc., a self-help training center.[83] Financial hardship, leadership loss, and personal conflict left NBWHP without a clear mission; in 1990, the staff and the board decided that self-help was "no longer central to [the] NBWHP's mission."[84] Instead, it focused its energy on shaping public policy rather than personal empowerment. To this end, the organization opened an office in Washington, DC, devoted to policy initiatives. According to historian Hart, the establishment of the public policy office "signaled the slow collapse of the Project's grassroots programs."[85] For Avery, the NBWHP's abandonment of self-help led to the dissolution of the organization she had built and nurtured. In an interview with Hart, she noted, "I felt the organization was the Self-Help part." Without self-help, she insisted, "the magic was not there." The name change to the Black Women's Health Imperative in 2001 only punctuated the critical shift that had taken place nearly a decade earlier.[86]

The National Black Women's Health Project was the foremost Black women's health organization of the 1980s. It brought publicity to the urgent health needs of Black women and a process to heal their wounds and organize their outrage. Two different models of self-help then provided the bedrock of the NBWHP's approach to improved health in the Black community. Byllye Avery, coming up through the women's health movement, never lost her appreciation for self-exam as the foundation for women's empowerment even as she understood the power of Black and Female. Indeed, in some ways she came to appreciate an embodied version of self-help more through the years. Although she once rejected menstrual extraction as too radical, by 1991 she had recommitted to self-exam and reconsidered menstrual extraction. Concerned that the reproductive policies of the oppressive Right disproportionately threatened the reproductive autonomy of Black women, she urged a return to gynecological self-help methods. As Avery put it:

> We must start training our sisters in gynecological self-help, so they will be able to maintain their health and teach self-care to their families. Women must learn to perform safe, mentrual [sic] extraction, catch babies, and provide general well-woman care. Looking at one's cervix is indeed a revolutionary and empowering action. It provides insight and powerful knowledge of what is at the other end of the speculum.[87]

In 1992, the NBWHP validated this approach to self-help by producing *It's OK to Peek*, a video promoting the value of gynecological self-exam.[88] Allen, by contrast, offered a vision of self-help that focused less on the physical body, looking to heal instead Black women's psychic wounds. She insisted that by bearing witness to each other's pain, common to all Black women and yet unique to each person, Black women would eventually be agents for social change in their communities. Both Avery and Allen sought to increase Black women's empowerment by insisting that they could look deep inside themselves and share what they found with other Black women. Working together, Black women could be for each other a buttress against the onslaughts of their racist and sexist society.

Bay Area Black Women's Health Project

In the early and mid-1980s, groups of Black women across the country came together to share their secrets, heal their pain, and secure their health. For some of these women, the model of Self-Help Groups promoted by Allen and the NBWHP provided an invaluable link to other Black women and a lifeline in the midst of personal despair. The Bay Area Black Women's Health Project provides a glimpse into the power and joy self-help afforded some women.

When Felicia Ward returned to the Bay Area from Spelman, she connected with the Bay Area Black Women's Health Project (BABWHP), a group that predated the conference. These women, including Sholey Malawa, Tandy Iles, and Zakiya Somburu, did not share a unified vision for the group.[89] Some wanted a storefront, providing communal space and informational materials, while others wanted to influence health policy. Ward just wanted to help Black women "not be crazy."[90] She hoped to replicate the power and the potential she had felt in Atlanta. After consulting with Allen, Ward sought out RC training and created Woman Rise, to develop Self-Help Groups among Black women. She launched her own Black and Female workshop, attended by about thirty women, to create interest in the process. The goal of Woman Rise in its earliest incarnation was simple. It provided a forum for Black women to come together, share their stories, and break the silence. Ward organized several Black and Female retreats and facilitated many Self-Help Groups under the auspices of the BABWHP.[91]

The BABWP has left only a thin paper trail, and some of the women involved have died (Somburu) or declined to contribute to this history (Iles and Malawa). Consequently, this portrait is based on an interview of a group of women who gathered in September 2017 to share their experiences with self-help as conceived by Allen and facilitated by Ward. A few published testimonies supplement the accounts from the group interview. Their stories illuminate the power of self-help to connect Black and racially "mixed" women together and to fortify themselves against the assaults of racism and oppression. As the stories of these women illustrate, these groups could be life changing.

When building her first Self-Help Group, Ward reached out to Carol Granison, a woman she knew from her Oakland ashram. Granison, a member of the Black Panther Party and a satisfied graduate from EST, believed in both social change and self-improvement. Although they did not know each other well, Granison had donated to fund Ward's trip to the Black Women's Health Conference at Spelman. "This is all I have," she thought as she handed Ward seven dollars. "You got to go to whatever this thing is." Ward, upon her return to Oakland, shared her newfound sense of purpose with Granison and asked her to join her new group, Women Rise. Granison eagerly agreed.[92]

Before Ward received formal training from Allen, the women improvised. At one point they sat naked together, to share their vulnerability and challenge their shame and sense of propriety. They did not, however, search for their cervices—"no, we did not!" They built up relationships of trust, allowing, for example, Granison to cry over her mother's death thirty years earlier, for the first time.[93]

Ward also facilitated groups for young women like Mandolin Kadera-Redmond, who joined a group when she was about eleven. Her mother was white and her father was Black, and she identified as mixed. Although her parents met in Oakland, they had started their family in Minnesota, her mother's home state. Her parents returned to Oakland in 1985, bringing their four children with them. At this point, addiction and family violence created significant instability within the family, and they moved repeatedly. According to Kadera-Redmond, they were "basically homeless."[94]

In search of stability, Kadera-Redmond and some friends, many of whom were also "mixed," began visiting the Bay Area Black and Female office in Oakland, where she met Ward. The friends knew that Ward ran groups for Black women, and they decided that they needed a group too. Ward was happy to oblige. The group of preteen and later teen girls met together once a month for several years. Kadera-Redmond was initially attracted to the group because it provided a refuge from her parents and her siblings. More specifically, it provided support as she tried to cope with the trauma and uncertainty around her: "I was just trying to be a good kid and go to school and take care of my siblings and hold it together and not freak out. And this gave us an opportunity to say all that and then talk about boys and talk about the things that were not okay at home. . . . [It was a place] to talk about what it was to be mixed and that your mom doesn't know how to do your hair, to talk about what it was to live in violence and to be hugged." This group provided an opportunity to share the vulnerability of her circumstances and gave her unconditional emotional support inside the maelstrom.[95]

When Kadera-Redmond was in ninth grade, her mother died, and her father's addiction left him unable to care for his family. She and her siblings returned to Minnesota, where she lived with her mother's white family. Grieving and cut off from her support networks, she and her sisters struggled. At a low point, a mother figure from Oakland reached out and invited her to a Sisters and Allies retreat in Minnesota. Sisters and Allies, a spin-off from Black and Female, facilitated Allen's self-help process in mixed-race groups. Kadera-Redmond attended, eager to build a new support system with already familiar tools. Through this retreat, Kadera-Redmond reconnected with the self-help process and joined new support groups that sustained her through high school until she left Minnesota for college in Oregon.[96]

A college degree, a marriage, a child, and a divorce later, Kadera-Redmond returned to Oakland in 2002 and "immediately" reached out to the women who had provided emotional support in her girlhood. "I connected back with this group . . . out of a pure place of conscious adult decision making," she said. ". . . I had family . . . other places, but I came here because I knew I'd be safe. I knew I'd have support. I knew I would be able to thrive." And she has thrived since her return to Oakland. She has credited her time with these self-help groups for giving her the skills to stay connected with her daughter through her teenage years, and to understand her sister's current struggle with mental illness: "I was trained. I know how to listen. I know how to just sit in uncomfortable things." These skills have allowed her to offer support and be supported in turn.[97]

Rita Shimmin, who we originally met when she worked at Lyon-Martin Women's Health Services, also participated in the BABWHP's Self-Help Groups. She became connected with the group when she was at a public library, where she researched the consequences of hysterectomies. There, she struck up a conversation with a woman who invited her to a self-help group. This group offered her support and encouraged her to attend a Black and Female retreat. The retreat was unlike anything she had ever experienced. As she described it, "I lost my mind. It was so fabulous." Shimmin likened the experience to being a biscuit rolling around in brown gravy: "It was just fabulous." After the retreat, Shimmin approached Ward and said, "I want help." What Shimmin appreciated most, what made these groups "life-changing," was the "experience of being allowed to be intense. It was really important to be held and to witness, to hold and be witnessed, and witness both, all that together."[98] Shimmin was committed enough in the process that after Allen

238   CHAPTER 7

left the NBWHP and founded Be Present, Inc., Shimmin joined her in this new organization.[99]

Gladys Fermon joined a BABWHP Self-Help Group after her father died. A longtime twelve-stepper, Fermon needed a different kind of emotional support to process her grief: "I needed to be held by a black woman, not in a sexual way but like a mother. I needed to be shown that I was lovable even when I was crying." In this group she found the support she craved. She found the people who would listen to her as she cried and witness her sorrow. The bonds of support and trust across difference were central to the power of this group. Fermon was attracted to the BABWHP because she wanted to join a group of Black women—"a community of my own kind"—but she discovered that these women interacted in ways unfamiliar to her. She marveled that they were "so at ease with one another, laughing, talking, and hugging." Fermon eventually decided to pay her experience forward. After local training, she, too, initiated and facilitated her own groups under the auspices of the BA-BWHP.[100] Fermon's account highlights that these groups were not meant to substitute for formal therapy or recovery. Instead, they provided a forum for Black women to support each other.

Fermon introduced Yvette Aldama to the BABWHP. The two had met at a twelve-step program after they had left residential recovery. They attended a Black and Female retreat together, and Aldama described it as "the first time that I had actually felt safe." For Aldama, the space was powerful because it required nothing specific from her. She said, "I could come into the space, and I could be quiet or sad or pissed or angry or not know and still be held in the room. . . . It's about being heard, but it's about me speaking me and telling my story. It's about me."[101]

At this retreat, Aldama met Ward and found a new calling. Aldama had sought treatment from crack addiction and engaged in professional and lay-led therapy, but she credits Ward and the self-help spaces she created with saving her life by creating a safe harbor. So inspired by the refuge self-help provided her, Aldama sought leadership training and developed groups for other Black women.[102]

As Aldama's story highlights, crack cocaine (and the policing and mass incarceration it resulted in) ravaged African American communities on the West Coast at roughly the same time that Self-Help Groups connected to the NBWHP were taking root. Although crack had been discovered in US cities in the early 1980s, it wasn't until the mid-1980s that it settled in. Oakland was one of the hardest-hit cities in the nation.[103] Granison pointed out that "nobody was untouched [by crack cocaine]. No community was untouched."[104] Nevertheless, these groups never organized around a particular issue like addiction or domestic violence. They came together to share their varied lives as Black women. Allen had envisioned a process where Black women would connect across their differences and through the pain inflicted by a sexist and racist society. The process focused on the wounds. According to Ward, "The wounds [were] the same," even if their immediate causes varied.[105]

Finally, Rachel L. Bagby, a recent Stanford Law School graduate, creative writer, and musician, sought connection in her life. At a friend's suggestion, she attended a Black and Female workshop, framed as a place for Black women to share their stories, heal their trauma, and grow stronger together. Bagby said of her experience, "We told one another the stories that we dared not tell anyone else, not even ourselves, not completely."[106] Allen, who facilitated this workshop, reiterated its philosophy, that systemic racism as well as personal trauma and shame sapped Black women's strength and health. Allen explained that by collectively holding "any sister's pain, any sister's anger, any sister's shame, any sister's story," both the hearer and the heard would be healed.[107] Bagby felt called to share her stories of shame and pain and trauma:

> We were encouraged to feel what we had buried deeply within us. We were encouraged to release, to talk, to express, to tell stories and feel feelings, to be heard and loved beyond all that we had suffered and in spite of and because of it, anyway. We were planting freedom in one another's ears. . . . Such a feeling I could not explain—to know that I was received by at least several sisters whose eyes said, we love you, as we love ourselves, *regardless*. . . . The hugging sistahs hugged. The rubbing sistahs rubbed. The tissues-bringing sistahs gave one another tissues. . . . Somehow, we meant it when we agreed that we were there to be honest and present with our feelings.[108]

These women testified to the importance of self-help in their lives and to the power of other Black women in their individual experiences of healing. Self-help forged bonds that nurtured resilience and hope. They did not connect through a shared search for a cervix, but like other versions of self-help, they saw the group as a place to escape the burden of their shame, share their pain and despair, rely on other women as resources, and create together a haven from personal and social storms.

Although many of the women involved in groups sponsored by the BABWHP may have identified as feminist, the groups themselves did not rely on or develop a feminist framework. Indeed, one of the participants believed that seeing this work through a feminist lens would "exclude her from the conversation." As she put it, she focused on "figuring out how to pay my rent and stay in a marriage." Feminism was "the last thing on my mind." And yet, from Ward's perspective, the work was feminist without the explicit label. "Why isn't everything we said feminism? Every single thing that was expressed, the way we went about our work was the work of what I understand feminism to be."[109] These groups gave Black women a place to unburden themselves, allowing them to shatter the conspiracy of silence around their lives. By providing safe harbor and fostering networks of support, the Self-Help Groups of the BABWHP empowered Black women.

Consistent with Allen's goal for Black and Female, Ward was committed to "social change" in addition to interpersonal support. Nevertheless, she did not "prod" the groups to take on activist projects. As she put it, "Effective collective empowerment . . . can only come when members feel empowered as individuals."[110] She noted that some Black women experienced generations of abuse that required significant time to heal before they can turn their focus outward. Nevertheless, she believed that by creating an environment for Black women to support other Black women, she strengthened Black communities. One story, one group at a time, Ward aimed to "empower people to . . . change what's going on in their lives."[111]

The BABWHP lasted about twelve years. It was always an organization with competing objectives, with some members focused on physical health projects while Ward developed and nurtured the Self-Help Groups. When the NBWHP abandoned its support for Self-Help Groups in favor of a policy-oriented focus, the Bay Area group incorporated independently to preserve the organization and its name. Ward never really saw the point, however. "I don't even believe in institutions," she admitted. She fervently believed that "wherever three shall gather in our name is a Black Women's Health Project group." Holding space for women to tell their stories required no money. In time, however, the group dissolved.[112] Ward felt devastated by the national group's abandonment of the grassroots groups, which she understood as women-led organizing: "I so wish they'd understood the power of what we were doing, not only here in the [B]ay [A]rea, but across the nation, within our homes, sitting in circles inside our living rooms, house by house, woman by woman, family by family. . . . We were preparing for something bigger than all of us. For one brief shining moment we had the chance to change the world entire."[113]

Black Women's Self-Help Collective

Although most Black women who joined self-help groups in the 1980s likely followed the model created by Allen and the NBWHP, others were inspired more directly by the larger women's health movement and especially the movement for gynecological self-help. Some of these women, like Avery herself, had joined self-help groups, worked at women's health clinics, and developed feminist health materials. But like Avery, other Black women created their own organizations where the needs of Black women came first, believing that they, like all women, would benefit from knowing their bodies.[114] One such group was the Black Women's Self-Help Collective of Washington, DC.[115]

In the 1970s, Washington, DC, a city with an African American majority population, inspired and nurtured a variety of initiatives focused on "social, political, and economic change." Organizations for racial justice, including the Black Panther Party and the Student Nonviolent Coordinating Committee, were active in the city, bringing men and women together to foster civil rights organizing and to empower Black communities.[116]

Feminists, both white and Black, also organized in Washington, sometimes together. The Washington, DC, Rape Crisis Center provides one example.[117] Still, according to the historian Anne M. Valk, because "few explicitly feminist organizations in Washington made black women feel welcome," feminist groups in the city "remained overwhelmingly white."[118] The radical lesbian group the Furies, for example, was exclusively white. Nevertheless, Black feminist groups did organize. A group of Black women founded a Washington branch of the National Black Feminist Organization in 1974 to address the specific oppressions experienced by Black women.[119] The Black Women's Self-Help Collective (BWSHC) was an explicitly feminist group created to meet the health needs of Black women.

The BWSHC was initially organized by a small group of college-educated, Black women who had originally known each other through their work in the African People's Socialist Party in Gainesville, Florida. Ajowa Ifateyo, Linda Leaks, and Faye Williams, all in their twenties, had each moved north separately, but their commitment to feminist politics and their determination to organize a Black women's feminist movement brought them back together in 1981. Although they each had their own particular political projects, they all worked to plan the first Take Back the Night rally in DC. There they met Mary Lisbon, a twentysomething activist who had recently left the National Alliance of Black Feminists in Chicago and was looking for new political projects.

Williams learned about self-exam while she was involved with the then white-majority Tallahassee FWHC in the late 1970s. In Tallahassee she allegedly refused to perform self-exam in a group as a condition of her employment, but she nevertheless believed that it held promise for Black women in other circumstances.[120] After arriving in DC, she introduced self-exam and self-help to her compatriots. They needed little convincing. Lisbon, for example, eagerly accepted Williams's offer to show Lisbon how to find her cervix. The moment changed Lisbon's life.

So, we couldn't see it at first, but when she opened the speculum, my uterus
came out right over the ribbon. It looked like the sunrise, and I just . . . thought
it was the most amazing thing I had seen in my whole life. . . . She was talking
about organizing black women around this and I was just like, "I'm in."[121]

The others were similarly convinced, and they agreed to share their zeal for
self-exam and the larger self-help movement with the larger community of
Black women in Washington, DC.

To launch the BWSHC, the group hosted a well-publicized "rap session"
on "Black women's sexuality" in March of 1982.[122] Flyers circulated at the
event identified the collective as

> a group of sisters who see the need for Black Women to grab ahold of the
> medical information denied us about our bodies, and to use that information
> to help ourselves—without the unnecessary anxiety and tension of not know-
> ing when things do go wrong, the unnecessary and outrageous expense of
> doctors and wasted precious time and energy waiting in doctor's offices and
> clinics. SELF-HELP IS POWER![123]

This framing of self-help echoed the FWHC's vision of the concept. But by
calling for a collective founded by and for Black women, the organizers acknowledged that Black women needed a forum that identified and centered
their health needs and developed bonds of trust and support between them.
The BWSHC aimed to provide space for Black women to "talk as freely and
uninhibited as possible" about their health and their "oppression as women
and why we are always in competition with each other." As they made their
case: "We believe it is absolutely necessary for black women to come together
to solve our problems and to bridge the gap that exists between us."[124]

The event attracted roughly eighty Black women. While most of them did
not participate in any further BWSHC activities, some became stalwart members of the collective. A group of about twelve women met regularly through
the spring and summer of 1982 to build an organization, grappling with the
goals and structure of the enterprise.[125]

From the beginning, it proved difficult to precisely define the mission of
the BWSHC. Many founders imagined it primarily as a skill-building and
information-sharing group focused on Black women's bodies and their
health. They saw the group as a response to the long-standing neglect and exploitation of Black women by medicine and other health care fields. But they
also saw the BWSHC as place of support for Black women, an organization
to foster "sisterhood" and "consciousness raising" among them.[126] The tension
between these different goals—focused on health and knowledge building on

the one hand, and support and political sisterhood on the other—ultimately
contributed to the group's undoing.

Promoting a Health-Centered Agenda

The founders of the BWSHC saw their organization as part of the larger
women's health movement, but they noted that the larger movement had
failed to influence "the day-to-day health care of Black women." BWSHC
members sought to provide "the catalyst that hopefully will get Black women
politically, socially, and emotionally involved in their health care." The group
acknowledged Black women's common struggle for reproductive rights,
understood broadly; but they insisted that Black women also needed to focus
on other vital health issues. In a publicity piece, Rosa Brunson framed the
BWSHC as both a support group and an incubator for social action. She
stressed that as a "Black women only" space, the BWSHC "provided a setting
where [sisters] can feel comfortable talking about their bodies, [and] sharing
their pain and fear." But the BWSHC also strove to encourage Black women
to be savvy health consumers, assuming responsibility for their health and
fighting to preserve their rights as medical patients.[127]

Some members wearied of the group's educational approach. By July 1982,
just four months after the group's creation, founder Faye Williams exhorted
her "sisters" to recommit to skill building and information sharing focused
on their bodies. She noted the various ways Black women carried disproportionate illness burdens—high rates of hypertension, low life expectancy, tremendous infant mortality—that demanded attention. "We all need to become
more educated about women's health. *We all need to get to know our bodies
and each other's.*" She argued that Black women owed it to themselves and to
each other "to better care for ourselves."[128]

Williams's plea found a receptive audience among the founding group and
a few new recruits. Others left. By the end of July, the members of the BWSHC
recommitted to become health educators for each other and the larger Black
community. The bimonthly meetings always included some kind of health
presentation on topics generated by the membership. These included vaginal
health, nutrition, sexuality, fibroids, menopause, hypertension, and "diseases
of black folks,"[129] among others. All members were expected to attend the
meeting having completed some assigned reading, and two members would
present further material and facilitate discussion. Whether the group should
focus so much of their effort on physical health, however, would prove a recurrent site of tension.

The BWSHC and Self-Exam

From the beginning, self-exam occupied a central place in the BWSHC's mission and its bimonthly meetings. Members believed that self-help empowered Black women, giving them symbolic access and actual knowledge about their bodies that would enable greater control over their lives. Lisbon regarded the moment when she saw her cervix for the first time as one of the "most empowering" moments of her life. It made her feel that "if we could take control of our bodies, we could take control of the world."[130] Ifateyo viewed self-exam as a check against the control of women through the submission of their bodies to medical surveillance. She also found self-exam especially important for Black women.

> Black women never really owned our own bodies. This was a way of owning our bodies. . . . In general, women don't have control over our bodies. But as black women, we have the added control of slavery and other things that made our bodies tools, economic tools, for the furtherance of capitalism. . . . And so to me, that speaks to the political aspect of the self-help. Self-help wasn't just gynecological, but it was also taking control of our health, our diabetes, our hypertension, the way we ate so that we can survive in America. America was killing us. If it wasn't through poverty . . . [it was through] dealing with racism all the time. All of this stuff was just really weighing on us. And so, self-exam was just one step, but it was also, how do we survive and thrive in this country, in a racist country?[131]

For Ifateyo and other BWSHC women, self-exam served as an important tool in Black women's struggle for survival and health. While they understood that self-exam was only one step in the empowerment of Black women, they considered it a necessary step.

As part of the project, the BWSHC took self-exam to a variety of settings, including prisons, social justice workshops, health fairs, and meetings held by Black women's groups. Lisbon described a presentation on sexuality delivered at a rehab center for substance abuse. At the beginning of the presentation, women from the BWSHC demonstrated self-exam. Many of the women in the audience initially recoiled, saying, "I'm not interested. I don't want to see that. No. No." But they looked anyway, and, according to Lisbon, the experience released something in them and allowed them to speak freely about their bodies and their sexuality. "They knew we had their back, that we would share something as intimate as that in a nonthreatening way that they could then speak up as well. . . . The women took over the discussion."[132] Lisbon and the others believed that a self-exam demonstration provided such an unexpected and total challenge to bodily shame and privacy that it cut through women's—especially Black women's—fears and defenses and invited them to share their secrets and concerns. By encouraging women to speak their truth, self-exam helped break the silence among Black women.

Cervical self-exam was also on the agenda for every meeting of the BWSHC. By October of 1982, however, some members of the group wondered why. They claimed that it felt rushed and repetitive, and some members believed its continual inclusion squeezed out other agenda items and the opportunities to "rap." Some members did not see the point of repeating the procedure, and others feared that new members would be shocked at the spectacle of self-exam had they not expected it. A few of the members were also uncomfortable with self-exam and always felt pressured to participate.[133] Moreover, some members argued that the focus on vaginal self-exam promoted a vision of self-help that was too narrow. Reflecting perhaps the earlier critique of the body-centered nature of the group, some members wondered why economic or emotional self-help failed to receive the same focused attention as vaginal self-exam.[134]

Proponents of the practice doggedly reiterated its benefits and insisted that its repetition was necessary for skill building, information sharing, and knowledge creation. They framed it as a step toward empowerment and bodily control. Despite the disagreements, the BWSHC continued to perform self-exam at their bimonthly meetings, except for a brief hiatus.

Some members of the BWSHC interpreted the discomfort with self-exam as a deflected response to the collective's focus on sexuality. From the initial meeting, the group had committed to breaking the silence around Black women's sexuality.[135] The members themselves proudly identified as heterosexual, lesbian, and bisexual, and they insisted that sexuality should unite Black women rather than divide them. They scheduled two presentations on sexuality, occupying two meetings in October 1982. Part one, likely focused on sexual anatomy, appears to have avoided controversy.[136] Part two, by contrast, included a discussion about "sexual roles of Black women," and culminated with a demonstration of masturbation to orgasm. The meeting minutes only hint at the schism this caused, but Lisbon and Ifateyo both remember the masturbation demonstration as a moment that fractured the group.[137]

In this telling, some members' discomfort with self-exam reached a tipping point when dictates of sexual propriety were so baldly transgressed. The shock of the masturbation demonstration caused the women of the BWSHC to reassess their mission, their understanding of self-help, and the value of self-exam, particularly as a regular part of their bimonthly meetings. Even as a health-centered self-help group, the BWSHC members struggled to reach consensus on their understanding of self-help and the value of self-exams.[138]

By insisting on the power of self-exam, the BWSHC differed from most other self-help health projects embraced by Black women. While some of the Self-Help Groups created by the National Black Women's Health Project included exposure to self-exam, none appeared to place it centrally on its agenda. It is perhaps not surprising that some Black women were shocked by self-exam. Other Black women's self-help groups emerging at the time, even those focused on health, tended to see health through a much wider lens. Indeed, many such groups, especially those developing out of the NBWHP, believed that Black women could not adequately address their physical health until they faced their emotional wounds caused by living under racial and sexual oppression. Self-help provided emotional support as a necessary first step to convincing women that they deserved better.

The BWSHC also differed from some of its self-help contemporaries by promoting a feminist—a Black feminist—agenda. Although the NBWHP identified as a feminist organization, not all the women involved, especially those involved in groups scattered across the country, identified as such. But for the BWSHC, feminism was central to the organization's value. Linda Leaks, one of its members and an antiviolence activist, made the case for the importance of feminism to Black women, insisting, "Feminism is the only existing ideology . . . that incorporates, in words and practices, the particular problems that black women face. The term feminism, itself, implies womanhood, and places primary importance on the liberation of women as the precondition to any other kind of liberation." For Leaks, a veteran of Black nationalist and socialist movements, Black women needed feminism to gain their own liberation; her Black nationalism did not preclude her feminism.[139]

Despite their differences from other Black women's self-help groups, the BWSHC eagerly connected to other health movement women. Several members of BWSHC attended the Black Women's Health Conference at Spelman in June 1983, joined by Loretta Ross and Nkenge Touré, colleagues of Leaks from the DC Rape Crisis Center.[140] They appreciated the "unity" Black women at the conference displayed, putting aside their differences to come together for a common cause. Despite their appreciation for the event, they decided not to affiliate with the larger organization.[141]

Purpose Lost and Found

In July 1983, Faye Williams, one of the founders and driving forces of the BWSHC, suffered a breakdown and returned to Gainesville to recover.[142] Wil-

liams had a clear vision for the group and a forceful personality. Her absence
gave other members of the BWSHC time and space to consider their own priorities. They committed the rest of the summer and fall of 1983 to rebuilding
the organization. They suspended their health presentations and self-exams
while they focused on the organization's purpose and structure.

A July 1983 brainstorming session, however, revealed how significantly the
members' vision for the organization diverged. Many members hoped the
BWSHC would increase its health activism, reaching out through newsletters, leaflets, and programming to a broader Black public. Others encouraged
members to train as lay health workers for the community, providing an array of services, including midwifery, mental health counseling, gynecological
exams, and reproductive health care. Some members wanted the BWSHC
to found a clinic. Alongside these outward-looking proposals, other members focused on the well-being of the members themselves. These members
wanted the BWSHC to serve as a support group, providing more time for
"rap sessions" and building love and support for the members.[143] Some of
these suggestions clearly spoke only to a few members, and other suggestions
seemed too ambitious for a small organization experiencing significant challenges. Still, the members believed that the group could eventually agree on a
mission that served most of the members' needs.

The question of whether the BWSHC should be a support group—perhaps
akin to the groups nurtured by Allen and the NBWHP or an activist group—
proved to be a perennial sticking point. In the fall of 1983, the membership
continued to wrestle with their mission and their goals. Although they easily
agreed to remain a collective of Black women, everything else about the group
seemed to be up for consideration.

After months of wrangling, in November the BWSHC approved a statement of purpose. The group recommitted to its identity as a lay health collective focused on improving the health of Black women through self-education
and skill building. The members also agreed to share health information with
others in the Black community. The group continued to feature self-exam
in its work as a tool for empowerment, self-discovery, and bodily control.
Their focus on self-help recognized the history of exploitation and oppression
Black women experienced through institutions of medicine and other health-
related fields, but the group did not reject medicine. Indeed, the BWSHC
insisted on the "right of every Black woman to have access to the best medical
and health care services." Self-help, however, enabled women to make informed decisions about their bodies and their health care.[144]

The statement of purpose also confirmed the BWSHC's feminist politics.
Black women, they argued, experienced the "triple struggle against racism,

sexism, and classism." Feminism, they believed, provided the political tools to secure the "political, social, and economic equality of all Black women." Although the group "network[ed] with people of other races and nationalities," the group was "open only to women of African descent."[145]

The statement of purpose reflected the members' commitment to instilling positive views of Black women's sexuality, replacing the myths and the stereotypes that damaged their self-image. The BWSHC vowed to encourage Black women to explore and define their own sexuality outside the destructive influences of racism and sexism. The group also vowed to fight for the elimination of homophobia, seeing it a corrosive force that caused "unnecessary antagonism among Black women and with the Black community." The collective agreed that an open discussion of homophobia helped build a "unified Black community."[146]

At the end of the document, the BWSHC affirmed its role as a support group:

> [The] Black Women's Self-Help Collective endorses and encourages Black women to support each other. We are a support group open to Black women to discuss their problems—whether they are health related, job related, or concerning interpersonal relationships. All of the above are important to us as Black women and in some way affect our physical, and mental, and spiritual health.[147]

This commitment to providing emotional support to the members of the BWSHC responded to the perpetual demand by some of the members; its location at the end of a document, invites speculation. Does its presence at the end mark it as an afterthought or a concession? By contrast, perhaps its location marks it as a conclusion, highlighting the importance of support to the group's mission. Regardless of the intention of the statement of purpose, the failure of the BWSHC to meet the emotional needs of its members likely led to its dissolution.[148]

In the wake of the new statement of purpose, the BWSHC intensified its health study presentations, continuing with topics covered in previous years like sexuality, lupus, and nutrition, while also moving into new areas including aging, mental health, and herbal remedies. The BWSHC encouraged members to acquire and share specialized skills, including first aid, midwifery, and lay health worker training offered at the Washington Free Clinic. The group also, with some grumbling, began to perform self-exams again during their bimonthly meetings,[149] and they presented self-exam to new audiences, including providing a demonstration with the Salsa Soul Sisters, a group of lesbians of color in New York City.[150]

Despite their invigorated educational programming, the group was again vexed by its inability to meet simultaneously the emotional and educational needs of its members. In December 1983, Ajowa Ifateyo, who in October had taken leave from the organization, shared her concerns about how the group functioned. She explained that over the course of the summer and fall she had been struggling personally, but she confessed that she had not shared her struggles with the BWSHC. Why, she wondered, if the BWSHC conceived of itself as "a support system for Black women" did she feel compelled to leave the group when she most needed support from her sisters? She wondered how and whether the group could "support individuals who are struggling with emotional problems." She worried whether, in its quest to gain and share knowledge about health and embodiment, the group "lost the support aspect."[151] Likely as a direct result of this letter, the group promised to discuss whether the BWSHC could "really be a support group" as well as a political and education group at their December 18, 1983, meeting.[152] The topic was not, however, addressed at the meeting.[153]

Throughout 1984, the group's membership declined precipitously. From a height of twenty to thirty, the membership roster listed only ten active members in May 1984, with another five women listed as "inactive." Only four to eight members typically attended the meetings. Desperate to resolve the group's interpersonal issues, the BWSHC held a workshop in July focused on improving the group's internal dynamics. The question of whether the group was or should be a "support group" again emerged as a point of conflict. Several members apparently yearned for increased emotional support from the other members. Those members who valued the group's educational mission resisted allowing the BWSHC to become primarily a place for women to "rap." (Some also feared that a few members' emotional needs required more expertise than they could supply.)[154] To resolve the issue, the facilitator noted that the group had already committed to acting as a support group in its statement of purpose: "We are a support group open to Black women to discuss their problems." She suggested a variety of options to help the BWSHC to meet the commitments outlined in its statement of purpose.[155] But the conflicts continued.

In what appeared to be a last-ditch effort to bring the group together, Audrey Sartin and Lauren Austin, two long-term members, cowrote a letter, pleading with the group to be more sensitive to the members' emotional needs. Both women described moments when the group ignored or dismissed their emotional needs. Sartin, one of the women who attended the group's first meeting, described how she had recently attended a meeting "seeking some form of support and encouragement, but [instead of support, she] encountered a void of uncaring and disinterest that [she] could not cross over." Both women shared their distress at the group's unwillingness to deal with "another sister's emotional needs," in the interest of staying on task. Sartin and Austin emphasized the political importance of building tender bonds between Black women. After reminding the group that the "personal IS political," they claimed that "our responsibility as womanists is to maintain emotional sensitivity to and in each other. Only through this trust and understanding can the work, the outreach, the political part be done. This is the major idea separating us from the capitalist patriarchy."[156] Echoing the ideas of Self-Help promoted by the NBWHP, these women tried to connect emotional labor with political goals, but their efforts were not enough to change the BWSHC's dynamics.[157]

It is unclear how the BWSHC ended. By December 1984, few members remained. Although an agenda was set for a meeting in January 1985, it is not clear whether the group survived into the new year.[158] Disagreements over the primary goals of the group apparently led to its decline.

Over its life, the BWSHC put the health of Black women at the center of its own agenda and onto the agenda of the larger women's health movement. Armed with an explicitly feminist politics, the organization brought women together to educate each other and to empower themselves to demand and receive better from the society around them. For many of the participants, the experience was formative. As Rosa Brunson described in her farewell letter to the group, the BWSHC affirmed her worth, power, and rights. It provided a community that linked her to other Black women, past, present, and future. She acknowledged the struggles, both political and personal, that characterized the group, but she nevertheless honored the "sisters of Black Women Self-Help Collective who dare[d] to walk in the spirit and tradition of sisterhood."[159]

The Black Women's Self-Help Collective used self-help as a guiding strategy to secure better health and to foster personal empowerment for the women involved. They came together as feminists and sisters in a larger struggle for self-determination. Self-exam, for many of the women involved, encouraged self-knowledge, skill building, and bodily acceptance. For many of the members, Black women needed self-exam to help them claim their bodies as their own. Despite its value as a tool of empowerment, however, the speculum did not provide the emotional support and connection many members sought.

The Washington, DC, Black Women's Self-Help Collective and the Bay Area Black Women's Health Project sought to meet the health needs of Black women through self-help, but they approached it from different perspectives. The Bay Area women believed that the first step toward health and healing depended on creating spaces for women to share their pain and to support each other. Any other approach to health would only paper over Black women's significant wounds without encouraging them to heal. The Washington, DC, women also believed in creating an atmosphere of support and sisterhood for Black women. And yet, their focus on health education frequently interfered with their ability to nurture interpersonal relationships. Moreover, the support needs of some of the members may have required expertise that the group could not provide. As a result, the group's inability to meet the emotional needs of its membership hobbled its effort to effectively nurture Black women's health.

Black women and other women of color were involved in the women's health movement from the beginning. Initially, however, they worked in organizations with few other women of color. As they worked to meet the political and health needs of "women," or "lesbians," some Black women yearned to build a movement that put their particular health needs at the center. They strove to work with Black women, for Black women. By the early 1980s, Black women across the country gathered to identify and enact their own health agenda.

Self-help was the primary tool of this health movement. Some groups embraced gynecological self-exam, highlighting it as a crucial tool for increasing Black women's ownership of their own bodies. Others embraced Black and Female—a version of self-help created by a Black woman and specifically endorsed by the National Black Women's Health Project—for its ability to speak to Black women's trauma. Still others, relying on generations of self-help traditions in some Black communities, gathered to educate themselves about mental illness, swap tips to cope with lupus flare-ups, and support their effort to exercise. Despite these significant differences, Black women's activism demonstrated that Black women's wounds, inflicted by historical and contemporary experiences of racism, sexism, and oppression, required the recognition of other Black women for healing. With each other, they could "rest a moment in the cradle of some safe arms."[160]

"The Challenge of Change": Feminist Health Clinics and the Politics of Inclusion

In 1981, the Santa Cruz Women's Health Collective (SCWHC) vowed to "confront its racism." Over the course of its history, the SCWHC had remained an organization of mostly white and middle-class women. Urged on by the few women of color in the group and by their desire to better serve the women of Santa Cruz, SCWHC members committed to personal introspection, frank conversation, and structural assessment in order to forge a truly inclusive institution. The process of change proved more contentious than most of the white women foresaw. Laura Giges, a member since 1976, described the white women's vision for the process: "Somewhat naively, we had thought that we could change who we are and who we serve without affecting how we work and how decisions get made." They underestimated the change required of them and the organization they built and sustained.[1]

In telling the history of the SCWHC's confrontation with racism while the end was uncertain, Giges recognized the anger, pain, and frustration women of color and white women experienced, but she remained optimistic about the pathway ahead. As she wrote, "Recognizing that we needed new ways of working together, we began to let go of the feelings that we knew what was right for the SCWHC. As the 'we' of the SCWHC was changing, new ways of working together would emerge." Working together, women of color and white women were "giving birth to a new collective."[2] Giges's prediction was only partially true. White women and women of color struggled together to create a health center more responsive to the women who needed its services most. The collective, however, failed to survive the rebirth.

In the 1970s, many health feminists peered between their legs and believed they saw a pathway to liberated sisterhood. They believed they wielded a tool that showcased women's shared oppression and revealed their shared power. Some of them were so inspired by their vision that they imagined and created women-centered health clinics based on the principles of self-help. They were joined by other health activists who aimed to bring feminist principles to community health care. These women believed that their clinics and the politics that guided them benefited all women.

Although women of color participated in many feminist health projects, the women who founded feminist health clinics were for the most part white.[3] These activists' enthusiasm for their projects, their analytical focus on gender, and their unexamined racism left them unable to see why their clinics primarily attracted white women. Women of color in communities with women's health centers often viewed them as "white" establishments. Over the years, many of these clinics wrestled with their own whiteness. The women involved had long counted racism, along with classism, capitalism, and imperialism, as key obstacles to the liberation of all people.[4] Many of the clinics took racism seriously as a topic for education and, perhaps less frequently, action. And yet, many of the clinics remained largely white organizations. In the late 1970s and early '80s, some of them—often urged on by women of color staff and collective members—worked to make good on their promise to meet the health care needs of all women in their communities and to diversify their staffs.

These efforts provoked a variety of results. In perhaps most of them, white women and women of color alike emerged bruised from their attempts to identify, confront, and ameliorate the racism built into their institutions. In some clinics, the process forged an organization and a clinic more responsive to the communities they hoped to serve. Others suffered from the recriminations of failing to meet their new goals. In each case, the effort sparked profound change within these organizations. To survive (and not all did), the organizations required a new politics and sometimes a revised mission from that which animated the clinics at their beginnings.[5] By changing the "we" at the core of the clinics, they transformed many of their political commitments.

This chapter examines the efforts of feminist health clinics as they acknowledged the exclusivity of their practices, confronted their own racist policies, and committed to a more inclusive organization. In particular, it focuses on the efforts of the Santa Cruz Women's Health Collective (SCWHC) as it attempted to redress its whiteness. In Santa Cruz, the effort to diversify the SCWHC and its health center provoked decisions that forever changed the nature and direction of both. The experiences of the SCWHC and other women's health organizations and clinics highlight the intellectual and political commitment to diversity and the personal introspection and political realignment that commitment required.

Whose Women's Movement?

Both contemporary and historical accounts of so-called second-wave feminism have frequently framed it as a movement of middle-class, white women in the interest of middle-class, white women. This critique threatens to "whitewash" the movement, dismissing the contributions of women of color as participants in predominantly white groups, as organizers of and activists in their own communities, and as beneficiaries of legal and social change. As the sociologist Benita Roth explained, "Early Black feminists were involved in political relationships with early white feminists, and influenced each other's thinking. . . . White feminists remained, however fitfully, in dialogue with women of color as they mobilized."[6]

Many feminists in the late 1960s and early '70s were aware of their own race and class position. Indeed, many early women's liberationists came to feminism from their work in the civil rights movement.[7] Moreover, many feminist groups—even those composed of white, middle-class women—often placed an examination of race, class, and sexuality at the center of their analysis. This theoretical attention to axes of inequality, however, did not always provide a clear pathway for how women with diverse perspectives could work productively together. As the historian Winifred Breines has characterized it: "Even amid the thrill of sisterhood and solidarity, activists recognized differences among women. . . . They did not ignore differences but they, like most others of that time, were not particularly successful in negotiating them."[8] Early white feminists' efforts to confront their own racism frequently generated anger, angst, recriminations, and guilt but little organizational change.[9]

Even as some predominantly white groups failed to act on their racial and class analysis, women of color frequently organized to address their needs and the needs of their communities. In the 1960s, for example, Black women activists continued their fight against racial oppression. Breines reminds us that after white folks were ejected from the Student Nonviolent Coordinating Committee, Black women stayed and fought for racial justice.[10] Black women also joined Black Power organizations, especially the Black Panthers, and they frequently challenged the sexism they found there.[11] Indeed, according to the historian Kimberly Springer, Black women sympathized with the goals of women's liberation to a greater extent than white women.[12] Some Black women organized around women's issues while strategically rejecting, or at least avoiding, the feminist label.[13] Black women also formed feminist organizations, including the National Black Feminist Organization (1973), the Third World Women's Alliance (1969 and 1971), and the Combahee River Collective (1974).[14] According to Breines, while Black feminism "never became a mass grassroots movement like the white women's movement," she argued that "black feminism developed its own track, in reaction to black nationalism and white feminism, with major insights and contributions of its own."[15] Roth identified a similar trajectory for Chicanas. In the 1960s and early '70s, women simultaneously participated in the Chicano movement and created a feminist critique of it.[16]

Although white women and women color frequently organized separately, a few events brought them together. In *The Trouble between Us: An Uneasy History of White and Black Women in the Feminist Movement* (2006), Breines described the development and actions of the Coalition for Women's Safety, an interracial group founded in response to the murder of Black women in Boston. In the first six months of 1979, twelve Black and one white woman were murdered in two predominantly Black neighborhoods. In response, Black feminists and other community activists organized in protest, demanding more police attention be focused on each murder and on the deadly violence against women of color as a group. They were joined by white women from various women-centered organizations, creating the multiracial, multiethnic Coalition for Women's Safety to publicize the murders, police neglect, and the media's disregard for the lives of Black and brown women. This organization held together in part because participants understood the particular oppression at the intersection of race, class, and gender and because white women supported Black women's leadership.[17]

Organizers understood the significance of the Coalition for Women's Safety for coalitional women's activism. At a 1979 Take Back the Night march, rally speakers marked the importance of the occasion:

> The brutal violence directed this year specifically against Black women has catalyzed an awareness among white women of what Third World women have known all their lives—that women of color are singled out as targets of violence both because of their race and their sex. White women have begun to learn from Third World women to organize against the violence particularly affecting women of color.[18]

According to organizers, the success of this coalition depended on white women providing support for rather than leading women of color.[19] Other

factors may have also supported its success, including the horror of its pre-
cipitating events, its clear animating cause, and its fairly evident path forward.
Most significantly, it did not require white women to consider the goals and
structures of their own political commitments through the eyes of women of
color. White women did not have to change their priorities or relinquish their
hard-fought power.

Coalitional Politics and Reproductive Rights

In the late 1960s and into the '70s, the fight for reproductive freedom frequently brought white women and women of color together to demand access
to reproductive health care and protection against medical abuse. Women of
color frequently defined the problem, revealing and highlighting facets unno-
ticed by white activists. In Washington, DC, for example, the largely white DC
Women's Liberation Movement and the interracial but largely Black Citywide
Welfare Alliance, a group of welfare rights activists affiliated with the National
Welfare Rights Organization, joined forces in 1969 to protest DC's limited access to abortion and contraception, particularly for poor women. According
to the historian Anne M. Valk, collaboration between these groups "created
a movement, and a consensus, that asserted women's rights to control their
fertility."[20]

In 1967, Washington, DC, abortion laws were fairly liberal, but access, especially for poor women, was limited. Therapeutic abortions were legal; however, they required approval by three physicians who agreed that pregnancy
threatened a woman's health. At DC hospitals charging high rates for abortion, women found the approval process easy. At public hospitals with low
abortion fees, by contrast, few women could access the procedure. Physicians
at the public DC General Hospital provided only eight therapeutic abortions
in 1967 but treated more than five hundred women for the complications of
legal and illegal abortions performed elsewhere. This contrast highlights the
demand for abortion among poor women and the obstacles to their access. At
the same time, physicians at two of DC's private hospitals provided roughly
170 abortions each month. Although not central to either the DC Women's
Liberation Movement or the Citywide Welfare Alliance, health care and abortion rights "established points of commonality" between their organizations.
Even in this example, however, the two groups differed in their analysis of
the situation. For the Citywide Welfare Alliance, poverty and the structure
of the welfare state created the problem, forcing poor women to secure an
underground abortion and threatening public aid recipients into using birth
control. For the DC Women's Liberation Movement, obstacles to abortion

and contraception represented compulsory motherhood and the foreclosed opportunities for other forms of life work.[21]

White feminists and women of color also came together to demand an end to sterilization abuse. In California, the Chicana rights movement mobilized around sterilization abuse as a core issue. Chicanas—joined by a radical, majority-white feminist group, the Coalition for the Medical Rights of Women, and a coalition of other multiethnic organizations—petitioned the California Department of Health to establish guidelines aimed at preventing sterilization abuse. Their demands included a fourteen-day waiting period between consenting to sterilization and surgery, a standardized process for education and informed consent, and a minimum age requirement of eighteen. Their efforts succeeded, and in May 1977, the California Department of Health adopted the activists' recommendations, creating comprehensive guidelines to protect vulnerable women against coercive sterilization.[22]

In June 1977, the United States Supreme Court upheld the constitutionality of the 1976 Hyde Amendment, which prohibited the use of federal funding for most abortions. This ruling decreased the accessibility of abortion and constricted the reproductive choices of poor women. In the aftermath of the decision, more than one hundred women—many of whom identified as socialist feminists but representing a variety of feminist organizations and perspectives—came together in a New York City basement and founded a new reproductive rights group. Though originally conceived as a coalition of activist groups, the Committee for Abortion Rights and Against Sterilization Abuse (CARASA) proposed a reproductive rights agenda at odds with some long-standing single-issue groups like the National Abortion Rights Action League (NARAL). According to the historian Jennifer Nelson, the women who founded CARASA "wanted to secure reproductive control for the least-advantaged women—the poor, the young, and women of color . . . [the] women who had the least control over their reproduction."[23] The women of CARASA, while largely white and middle class, listened to women of color and understood that welfare benefits and subsidized child care were reproductive rights issues as much as access to abortion and freedom from coercive sterilization. CARASA took seriously the complaints issued by many Black women and Latinas that birth control efforts had often focused on getting women of color to reduce their fertility rather than encouraging their reproductive autonomy. Between its 1977 founding and its 1982 disbandment, CARASA, often in coalition with other organizations like the multiracial, multiethnic Committee to End Sterilization Abuse, demanded and created an inclusive movement for the reproductive rights of all women.[24]

These examples show that when confronted with clear infringements of reproductive rights, white women frequently allied with women of color to increase reproductive freedom. But sometimes multiethnic and multiracial coalitions crumbled explicitly over issues of race and racism. The Reproductive Rights National Network (R2N2) provides a case in point. Founded in 1979, R2N2 was a multiethnic and antiracist coalition of several local and national reproductive rights organizations.[25] In its early years, it had the reputation of working together better than other multiethnic groups, including CARASA. Despite its commitment to reproductive justice for women of color, Black women in the organization repeatedly claimed that while white women pledged their support, they proved unwilling to relinquish their power.[26] As a result, Black women consistently called upon white women to confront and address their racism; white women failed repeatedly to meet the challenge. In the aftermath of an explosive conference in November 1984, the already ailing R2N2 collapsed, allegedly because of the "inability of White women in the Network to appreciate what our work and responsibilities were as part of a Multiracial organization."[27]

In CARASA and R2N2, white women worked with women of color to secure and protect the reproductive rights of the women with the fewest reproductive options and who were the most vulnerable to medical abuse. Sometimes, however, white, middle-class women fought for the rights of women like themselves, even when those efforts put the reproductive lives of women of color at increased risk. As the historian Rebecca Kluchin describes, some feminist organizations like NOW and NARAL opposed mandatory waiting periods and age minimums for sterilization, believing that they constrained (white) women's reproductive choices and would ultimately be used to erode women's access to abortion.[28]

Women of color, organizing among themselves, also fought to secure reproductive rights, sometimes against the political positions of the men they were aligned with. Nelson, for example, describes how the Black Panther Party, once opposed to all forms of reproductive control as "genocidal," came to support a reproductive rights agenda that decried sterilization abuse and demanded access to abortion and voluntary contraception under the leadership of Elaine Brown and other—frequently feminist—women.[29]

Clearly, white women and women of color organized separately and together to secure health care and reproductive freedom. When they joined together in coalition—often to assert and protect the reproductive rights of the women most vulnerable to abuse and least able to access compassionate care—they succeeded best when they focused on a concrete goal.

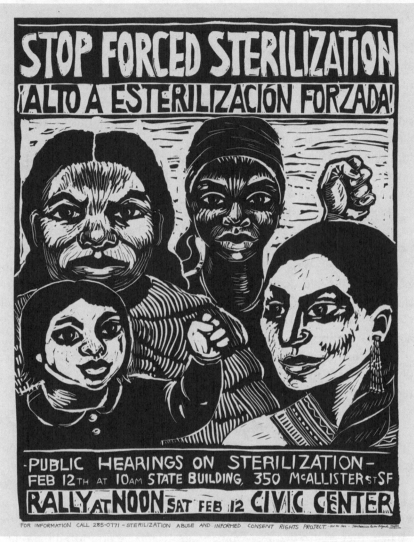

FIGURE 8.1. Women of color from different communities led the efforts against sterilization abuse. White women sometimes stood with women of color, supporting their efforts, and sometimes they fought restrictions on sterilization. Linocut by Rachael Romero, SF Poster Brigade. Retrieved from the Library of Congress.

Consequently, many of the most successful coalitions during this era were short-term organizations that dissolved after their objectives were achieved. Less-focused organizations tended to split apart in acrimony over accusations of racism and an inability to forge a long-term mission that reflected the priorities of all the parties.

Building a More Welcoming Movement

Moments of convergence between the movements for reproductive freedom and women's health occasionally created space for white women and women of color to work together. The broader women's health movement faced a different set of challenges. Its goals were typically more diffuse—liberation, self-knowledge, empowerment, feminist health care—and its timeline unbounded. In many women's health organizations, the politics of diversity and inclusion posed significant challenges, frequently leading to crisis about each organization's very structure and mission. The example of the Rising Sun Feminist Health Alliance is instructive.

Founded in 1978, Rising Sun arose to create a network of women's health organizations on the East Coast to provide moral support, swap best practices, and share resources. Unlike the Federation of Feminist Women's Health Centers centered on the West Coast, Rising Sun connected member organizations that differed significantly in scope, mission, and politics. Membership shifted over time; in 1979, it included the Boston Women's Health Book Collective, HealthRIGHT, and the New Hampshire Women's Health Center, among many others.

At its founding, original members noted that the organization lacked diversity, and so they invited organizations run by women of color to send representatives to their July 1979 meeting. Although the extant record does not describe the dynamics of the July meeting, an October 1979 debriefing conversation suggests that the July meeting ended in rancor and confusion. The conversation revealed several tensions that women's health organizations encountered as they tried to diversify their organizations.

Some women wondered whether creating a women's health movement attentive to more women's needs required white-majority organizations to abandon their focus on reproductive care, especially as it benefited healthy women. They argued that well-woman care—care that prioritized reproductive health rather than illness—always implicitly privileged middle-class women who had other means to access health care for illness. These women viewed wellness as a classed and raced privilege. Other health activists, white women particularly, frequently resisted this framework because it dismissed and denigrated the work that had animated their efforts—abortion counseling and provision, for example—and elevated as crucial the "survival issues" of poor women and women of color. Their frustration simmered as they noted that Black women disproportionally sought abortions even as they failed to spend their political capital fighting for it.[30]

This discussion introduces some of the dilemmas white women confronted as white-majority organizations "reached out" to communities of color. Women's health organizations were proud of their achievements and believed that their work already benefited white women *and* women of color alike. As a result, they resisted setting it aside in order to attract women of color to their organizations. Because of their investments in the organizations they created and nurtured, white feminist activists frequently hesitated to relinquish power to newly recruited women who did not share the same vision for the future of women's health organizing.

Women's Health Clinics: Serving Which Women?

Health activists who founded feminist health clinics generally began from a belief in women's common need for reproductive health care and bodily knowledge. By founding a clinic and welcoming all women—or so they thought—this largely white group of women believed they increased the autonomy of all women. As they built their health centers and clinics, however, their decisions, big and small, signaled their commitment to some women in their communities and not to others.

Women's health organizations in Seattle provide one example of how feminist activists understood, at least on some level, the health concerns of women of color but still failed to design a clinic that directly engaged with them. Feminists associated with the University of Washington Young Women's Christian Association (UW YWCA) decided in 1971 that the medical marketplace in Seattle—even the vibrant community-clinic marketplace—was insufficiently attentive to the needs of women, so they planned a women's health clinic infused with feminist principles. When the founders sought input for what became the Aradia Women's Health Clinic, members of the community asked for broad-based medical reforms that addressed the medical abuse of "Third World People," the health needs of prisoners, and the "forced sterilization of welfare recipients." These demands, however, exceeded the vision of the founders; Aradia opened in 1972 in the mostly white neighborhood around the University of Washington, limiting its attraction to volunteers and clients of color. According to one of its founders, only a "small number" of women of color worked at the clinic, and it served a disproportionately white clientele.[31]

Aware of the shortcomings of the Aradia clinic to address many of the issues raised during the early planning discussion, a group of women associated with the UW YWCA, some white and some women of color, formed a Third World Women's Resource Center (TWWRC) in 1972 to eliminate "racism wherever it exists by any means necessary." One of its projects proposed to use the Aradia clinic to train "Third World Women" to provide family planning services and educational resources to the "Third World" community. Its planners imagined this "Third World Women's Preventive Medicine and Health Education Center" joining a new community center, El Centro de la Raza.[32]

According to historian Nelson, the Aradia clinic, the TWWRC, and the Third World Women's Preventative Medicine and Health Education Center demonstrate that Seattle feminists "were attentive to the ways in which race and class affected women's reproductive health access," and were compelled to act creatively to meet the reproductive health needs of women of color. And yet, this effort might provide a different lesson; it is unclear whether the Third World Women's Preventive Medicine and Health Education Center ever proceeded beyond the planning stage. Perhaps the project never recruited sufficient numbers of women of color to the Aradia clinic for training. Perhaps it never attracted sufficient funding. Perhaps it enjoyed a brief tenure before closing, like so many other health experiments of the time. Regardless of whether it actually served clients, this story might also be read as white women advocating for and with women of color on the side while devoting their primary labor to a clinic that met the needs of white women.

As the example of the Aradia clinic shows, the need to locate a clinic in a particular place highlighted the difficulty of creating an institution available to all women, especially in large cities with neighborhoods defined by economic and racial segregation. In *Finding the Movement* (2007), the historian Finn Enke has described how resistance to a Feminist Women's Health Center in Detroit led to the clinic's relocation in 1977 to the suburban outskirts of the city, leaving downtown Detroit without a clinic providing "safe, affordable sexual health care and abortions." To fill this void and serve the needs of the women left behind, especially women of color, three Black women who had trained at the Detroit FWHC—Faye Roberts, Pam Carter, and Janette Salters—sought its help creating a new feminist clinic downtown. The original FWHC offered "support," but, citing their own all-consuming battles to survive, they declined to collaborate further. They also argued that "the women we serve would not be comfortable" downtown. Consequently, Enke concluded, the Detroit "FWHC . . . became part of an urban topography in which bodily autonomy was an economic privilege."[33]

Confronting the Unsustainable Whiteness

These decisions concerning location forced some clinics to confront the limits of their efforts to serve women after they brought their vision to life with bricks and mortar. But location was not the only way a clinic signaled its welcome. By employing white, monolingual English speakers for the most part, these clinics frequently gained the reputation as white clinics meeting the needs of white women. In the mid- to late 1970s, some clinics confronted their whiteness and attempted to change their image, staff, and outreach.

The Berkeley Women's Health Collective (BWHC) provides an early example of a clinic attempting to diversify its clientele and staff. Founded by white women in 1971, the BWHC strove to be an institution by and for all women; but in the summer of 1976, the collective that governed the clinic finally confronted its failure to attract women of color. To address this situation, the collective resolved to change its hiring practices. Whereas it had always hired paid staff by promoting collective volunteers, the collective understood that this policy supported the clinic's overall whiteness. The leadership agreed to hire staff from outside the collective, providing a mechanism to hire a more diverse staff. In May 1977, the collective pledged to "attempt to establish and maintain a minimum of 50% third world women and 50% lesbians on the paid staff." By the end of 1978, they had finally achieved this mandate, but the battles over diversity and the change it demanded continued. Long-term collective members bemoaned the changes that new staff members brought in their wake, and they accused the newcomers of dismissing the clinic's history and its politics.[34] Perhaps reflecting ongoing tensions, in 1983, some members of the BWHC founded the South Berkeley Women's Clinic against wishes of other collective members.[35] The creation of the clinic and the opposition to it demonstrate the BWHC's ongoing struggle to be a welcoming place for all women.

The BWHC's awareness that it hadn't provided a clinic for all women, its mechanism to diversify, and its wistful nostalgia in the wake of success were not unique to this clinic. Rather, they illustrate the efforts and aftermath common to many feminist health clinics as they tried to make good on their promise to meet the needs of all the women in their communities.

In New York City, St. Marks Clinic similarly confronted its lack of diversity, at least among its volunteer staff. Founded in 1973, the Women's Health Collective of St. Marks Free Clinic offered health services once a week to women who did not need reproductive health care. It primarily served a lesbian clientele, and it sometimes called itself a lesbian health collective, but it tried to avoid an identity-based approach. It focused instead on providing health services to women beyond their reproductive needs.

The Women's Health Collective at St. Marks struggled over a variety of issues, including the scope of services, the composition of the board, and the place of alternative treatment modalities. These differences caused St. Marks to split into two clinics in 1980, both retaining the name. Both before and after the split, the Women's Health Collective (WHC) struggled internally over issues "concerning racism and collectivity."[36] As they described the situation in March 1980, "The group is trying to explore and change our practices that lead to [the] isolation of coll[ective] members who are ♀ of color and of diverse cultural backgrounds."[37] According to Loretta Mears, one of two Black members in 1979 and 1980, "We had workshops all the time to try to work it through because we didn't assume that it was unresolvable back then. We had hope."[38]

To change the climate of the clinic, the WHC of St. Marks launched a series of antiracism discussions.[39] These meetings were designed to "address racism as it affects the way we treat each other and patients."[40] Some WHC members apparently balked at devoting so much time to antiracism efforts. For example, at the June 1980 meeting, the members disagreed whether these meetings would include discussion of "other divisive tendencies such as class bias, age bias, etc." This recommendation was likely controversial, seen as an attempt by some white women to avoid discussing racism. It was also likely an indirect complaint that women of color were unwilling to listen to the grievances of white women.[41] Apparently, attendance at these meetings was low;[42] only four women attended the July 1980 meeting.[43] As a result, the WHC organized two all-day workshops to help "white women . . . overcome their racism," and required that all white women in the collective attend one of them.[44] Only white women were required to attend because "we do not believe that those of us who are women of color should be obliged to take part in the process of white women's struggles with their racism." The women of the collective continued to address their own racism and to organize antiracism efforts through the fall of 1980.[45]

Finally, the WHC took concrete steps to increase the participation of women of color by placing a moratorium on accepting new white lesbians into the organization. The WHC members agreed in May 1980 that the "overwhelmingly white" staff was already large enough to offer services two nights a week, and thus they could limit the participation of new members to women of color. Because of their pressing need for doctors, they still accepted white physicians.[46] By October, however, their optimism had faded, and they faced significant staff shortages "for all jobs on all nights."[47] In November 1980, the WHC considered opening membership to white women if they were Jewish, to address the "growing expression of anti-Semitism throughout the world" and to recognize the paucity of Jewish lesbians among the membership. This recommendation was rejected.[48]

By April 1981, staffing shortages stretched the all-volunteer clinic staff too thin. Several health workers threatened to quit if staffing didn't increase. To

respond, the WHC ramped up its health care trainings for "[3rd] world lesbians" and lifted the moratorium on new white women volunteers if they
brought health care skills to the group. Nevertheless, they did not abandon
their policy altogether, insisting that the "collective policy is still to establish
periods of moratorium of hiring white lesbians as necessary."[49]

After this moment, the WHC learned they were to be evicted within
months, and its focus turned to finding and remodeling new clinic space.
The clinic reopened in a new location in June 1983. In the flurry of displace-
ment, construction, and financial instability, survival led the WHC's agenda.
And yet, by October, the clinic began once again to recruit women of color as
volunteers and patients. In its 1985 statement of philosophy and function, it
highlighted its commitment to lesbians of color: "The Collective recognizes
and acts upon the need for Women of Color and Third World Women in
positions of action and leadership in the organization."[50] And by April 1986,
St. Marks once again had organized workshops as part of its commitment to
antiracism.[51]

On the one hand, that antiracism was a continual topic for workshops and
conversation might be read as a failure of the WHC to sufficiently change its
model to fully welcome and accommodate women of color to its staff. On the
other, long-term members of the WHC and new volunteers alike remained
committed to the struggle. The women who volunteered at St. Marks understood that inclusion and antiracism were long-term projects that required
constant attention and effort.[52]

Diversifying a Clinic: The Santa Cruz Women's Health Collective

Across the country from St. Marks, the women of the Santa Cruz Women's
Health Collective (SCWHC) and health center were experiencing their own
struggles trying to diversify their membership and their clinic's clientele. At
its founding, the SCWC was composed exclusively of white and middle-class
women.[53] Over time, a few women of color and working-class women joined,
but the SCWHC remained overwhelmingly white through the 1970s. Indeed,
it had the reputation among some in the community as a "white clinic," an
insular institution that did not speak to the needs of women of color.[54]

The founders reflected the relative homogeneity of the surrounding community. In 1970, the residents of the city and county of Santa Cruz were predominantly white. Nevertheless, roughly 10 percent of the county's residents
identified as Hispanic, according to the census. Within the city's limits, Hispanic workers filled many of the service jobs associated with tourism; outside the city, Hispanic agricultural and factory workers built significant com-

munities in the south (Watsonville) and the north (Davenport). Over time, these communities grew, composing roughly 20 percent of the residents of the county in 1980 and 1990. The city roughly reflected the demographics of the county.[55]

From its founding through the late 1970s, the SCWHC worked to articulate a political mission, adopt a governance structure, develop and deliver educational materials, and provide clinical services. The members struggled to execute and refine their mission while regularly encountering new challenges. In the face of what clearly felt like monumental effort, the collective's racial and ethnic homogeneity failed to animate most of its members. Only with the pressure of the few women of color within the SCWHC and in the wake of restructuring forced by financial crisis did the SCWHC acknowledge that it had failed to meet the health needs of the women of Santa Cruz because it had focused primarily on the health needs of white women.

Jane Reyes, one of the first woman of color to join the SCWHC, initially became acquainted with it as a client.[56] In 1973 or 1974, Reyes needed an abortion and was relieved to find the collective's abortion referral service. As she recalled it, collective members left Santa Cruz at 4 o'clock one morning to drive a carload of women seventy-five miles across the coastal mountains to Oakland for an abortion. She remembered sharing the cramped space with "5 women trying not to puke." Despite what sounds like a difficult ride, Reyes found the experience "so supportive and wonderful" that when she earned her LPN license a few years later, she returned to the SCWHC as a volunteer and member.[57]

The culture and the politics of the SCWHC differed from anything Reyes had ever encountered: "I grew up in Oakland, and socialist feminists from East Oakland? You know, you just didn't think about that. Like you were what you were and you [did what you] had to . . . [to] survive." She found much of the language and the politics of the collective unfamiliar, challenging, and sometimes alienating. When she told her friends outside the SCWHC about her experiences, she would often joke that she spent the first eighteen months listening to all the acronyms, wondering, "What are they talking about?" Nevertheless, she enjoyed the experience and was enriched by it. At the SCWHC, Reyes discovered herself and her "feminist roots." She had always sought "equal rights and justice for all," and on many fronts, the mission of the SCWHC matched her personal commitment and ambitions.[58]

Despite her connection with the SCWHC, Reyes's perspective as a woman of color frequently differed from the prevailing views of her colleagues; her experiences illuminated issues invisible to many of the members. She urged the collective members to consider perspectives outside their own, but she was nonetheless relieved when another woman of color, Nancy Lim, joined the group. According to Reyes, "Having another woman of color to [offer] the same perspective . . . was really affirming." For her, it was crucial to have another woman in the collective "willing to talk about differences."⁵⁹

From the beginning, Reyes pushed the SCWHC to diversify its membership, in part as an effort to diversify the clinic's clientele. She insisted that "if we're going to call ourselves the women's health collective, then we have to represent all of the women in this county and we have to get more women from different ethnic groups in the county to work here."⁶⁰ The SCWHC agreed with Reyes's vision in principle; it denounced white supremacy and supported inclusion. It supported "all women and groups struggling against sexism."⁶¹ Nevertheless, the SCWHC did not initially develop an understanding that sexism played out differently for white women than for women of color. Despite Reyes's pressure, the collective remained a mostly white organization through the end of the 1970s. Longtime SCWHC member Laura Giges noted that while most of the women in the collective had been aware of its homogeneity, "periodic discussions about racism and affirmative action . . . seemed to exist in a vacuum with little translation into change."⁶² The members of the SCWHC appeared unable to imagine their way to a more inclusive organization, particularly if it required rethinking their priorities and policies.

Early attempts to diversify the SCWHC proved fraught. In 1978, the SCWHC described its struggle to expand its membership. Incorporating new members into the group always created tension between established members who had a clear vision for the SCWHC and how it should be governed and new members with "fresh observations and criticism." The SCWHC believed that these difficulties would be compounded by recruiting "many different kinds of women" instead of seeking out women already committed to feminism and collective governance. As they described the situation, "[Some women enter the group] on a more common ground with us, and are . . . generally more comfortable. . . . [In contrast,] women from various minority groups who join the collective often feel isolated and invisible as a group." The SCWHC understood the depth of the problem, and they wondered whether the collective structure could accommodate increased individual difference. But the members concluded that the challenges of diversity could be addressed through an intense commitment to "discuss problems, to compromise, and to accept one another's differences."⁶³ This statement reveals the anxieties the efforts to diversify the SCWHC produced among some of its members. Would diversity endanger the collective? Could more talk create consensus across difference? If difference required compromise, who should give in and on what grounds? Did differences of opinion reflect individual differences or perspectives common to newly included communities? These questions, not articulated outright, simmered just under the surface.

In retrospect, former collective members offered various explanations for the SCWHC's enduring homogeneity. Jody Peugh, for example, blamed the center's reliance on unpaid volunteer labor for its inability to attract women of color: "In the collective, we talked about wanting to . . . expand and be available to women of color, but . . . it just wasn't a place that people were attracted to come or could afford to volunteer or work for shit like that."[64] Peugh understood that the cost of volunteerism came at a higher cost to women of color, particularly those working for poverty wages in outside jobs. And yet, the belief that women of color didn't or couldn't volunteer was often used to explain why white feminist organizations remained predominantly white. Nevertheless, women of color, both middle class and poor women, had rich traditions of community involvement, volunteerism, and activism. In these instances, the women believed that they were working for a cause that reflected their needs. Peugh also believed that the collective structure of the SCWHC—a structure painstakingly constructed and highly valued by its founders—posed an obstacle: "There was something about the way we, us being a collective . . . that just seemed insurmountable [to women of color]."[65]

Reyes offered a quite different assessment. She didn't dispute that SCWHC members wanted to attract women outside the white middle class, but she noted that they found it unexpectedly difficult to "give up . . . cultural power." The members who had built and nurtured the SCWHC through their dedication and effort did not want to let it go. According to Reyes, many of these women "wanted to hang on" rather than cede the foundation they built to another group of activists who did not share their political commitments.[66] Clearly, members of the SCWHC believed in what they built and were proud of what they achieved. It was easier for them to hold on to what they might lose than to clearly imagine what the larger community might gain.

Committing to Diversity: Reckoning with Change

Sometime in 1980, SCWHC members vowed to confront their personal and institutional racism in order to create a more diverse organization. To begin to "unlearn racism," they invited two University of California, Santa Cruz, professors to facilitate trainings in early 1981. At these workshops, collective members explored their struggle to recognize their own racist beliefs and actions. Perhaps more crucially, these workshops identified the structural barriers to the meaningful inclusion of women of color into the SCWHC.[67]

Unexpectedly, policies for filling paid positions within the collective and health center became a focal point.

In flush times, collective members who sought paid positions nominated themselves and sought the SCWHC's endorsement. They explained what they brought to the job and why they needed paid employment. Sometimes these members invented their own positions, justifying their value to the collective and the clinic. When funds were plentiful, this system, while never perfect, worked well enough to keep most people mostly happy. After the 1979 budget cuts in the wake of Proposition 13, seniority became the sole criteria for distributing paid employment among collective members. In essence, SCWHC members earned paid positions through their long-term volunteer commitments. This process rewarded members whose politics matched the SCWHC, thus sustaining political homogeneity. It also preserved the preponderance of white and middle-class women; most women of color with the means to volunteer presumably gave their labor to organizations more visibly committed to their interests.

The members of the SCWHC struggled with the claim that their employment structure supported racial homogeneity. On the one hand, they believed it fair to reward volunteers for their service to the institution. On the other hand, they understood that their policies compromised their efforts to diversify. Their conversations forced the members of the SCWHC to question whether their beloved collective structure and policies contributed to their failure to "include and serve women of color." They began to wonder whether they had, against their explicit intentions, created a feminist health institution shaped around white women's needs "rather than health care for all women." Chagrined, SCWHC members confronted the exclusivity of their creation. They vowed to do better.[68]

As the first step in its newly invigorated resolve to diversify, the SCWHC launched the Bilingual Outreach Program, a project initiated by a "multicultural group of women." In the summer of 1981, the SCWHC used grant funding to hire two "bicultural/bilingual" health counselors to facilitate its outreach efforts in Latina communities. The SCWHC hired RosaMaria Zayas, a Puerto Rican woman with a long history of community organizing, and Carmela Saavedra, a "Mexicana farmworker and pre-med student."[69] The SCWHC also hired a third Latina to work as an office coordinator and translator.[70] Hiring these women of color allowed the SCWHC to increase its reach, building bridges and blazing paths between the Latinx community and the center's services. It also created unanticipated struggles within the organization.

From the perspective of some white women in the SCWHC, the new hires immediately challenged the structure and culture of the SCWHC and the attitudes of many of its members. Giges, a member of the SCWHC since 1975 and a member of the Bilingual Outreach Program, described the new hires as "disgusted and alienated" by the first few meetings they attended, and they refused to participate further. They objected to the tone of the meetings, the disapproval of showing anger, and the inability of the group to make crucial change quickly. The Latinas, nameless in Giges's account, dismissed consensus-based decision-making, insisting that they didn't have the time "to talk for hours and make no decisions," especially when they had a clear vision for the path forward. They insisted that if the SCWHC strove to serve all women, it required a thoroughgoing reorganization. They insisted that the SCWHC review "every aspect of how the clinic was run" so the white women could see how policies and politics that "worked for [them] might not work for Latina or African American women."[71]

But if decision-making by consensus alienated the new women, abandoning it left some longtime SCWHC members without tools for sharing their concerns and frustrations. As Marilyn Marzell, who joined the SCWHC in 1979, noted, the process for vetting disagreements—"the process to argue"—disappeared. Some of the white members of the collective found that their inability to confront disagreement across racial or ethnic lines left them hamstrung, unable to respond to accusations they found unfair and behaviors they found inappropriate. Marzell described how some members of the SCWHC had even cosigned a personal loan for one of the Latina members, despite considerable misgivings: "We didn't want to . . . cause any trouble."[72]

Several long-term white members of the SCWHC acknowledged that their approach to inclusion had been naive and inadequately sensitive to the personal and political transformation required to truly be a health center for all women. According to Marzell, white members of the collective did not have the language or the skills to partner with women of color to move the SCWHC forward.[73] Giges agreed that the SCWHC was unprepared for integrating women with different perspectives and possibly different goals. She recalled in 2000, "We had a very limited idea of what integration really meant."[74] In retrospect, many white members of the SCWHC marveled at their naivete: "We had thought we could change who we are and who we serve without affecting how we work and how decisions get made."[75]

While some, perhaps many, white members of the SCWHC acknowledged their role in creating dysfunction, some also believed that process had been complicated by the personalities of the Latinas the SCWHC hired. Many of the women interviewed for this book found Zayas charismatic and visionary, but also manipulative, and ultimately destructive. They insisted that she also alienated the Latinas she worked with.[76] Zayas may well have been disruptive. She was fired from her later employment as the executive director of the Community United in Response to AIDS/SIDA in San Francisco in 1992. Still, women of color were (and are) frequently dismissed as difficult when fighting to be seen and heard in white-majority spaces. The white women who painted Zayas as "difficult" failed to acknowledge how the context of recruitment—white women inviting Latinas into their organization—engendered the conditions that created "difficult" women of color as they confronted and condemned the policies and attitudes that thwarted their belonging.[77] These women's comments, however, clearly capture the wistfulness some of the white women felt, believing perhaps that the transition to a more diverse, welcoming health center might have proceeded with less rancor if they had hired someone who did not challenge the structures and mission of the SCWHC. Their comments suggest their underlying hope that some of the difficulty of the transition was caused by the new women's behaviors rather than their own disinclination to relinquish power.

Many of the white women felt unfairly judged as individuals and distressed that the new women dismissed the collective's carefully considered processes.[78] Peugh felt "heartbroken" because the new Latina recruits, while possessing "really good intentions and good hearts," seemed to have had no political connection to the clinic and no interest in its past. According to Peugh, they approached the work at the SCWHC as any other job, with "no commitment to the longevity of the organization," refusing to acknowledge and "honor" the accomplishments of the women who had created and nurtured the clinic from the ground up. Peugh believed that the Latinas dismissed the achievement of the longtime members "because we were . . . white girls."[79] Although her heartbreak in the face of critique and scorn is understandable, it reveals, perhaps, Peugh's inability to acknowledge some of the SCWHC's shortcomings. The SCWHC hoped to create a more welcoming environment for all women, but long-term members balked as women of color identified structures and attitudes that thwarted diversity. Moreover, Peugh's sense that the new women viewed their work at the SCWHC as "any other job" reveals more about her assumptions about them than about the Latinas' motivations. Zayas, for example, had been a community organizer in Los Angeles for eighteen years before moving to Santa Cruz, suggesting that her work with the SCWHC was part of a life committed to social change.[80]

The anthropologist Sandra Morgen observed a similar attitude in her examination of the Berkeley Women's Health Collective's attempts to diversify. At the BWHC, some collective members concluded that staff hired with federal Comprehensive Employment and Training Act (CETA) funds met "diversity requirements" but did not embrace the politics and the mission of the clinic. According to one BWHC member, the new women "didn't have the commitment," and they didn't understand the collective's value.[81] These comments may have captured the lack of political commitment on the part of some women of color hired to diversify white-majority clinics. Or these comments may reflect an unwillingness on the part of white health activists to recognize political commitments different from their own. Either way, it seems likely that newly hired women of color were not invited to bring their particular political commitments into the workplace; rather, they were expected to embrace a mission they had not been invited to shape.

Committing to Diversity: The Change Within

Although developing an outreach program to the Latinx community and hiring Latina workers helped diversify the SCWHC and the clinic's clientele, the members of the collective understood that they needed to do more. In August 1981, they convened another retreat to consider and implement their next steps. There the collective vowed that 50 percent of the center's paid staff would be women of color. As Marzell put it, "No more lip service."[82]

This decision threatened the seniority system that guided the assignment of paid positions within the SCWHC. Budget cuts in 1979 had eliminated most paid positions, and those that remained were occupied by members with the longest tenure. Committing to a paid staff composed of 50 percent women of color would require abandoning this reward for long-term service. Nevertheless, the SCWHC agreed that the plan provided the best pathway to enacting their political commitment to diversity. The SCWHC pledged half of its scarce resources to the salaries of women of color as a symbol of its commitment to diversity and inclusion.

After the August 1981 retreat, some members attempted to walk back their decision. They feared it would force out skilled, knowledgeable, and dedicated members while rewarding women with no demonstrated commitment to the center or its ideals. Plan supporters condemned those who second-guessed the decision, insisting that opponents should have presented their objections before the collective reached consensus. Supporters also identified "racist undertones" in the arguments against the new hiring policy.[83] Resentments and misunderstandings simmered without a public airing. Giges noted, "Our failure to fully challenge each other prevented us from hearing or understanding each other's feelings." For a group committed to productive criticism and the open exchange of feedback, this felt like a breakdown of their process.[84]

In retrospect, the SCWHC's decision to move ahead with its plan despite the simmering resentment and anger presaged the outcome of the plan's execution. The foundational commitments of the collective—indeed, the collective itself—would not survive the efforts to increase its appeal to a broader range of women.

It was unclear how the SCWHC expected to reach its goal, though its members understood that some currently paid employees would need to give up their paid positions or leave the collective. The SCWHC did not create a mechanism to enforce its commitment, and women who had given several years of labor and service to the organization were loath to relinquish their jobs and their paychecks. In late 1982, when the SCWHC had not reached its goal, it appealed to its board to enact their resolution. The board of directors, which had until this moment been titular, was tasked with firing some paid members to hire more diverse workers. Reyes became board chair at this tumultuous time. Although she and the rest of the board based their decisions on performance-based evaluations, she still found the decision-making wrenching. The board initially fired two women, both of whom had been with the SCWHC for years.[85]

Presumably feeling betrayed, these women did not go without a fight. In one instance, the fight was allegedly physical. Reyes recalled how she was attacked: "I had one woman come to my house . . . with her friends and she walked in and literally kicked my ass." (Reyes resigned from the board and the SCWHC shortly after this assault.) The fired women also fought back through legal threats. One of the women threatened to sue. In response, the board fired everyone, inviting them all to reapply for their jobs. (The two women who were originally fired did not apply for their old jobs.)[86]

In the aftermath, "everything fell apart." According to Marzell, one of the few SCWHC members whose tenure bridged the SCWHC's commitment to change and the transformed organization on the other side, the board's sudden power and drastic actions felt completely illegitimate: "Because there was no process, we had no process. . . . There was no reason for layoffs, other than that these women were not women of color. . . . There was no map. There was no guideline."[87]

Although some SCWHC members found the episode hurtful, "ugly," and "sucky," many of the people involved still defended the decision. They acknowledged that they were "bumbling and making things up as we went along," but they knew that the staff had to become more racially diverse and that they had no better path to that end. Peugh, for example, had "faith that we were doing the right thing somehow, even if the way we went about it was sucky. It's painful . . . but . . . we know it's right." (Peugh was not one of the women originally fired.) Marzell, in the thick of it, kept reminding herself that justice did not come easy.[88]

Others, however, were unable to understand the process as painful but necessary. Kater Pollock, who had been involved with the SCWHC since 1973, agreed that it was "absolutely crucial" for the SCWHC to confront its racism, but she refused to frame the firing of women who had "really put their hearts into" the SCWHC as difficult but necessary. Instead, she characterized it as "destructive" and largely a failure. She understood the desire to describe these events in terms of a positive outcome, but Pollock could not defend the decision.[89]

Some of the women of color involved remember this struggle with less anger or ambivalence. Reyes had been one of the major proponents of diversifying the SCWHC; she insisted that the firing was "absolutely" the right strategy, a big correction that enabled the clinic to survive: "When you're calling yourself something, you gotta represent everybody so that people feel comfortable and want to come."[90] Barbara Garcia, who joined the SCWHC's board in 1982, acknowledged the pain "integration" caused. Still, in her memory, the "white women who wanted the organization to change and the women of color who were changing the status quo" were "unified" in their goals. She had never before experienced such "tremendous unity between white women and women of color . . . struggling together around classism and racism." The novelty and the power of the experience changed her life.[91] Reyes's and Garcia's comments focus on the outcome of the struggle and the commitment to diversity despite the pain. Perhaps they never expected that inclusion would proceed without struggle. Garcia's position as a newcomer to the SCWHC likely also allowed her to focus on future gains rather than perceived losses.

An Integrated Health Center Reaches Out

Despite the chaos and discord, the SCWHC made good on its promise to meet the needs of more women in Santa Cruz. Formed in the fall of 1981 to mark the SCWHC's renewed commitment to diversity, the Bilingual Outreach Program (BOP) continued through and beyond the tensions. It brought bilingual health care, health information, and other crucial services to the underserved Spanish-speaking areas of Santa Cruz.[92] While the BOP was initiated by a "multicultural group of women," it was explicitly a project "for Latina women, designed by Latina women."[93] By their interest and actions, the outreach workers encouraged the neighborhood women "to organize and empower themselves with the SCWHC's resources."[94] Ultimately, the program hoped this information would allow Latinas to "have/take more control over their lives and the lives of their children and families."[95] The BOP began by literally knocking on doors in Latinx communities, especially those in northern Santa Cruz County, to assess their health care needs and desires.[96] Watsonville, in southern Santa Cruz County, was better known for its large Latinx community, but the organizers of the BOP felt that Watsonville was already well served by the publicly funded Salud Para La Gente.[97]

The BOP team dreamed of bringing health services into underserved neighborhoods. When they floated the idea of a mobile clinic to the communities, the women they surveyed responded enthusiastically. By the summer of 1982, the mobile health unit—funded through grants from the Ms. Foundation, the San Francisco–based Vanguard Foundation, and city revenue sharing—shuttled between Davenport in the north part of the county and two low-income neighborhoods in the city proper using Zayas's "elegant if ancient" nine-passenger Dodge van. Outfitted with a library, Spanish-language handouts, and a minilab, the van also offered basic health screenings, prenatal care, nutrition classes, and reproductive health counseling. Explicitly aiming to improve health care access for Latina women, the mobile health unit served as a link between the Latinx community and the bilingual services available at the SCWHC's clinic, WomanKind.[98] Nevertheless, economic and cultural barriers prevented many women from seeking care at the clinic.

The BOP identified the SCWHC's commitment to empowerment through bodily knowledge as one of the cultural barriers. Health counselors at WomanKind routinely suggested that clients get familiar with their own bodies by looking at their cervices during the gynecological exam, learning to perform cervical self-exam, or using a diaphragm for contraception. As SCWHC members Martha Ways and Deborah Abbott described it, these suggestions mistakenly assumed "that women [would] feel comfortable touching and examining their genitals. For many Latinas, religious or cultural influences [made] such genital contact an unwanted and alienating part of an exam."[99]

This statement honoring cultural difference likely captured some of the reasons why some potential Latina clients might feel uncomfortable seeking services at WomanKind. And yet, it also marks a significant reconsideration of self-help as the political foundation of their organization. Proponents of self-help originally understood that all women had been taught that their genitals were off limits. Self-help was an explicit challenge to patriarchy and its control of women's bodies as well as a tool for moving beyond it. Ten years after its creation, self-help, especially self-exam, was framed not as a tool for all women's liberation but a barrier to some women's access to feminist health care. This framing both suggests that the self-help movement was reckoning with the limits of a universal womanhood and notes a decline in the central-ity of women's liberation as a major goal of the women's health movement.

La Familia Center, the second initiative of the Bilingual Outreach Project, developed in the wake of the path blazed by the mobile health unit.[100] It began with the need in the Beach Flats neighborhood for a source of electricity for the mobile unit. The Beach Flats, filled with housing stock once meant for short-term visits by tourists, had become by the 1970s a low-income, largely Latinx neighborhood, home to many restaurant and hotel employees and other low-wage workers. A stone's throw from the city's famous boardwalk, it had long been without community services.[101] A local landowner responded to the call for electricity by donating a local building. The women of the BOP immediately saw the possibilities of this gift. In particular, they envisioned the building as a free health clinic for women, responding to the neighborhood's unmet health needs. Local health providers agreed to donate their time once a week, and a donor offered to support a renovation. While working on the project, Zayas and others dreamed bigger, seeing the building as an oppor-tunity to create a neighborhood center, offering community services, events, education, and support. As Zayas saw it, "The center [was] a place where people [could] come for support and problem solve with their own language and culture." Reconceived as La Familia and designed to "empower the com-munity," the enterprise quickly gained community support, with neighbor-hood residents donating their services.[102]

Described variously as a "self-help center," a "crisis intervention center," and a "community services center," La Familia Center opened in June 1983. It offered free, bilingual, multicultural crisis counseling, information, and re-ferrals six days a week, and medical services for women one night a week.[103] It was staffed by two coordinators funded through a community develop-ment grant, SCWHC outreach workers, and "apprentices" trained in counsel-ing, education, and advocacy. Within its first months, community members and workers alike considered it a "huge success."[104] Although rooted in the efforts of the SCWHC and the BOP, the broad focus of La Familia made the SCWHC's ongoing relationship to it unclear.

La Familia proved to be a flashpoint within the SCWHC, raising issues of governance and identity politics, plus accusations of racism. Over the next few years, as personal, professional, and political relationships within the SCWHC became increasingly strained, Latinx members of the SCWHC, who believed they had created La Familia and enabled it to thrive, began to see it as theirs. This sense of ownership increased as tensions within the SCWHC grew, and feelings of "us versus them" increased. La Familia eventually severed its ties with the SCWHC in 1985 and 1986, joining forces with the Beach Flats Community Center.[105] In 2022, both of these programs were part of Nueva Vista Community Resources, a program of Community Bridges. The health clinic at La Familia closed along the way.

Health Center Rebirth

The outreach efforts launched by the SCWHC were a partial success—more Latinas did come to the health center for services. But the departure of La Familia from the center's oversight suggests that the "integrated" organization failed to operate as one. As described above, the Latinas who created La Familia saw it as their project rather than the SCWHC's.[106] Nevertheless, building an organization more sensitive to the needs of women of color in the community, especially Latinas, demanded a new structure for its continued survival and possible success.

The SCWHC was born again on a radically different foundation. In 1984, the organization was in trouble. It faced many economic challenges; many of its members, exhausted, angry, and resentful, had quit. The remaining members understood that survival required significant change. In 1984, they recruited Ciel Benedetto to serve as the center's administrator. Reflecting the SCWHC's acquiescence to a hierarchical governance model, Benedetto quickly became executive director.[107]

Benedetto, a New York City native, had moved to Santa Cruz for college in 1974. Although she identified as a feminist, earned a degree in women's studies, and participated in several health-related projects, she had never been especially interested in the SCWHC. It had struck her as too focused on white women's issues and inadequately concerned about women most vulnerable to medical abuse and least able to access health care. Immediately after graduation, Benedetto worked for Interim, a Monterey County agency that sought to create alternatives to psychiatric institutionalization. The politics of the work appealed to her, but after five years, she could no longer bear witness to society's failure to adequately care for the mentally ill. She was looking for a change.[108]

When Benedetto came on board, the SCWHC lacked money, staff, and a clear mission. Nevertheless, Benedetto had a vision. She set two linked goals: she vowed to serve sick women, moving away from the primary focus on reproductive health, and she promised to further diversify the clientele. As she put it in her interview, "If you hire me, I will guarantee you that the women who come here will represent our community." She was especially committed to serving women who had the fewest options.[109]

Benedetto made good on her promises. Under her watch, the Santa Cruz Women's Health Center transformed from a small, collectively governed organization with a reproductive health clinic to a health institution with a budget of several million dollars. It expanded the scope of its practice, moving first into primary care and eventually into prenatal care and pediatrics. By 1995, the Santa Cruz Women's Health Center boasted a scope of practice from "newborns to seniors." As its services expanded, the Santa Cruz Women's Health Center intensified its efforts to reach the most medically underserved communities. To serve the Latina community in particular, it began to publish all its materials in Spanish and English, and it hired a nearly completely bilingual staff.[110]

Although the health center thrived, the collective overseeing its management did not. It never officially dissolved, but neither did it survive. In retrospect, many of the former SCWHC members argued that diversity itself forced the dissolution of the collective. Peugh, for example, claimed that there was something about the "collective process and some of the . . . commonality that allowed us to have collective process that just seemed insurmountable" with a more diverse group. In her opinion, if the SCWHC hoped "to include people that . . . had really different backgrounds," the members had to let the collective go.[111] Reyes, however, rejected this analysis of the decline of the collective, seeing it as a claim that people from different backgrounds couldn't sit down, talk with each other, and forge policies amenable to all. She believed that with education and shared goals, collective decision-making could continue, perhaps thrive, with any group of people. "You always have the choice of doing it or not doing it," Reyes declared. She suspected that former members blamed diversity for the end of the collective out of frustration that their ability to lead the organization "their way" dissolved.[112] Benedetto, who arrived at the Santa Cruz Women's Health Center after the collective had de facto dissolved, attributed its decline not to racial and ethnic diversity but a lack of political cohesion: "The spoke of the wheel was a certain brand of feminism at the time that held the nucleus." She noted that as the center diversified, not all the new women shared the founders' political vision and commitments. Instead, they brought with them different priorities, drawn from their identities or their personal experiences. According to Benedetto, the loss of the "nucleus," the singular political purpose, forced the dissolution of the collective.[113] In her interpretation, the collective could not survive the loss of political homogeneity.

While Marilyn Marzell felt overwhelmed by the effort to make the Santa Cruz Women's Health Center a welcoming place for a more diverse group of women, she was buoyed by the voice of the feminist civil rights activist

Bernice Reagon reminding her that the struggle ahead "ain't easy, it's hard."[114] By invoking Reagon, Marzell demonstrated her understanding that the journey would challenge the collective members personally and politically and test their commitment to meeting the health needs of all the women in the community. Reagon, who frequently worked in multiracial and multiethnic coalitions, has said, "Wherever women gather together it is not necessarily nurturing. It is coalition building. And if you feel the strain, you may be doing some good work."[115]

The Santa Cruz Women's Health *Collective* was clearly strained, perhaps broken, by its efforts to made good on its commitment to racial and ethnic inclusion. Its commitment forced radical changes to the SCWHC's mission, structure, and politics. Most significantly, the SCWHC abandoned its collective structure—a hallmark of its original vision to promote a politics of women's liberation. The surviving Santa Cruz Women's Health *Center* became a different kind of feminist enterprise, less committed to challenging patriarchy, contesting medicine as usual, and empowering women through self-help praxis. The center emerged as a feminist-inspired, comprehensive, explicitly multicultural health clinic, poised to identify and meet the health needs of the most marginalized members of the community.

In the 1970s, many feminists founded health clinics to demonstrate their vision for health care that met women's physical needs for medical care and reproductive control; some of these activists also believed that feminist health care could empower women to take control of their lives. The mostly white women who founded and nurtured these clinics believed that their offerings benefited all women. Their commitment to their vision sometimes left them unable to see why some women—especially women of color—viewed many feminist health clinics as white establishments for white women. To broaden their clinic's appeal, the white women running the clinics needed to identify and jettison the aspects of their original vision that discouraged the participation of a diverse group of women, both as clients and as workers. Moreover, white women in these clinics needed to confront and address their attachment to power and their own racism.

This process required struggle. To their credit, health activists, white women and women of color, frequently struggled together to create a more inclusive movement anchored by more diverse institutions. Surely many activists gave up—some finding white women's racism intractable, others because they could not abide the denigration of their life's work. But because women stayed despite their anger, resentment, and disappointment and new women with different commitments came on board, some feminist health organizations, including some clinics, transformed their structures and their missions to better meet the needs of various women in their communities. In the process, they abandoned some of their early animating commitments and guiding aspirations. The speculum no longer represented a pathway to women's empowerment and liberation. Instead, it promised access to health care for women who had the fewest options and the most pressing needs.

Conclusion

This book offers a history of women who imagined a world where women could control their bodies and the institutions they built to bring their vision to life. It is a history of dreams, fury, labor, identity, community, and compromise. It captures moments of radical possibility and highlights examples of limited vision. It's a history of women who vowed to make a difference, who left an enduring legacy, who came up short. It's a history of grit, determination, struggle, loss, and achievement. Outraged by their own ignorance and their inability to control their bodies, women across the country and beyond launched hundreds of political projects centered on women's health and reproduction. They peered inside their bodies, shared their deepest hurts, extracted their menses, developed feminist knowledge, and founded women's clinics. They created a movement animated by the belief that women could be liberated by wresting control of their bodies from the forces of patriarchal oppression.

The women of the movement promoted diverse goals. Some feminist health activists dared to imagine that women could foment a revolution. They overcame the obstacles that blocked women's access to knowledge about and control over their bodies—deference to medical authority, internalized bodily shame, acquiescence to male prerogatives—in their quest for female empowerment and women's liberation. They did not reject medicine outright, but they denounced its outsize role in healthy women's lives and the sexism that undergirded its knowledge production and practice. Other activists did not see health as the entry point to liberation or revolution. They worked to improve medicine itself, making it less sexist and homophobic and more responsive to its female patients and practitioners. They developed a woman-centered approach to medicine that gave women more input into their own care. Still others were "sick and tired of being sick and tired," but they didn't view medicine as either the primary problem or the most promising solution. They gathered together to identify and acknowledge the physical and mental harms of racist oppression in their quest for personal well-being and community health.

"Self-help" became a central practice for many health feminists. Building on longstanding traditions of self-care and community caretaking, feminist health activists developed new self-help strategies to meet their political and health needs. Some adopted the speculum—a medical tool associated with women's passivity and isolation—as an implement for women's empowerment and female bonding. It symbolized bodily self-determination in response to medical surveillance and control. For other women, especially Black women, self-help indicated a practice of self-disclosure and support to heal the wounds inflicted by racist oppression. Both models of self-help relied on women's shared knowledge, experiences, and vulnerability to empower each other and to forge bonds of sisterhood.

Some feminists established clinics to promote the value of self-help approaches and to meet women's health needs. The history of these clinics demonstrates how activists enacted their politics through health care practices. It also illuminates how a national movement functioned in local communities. In clinic spaces, self-help proved difficult to sustain, fitting uncomfortably alongside state funding requirements and medical practice protocols. In many feminist health centers, clinical services eroded the very model that activists, especially clinic founders, hoped to enact. The demands of clinical services also frequently overwhelmed activists and displaced their commitment to broader political projects. As services took center stage because of community demand and financial need, some activists wondered whether they were merely offering health services or whether they were facilitating social change; for others, improved health care and increased access to it was always their primary goal.

Abortion politics loomed large in the feminist health movement. While abortion's prominence discouraged some women from identifying with the movement, for many, access to safe, affordable, compassionate abortion undergirded women's liberation. Without the ability to terminate a pregnancy, women could not control their lives. Feminist health activists provided illegal abortions in Chicago, publicized menstrual extraction, and referred women to reliable providers. They also opened and nurtured feminist abortion clinics. Like clinics inspired by feminist self-help, a specifically feminist abortion provision proved difficult to sustain—at least, as its proponents envisioned it. Requiring collaboration with the state for funding and with physicians for services, clinic survival demanded that activists jettison some of their guiding principles. Feminist abortion care, once imagined as a challenge to medical care as usual, became increasingly similar to it. And yet, providing abortion care in a context of increasing antiabortion violence and legislation became an increasingly vital feminist practice.

As some health feminists struggled to enact their self-help politics within health care institutions regulated by the state, others complained that the movement's focus on women as a universal category created a movement primarily attuned to middle-class, white, straight women's needs, ignoring other groups of women. Lesbians and women of color pushed to expand the scope of the movement. Some lesbian health activists insisted that a feminist health movement focused primarily on "women" could never meet the needs of lesbians. They urged the movement to incorporate a critique of homophobia and heterosexism into the feminist critique of medical care. Feminist clinics across the country also developed lesbian-specific services. And yet, some lesbians felt diminished by the significant time and energy focused on the reproductive concerns of straight women; they directed their own activism toward creating a movement to identify lesbian health needs and to provide health services to the underserved lesbian community.

Women of color participated in the women's health movement from the beginning, discovering self-exam and directing women's health clinics. These activists believed that the movement worked for them, but they also prodded their communities and organizations to pay more attention to women's different experiences with illness, medicine, and oppression. They pushed their organizations to diversify. Other women of color—in particular, Black women working with new conceptions of self-help—developed understandings of health and illness directly connected to their experiences as Black women under conditions of oppression. Their pathway to health required that they share their wounds in order to change their lives.

By exploring the history of the women's health movement over four decades and beyond, we can see how the movement and the institutions it created transformed, responding to pressures and divisions within the movement and challenges external to it. This history shows how activists reconsidered their goals when confronted by increasingly conservative politics, decreasing state support, newly emboldened opposition, and changing community needs. Change left some activists disappointed, others betrayed, and still others gratified. But overall, feminist health activists responded to their changing circumstances ultimately by focusing their efforts on women and other people with the fewest health options.

The women's health movement highlighted the need for and the prom-

ise of the larger feminist movement. Activists argued that for women to secure their liberation, they needed to wrest control of their bodies, especially
their reproduction, from men: fathers, husbands, legislators, physicians. The
movement succeeded on many levels. It reclaimed, both rhetorically and in
practice, women's bodies from medical control and physician's gaze, giving
women permission and access to explore their own bodies and those of their
"sisters." It encouraged women to overcome bodily shame and demand bodily
autonomy as every woman's right. The movement nurtured new forms of
feminist knowledge, encouraging activists to examine medical information
with a critical eye and to create their own expertise through shared experience and practice. It developed new forms of self-help to empower women
to fight for their wellness and their liberation. It laid claim to a sisterhood
of common purpose and experience that brought women—some women—
together to protest and to strategize. It built brick-and-mortar institutions to
provide models of feminist health care and to meet the health needs of local
communities. In sum, it generated ideas, practices, and demands about reproductive justice and equitable health care that are yet unmet but continue
to guide health activism.

Legacies

In the fifty years since activists launched a movement to improve women's
health care, increase women's control over their bodies, and liberate women
from patriarchal oppression, the issues surrounding women's health have
changed significantly. Medicine, for example, is no longer a male bastion.
While only 7 percent of physicians were women in 1970, by 2019, more than
50 percent of medical students were female. In some fields—obstetrics and
gynecology and pediatrics, for example—women constitute the majority of
practitioners. In 1990, the National Institutes of Health established the Office of Research on Women's Health, signaling federal interest in women's
health issues. Women's health centers, designed to address women's health
needs including and beyond reproduction, have become commonplace in US
cities. The Affordable Care Act (ACA), passed by Congress in 2010, required
that health insurance plans provide pregnancy, maternity, and newborn care,
as well as preventative health screenings.[1]

From many angles, these represent significant landmarks in women's
health and can be understood as legacies of the women's health movement.
Nevertheless, many of these achievements undermine the primary goals of
many feminist activists. Some health activists denied that medicine could be

changed from within, even by women physicians. As outsiders to the medical establishment, they challenged medical prerogatives and the widespread medicalization of women's bodies, demanding less medical involvement in healthy women's lives rather than more. Women's health centers, advertised as sensitive to women's health needs, have co-opted a feminist vision of empowerment and deployed it to increase hospital revenue and medical access to (insured) women's bodies.[2] The ACA increased women's access to health care, especially preventative and reproductive health care. However, it blunted the feminist challenge to routine medical surveillance, overtreatment, and the increased profitability of screening exams. The feminist critique of medicine did not disappear with the increased access to health care.

Racial health inequities persist. The mortality rate for Black infants is more than twice as high as the mortality rate for white infants. The gap between Black and white maternal mortality is even more galling, with Black women dying of pregnancy-related causes three or four times as often as white women.[3] Black women also experience more heart disease, diabetes, and hypertension than white women. Access to health care will not eliminate these markers of inequality. As long as racist oppression operates through Black bodies, the ACA will not secure well-being.

The right to discriminate against trans patients in health care remains a political battleground. Under the Obama administration, the ACA prohibited discrimination based on gender identity. The Trump administration overturned this interpretation, claiming that the law's provision prohibiting discrimination based on "race, color, national origin, sex, and/or disability" was never meant to apply to gender identity. In May 2021, the Biden administration reversed the policy again, reinstating health care protections for transgender individuals. Access to health care for trans people hinges on political winds.[4]

In June 2022, the Supreme Court decision *Dobbs v. Jackson Women's Health Organization* overturned *Roe v. Wade* and left abortion regulations up to the states. *Dobbs* followed decades of successful efforts to erode legal, economic, and physical access to abortion.[5] This chilling ruling, denying women's and other people's right to bodily autonomy, highlights the continued power of misogyny and women's continuing struggle to control their lives.

And yet, this history of the feminist health movement should be read as evidence that determination, rage, and vision can create profound change. These activists believed they deserved better. They imagined new ways to know their bodies, control their reproduction, and secure their health outside of medical control. They built clinics to provide feminist models of health care, and they responded to demands for greater inclusion. As we consider the future of reproductive autonomy for women and other people in the wake of the *Dobbs* decision, this history gives me hope that the next generation of activists will envision and enact still new approaches to health, knowledge, and being with each other. Perhaps they will "change the world entire."[6]

Acknowledgments

Over the years I worked on this book, I accrued many debts. I am pleased to have the opportunity to acknowledge some of them and to publicly offer my gratitude.

This book relied on research and other forms of support provided by graduate students in the Departments of History; History of Science, Medicine, and Technology; and Gender and Women's Studies at University of Wisconsin–Madison. Bridget Collins, Bennet Goldstein, Scott Prinster, and Kathleen Robinson provided some of the initial research, digging into the feminist press using microfilm collections, print journals, and eventually online resources. Isobel Bloom joined this project at the end, and she cheerfully threw herself into cleaning up loose ends. Several other graduate students transcribed the oral histories—often recorded in coffee shops with country music, crying children, and coffee grinders blaring in the background. These included Ariel Baumwell, Jocelyn Bosley, Vicki Fama, Judith Kaplan, and Anna Piechowski. Each transcriber did an outstanding job with a challenging task.

Two graduate assistants deserve special recognition. Irene Toro Martinez helped me plan and execute three research trips after I thought that my research for this book was complete. She tracked down sources and people in San Francisco, Washington, DC, and New York City. She helped me design interview questions, taught me about AirDrop, and debriefed with me after interviews. A wonderful travel companion, Irene discovered places to see and meals to eat in these cities after the workday was over. Chapters 7 and 8 were especially influenced by her efforts. Emma Wathen worked on this project for nearly a year. She researched a variety of topics, interpreted statistical tables, provided editorial comments, and secured permissions. Emma also provided superb copyediting, improving my prose, checking my quotations, and correcting my endnotes. I was lucky to have them on my team.

Sabrina Jones, an undergraduate student at Humboldt State University, also provided research assistance. When I reached out to Professor Suzanne Pasztor, the chair of the History Department at HSU, asking if she could recommend a student researcher, she quickly identified Sabrina as an ideal candidate. Sabrina performed the research with creativity, giving me access to sources that enlivened this history.

Many scholars provided guidance on this book. Two anonymous reviewers of the proposal and the first draft provided encouragement and valuable commentary, sharing generously their time and expertise. The History Department at UW–Madison funded a book workshop in the fall of 2021. Susan Cahn, Finn Enke, Pernille Ipsen, Naomi Rogers, and Johanna Schoen read the manuscript, offered interpretive and structural advice, and clarified my approach. Their feedback and support reinvigorated my own enthusiasm for the project and helped me bring it home. This was a big ask, and I am grateful.

Colleagues at UW–Madison in the Departments of Gender and Women's Studies; History of Science, Medicine, and Technology; and History have listened to bits of this history over many years, and they have been curious, enthusiastic, and helpful. Comments from Tom Broman, Pablo Gomez, Florence Hsia, Emer Lucey, and Karen Walloch were especially generative. Conversations with scholars in the history of medicine community over the years, especially Charlotte Borst, Chris Crenner, Janet Golden, Jeremy Greene, Wendy Kline, Leslie Reagan, Susan Reverby, Naomi Rogers, Johanna Schoen, Elizabeth Toon, Arlene Tuchman, and Elizabeth Watkins have advanced and sharpened my ideas. Johanna in particular has cheered this project on for years, inviting me to share my work at interdisciplinary workshops, providing comments on individual chapters, and pushing me to get it done. Judy Leavitt provided invaluable feedback and support from the very beginning. Finally, I benefited from time spent as a Summer Humanities Fellow, a program of the Institute for Research in the Humanities. Conversations with program director Steve Nadler and the fellows Charo D'Etcheverry, Paola Hernandez, Daniel Kapust, Paul Kelleher, and Katrina Thompson developed new ideas and provided intellectual community.

This project allowed me to talk with many of the health activists featured in this history, and others whose stories influenced the history I tell. Most people responded enthusiastically to my requests for interviews and connected me with other people to meet. These people shared the struggles, triumphs, and disappointments that came with attempting to change the world. I was impressed with their candor, passion, and introspection. In addition to sharing their stories, they fed me dinner, gave me a place to stay, showed me the sights, and supported my efforts. Norman Bell, Carol Downer, Mary Lisbon, Val Loeffler, Loretta Mears, Kater Pollock, Joan Waitkevicz, and Linda Wilshusen also gave me documents to keep or copy. Teri McGinnis, then of Lyon-Martin Health Services, and Shauna Heckert of Women's Health Specialists, Chico, gave me access to administrative clinic records. These stories and sources made this history possible.

This project occasionally felt stalled, especially as I took on administrative work. At a crucial time, Lynn Nyhart insisted I share my work in public—work that did not yet exist—to jumpstart the project. So I did. Lynn also provided valuable feedback on several chapters. More recently, Claire Wendland has become my writing partner. Her disciplined approach to making time for her own scholarship has helped me make time for my own. We cheered each other's progress and encouraged each other after difficult days. Claire also provided fresh eyes, productive conversations, and thoughtful suggestions in the last weeks of this project. She kept me moving forward.

Funding for research came from the University of Wisconsin–Madison through an Evjue-Bascom Professorship in Gender and Women's Studies, and a Vilas Associates award. Support was also provided by the UW–Madison Office of the Vice Chancellor for Research and Graduate Education with funding from the Wisconsin Alumni Research Foundation. A Simon Visiting Professorship in the Centre for the History of Science, Technology and Medicine in 2010 gave me time to think about the big picture and provided new audiences for my ideas. Ten years later, a Feminist Scholars Fellowship from the Center for Research in Gender and Women at UW–Madison allowed me to finally produce a draft of the manuscript. The project also benefited from travel grants provided by the Schlesinger Library at Radcliffe and the Sophia Smith Collection at Smith College.

Some of this work has been published in earlier form. Parts of chapters 2 and 4 first appeared in "The Best Prescription for Women's Health: Feminist Approaches to Well-Woman Care," in *Prescribed: Writing, Filling, Using, and Abusing the Prescription in Modern America*, ed. Jeremy A. Greene and Elizabeth Siegel Watkins, 134–56. © 2012 The Johns Hopkins University Press. Reprinted with permission of Johns Hopkins University Press. A portion of chapter 5 also appeared in "Medicine and Health for Sexual Minorities," in *International Encyclopedia of the Social & Behavioral Sciences* (Elsevier, 2015) 110–17. Reprinted with permission.

At the University of Chicago Press, Karen Merikangas Darling has been quietly in my corner on this book for nearly decade, encouraging me and this project even when it seemed like it might never be finished. Thanks also to

Fabiola Enríquez for managing the early manuscript and to Johanna Rosen-bohm for her careful copyedits and thoughtful suggestions in its latter stages.

Librarians and archivists helped me track down a range of difficult to find sources. They were especially valuable at the Sophia Smith Collection of Women History, the Schlesinger Library, the Lesbian Herstory Archives, the LGBT Historical Society, the Sallie Bingham Center for Women's History and Culture, the Iowa Women's Archives of the University of Iowa Libraries, and the Archives of Labor and Urban Affairs at the Walter P. Reuther Library.

During my first year of graduate school, I realized that the history of celestial motion was not my passion. I panicked. Looking for a new place to land, I enrolled in a class ostensibly outside my historical interests, Women and Health in American History. Clearly a product of the women's health movement, this course changed the trajectory of my life. It led me to a career writing and teaching history at the intersection of health and gender. It also led me to Judith Walzer Leavitt, my dissertation advisor, colleague, and friend, whose pathbreaking scholarship shaped the field. Shortly after I discovered the history of women's health, I became a teaching assistant for another course inspired by the women's health movement, Women and Their Bodies in Health and Disease. This course showed me that people, especially women, remain hungry for information about their bodies. Teaching this course also introduced me to Mariamne Whatley and Nancy Worcester, whose activism, teaching, and scholarship continued the work of the movement. I dedicate this book to Judy, Mariamne, and Nancy.

Friends and family have engaged with this project and distracted me from it. Finn Enke, Nan Enstad, Mary Moore, Claire Wendland have been friends for years; during the epidemic they became a lifeline. Before and during the epidemic, Carrie Kruse and Ellen Pryor nudged me outside. Lisa Tetrault provided a weeklong writing retreat in Pittsburgh in the summer of 2019; COVID-19 ruined our plans for 2020. Although Sarah Pfatteicher is no longer my belay partner, her friendship continues to sustain me. My brother Bob Houck introduced me to some of the activists in Arcata; my sisters Emily Houck and Susan Houck gave me a place to stay during research visits in Northern California. My siblings connect me to my California home now that my parents are gone.

Lisa Saywell has been the center of it all for more than thirty years. She has supported this project in countless ways. The life we have built together, our shared joys, sorrows, and journeys, provides the foundation for everything beyond it.

Abbreviations

Archives

Materials from the archival collections listed below are cited in the footnotes using the following abbreviations:

A A W O : Alliance Against Women's Oppression records, Sophia Smith Collection of Women's History, SSC-MS-00699, Smith College Special Collections, Northampton, Massachusetts

A F W H C : [Atlanta] Feminist Women's Health Center records, 1973–2003, Sallie Bingham Center for Women's History and Culture, Duke University

A L F A : Atlanta Lesbian Feminist Alliance (ALFA) Archives, David M. Rubenstein Rare Book & Manuscript Library, Duke University

B W H B C : Records of the Boston Women's Health Book Collective, 1905–2003, Schlesinger Library, Radcliffe Institute

B W H I R : Black Women's Health Imperative records, Sophia Smith Collection, SSC-MS-00487, Smith College Special Collections

D F W H C : Detroit Feminist Women's Health Center records, Walter P. Reuther Library, Wayne State University

E G C : Emma Goldman Clinic (Iowa City, Iowa) records, Iowa Women's Archives, University of Iowa Libraries

F C : Femina Collection, McCormick Library of Special Collections and University Archives, Northwestern University

F W H C R : Feminist Women's Health Center records, 1973–2003 and undated, David M. Rubenstein Rare Book & Manuscript Library, Duke University

I G I C : International Gay Information Center ephemera files—Organizations, Manuscripts and Archives Division, New York Public Library

L H A : Lesbian Herstory Archives, New York City

R M P : Records of the Mautner Project, 1989–2010, Schlesinger Library, Radcliff Institute

R O S S   P A P E R S : Loretta J. Ross Papers, Sophia Smith Collection, SSC-MS-00504, Smith College

V F O H P : Voices of Feminism Oral History Project, Sophia Smith Collection, Smith College Special Collections

WCHC: Records of the Women's Community Health Center, Schlesinger Library, Radcliffe Institute

WHAM: WHAM! (Women's Health Action and Mobilization) records, Tamiment Library and Robert F. Wagner Labor Archives, New York University

WHRC: Women's History Research Center, *Women and/in Health* (Berkeley: Women's History Research Center, 1975), microfilm

Collections

All the people and organizations in the list below generously provided materials from their personal collections. Materials from these personal collections are cited in the footnotes using the following abbreviations:

CHICO FWHC COLLECTION: Chico Feminist Women's Health Center

DOWNER COLLECTION: Carol Downer

LISBON COLLECTION: Mary Lisbon

LMHS COLLECTION: Lyon-Martin Health Services

MEARS COLLECTION: Loretta Mears

WAITKEVICZ COLLECTION: Joan Waitkevicz

WILSHUSEN COLLECTION: Linda Wilshusen

Notes

Introduction

1. Margarita Landazuri, "Self Help," *Off Our Backs*, December 1971, 18.

2. For speculum quote, see "What Is a Free Clinic? Women in Imperial Beach," *Goodbye to All That* [San Diego], January/February 1973, 13. See also Evalyn S. Gendel, "It's Your Body, Not Your Doctor's," *Redbook*, March 1974, 88–89, 166; "Are Our Doctors Pigs?," *Rat*, June 19, 1970, 12; Stephanie Allan, "Some Horror Stories," *People's World*, September 1974, 7; Shirley McClure, "A Woman-Controlled Clinic: The Chico Feminist Women's Health Center," *Wildcat*, February 27, 1975, 12; and Sheryl Burt Ruzek, *The Women's Health Movement: Feminist Alternatives to Medical Control* (New York: Praeger, 1978).

3. Jonathan Engel, *Poor People's Medicine: Medicaid and American Charity Care since 1965* (Durham, NC: Duke University Press, 2006).

4. Jennifer Nelson, *Women of Color and the Reproductive Rights Movement* (New York: New York University Press, 2003); Rebecca M. Kluchin, *Fit to Be Tied: Sterilization and Reproductive Rights in America, 1950–1980* (New Brunswick, NJ: Rutgers University Press, 2009); Johanna Schoen, *Choice and Coercion: Birth Control, Sterilization, and Abortion in Public Health and Welfare* (Chapel Hill: University of North Carolina Press, 2005).

5. Beth Bailey, "Prescribing the Pill: Politics, Culture, and the Sexual Revolution in America's Heartland," *Journal of Social History* 30, no. 4 (Summer 1997): 827–56; Elizabeth Siegel Watkins, *On the Pill: A Social History of Oral Contraceptives, 1950–1970* (Baltimore: Johns Hopkins University Press, 1998). See also Barbara Seaman, *The Doctor's Case against the Pill* (New York: P. H. Wyden, 1969).

6. Leslie J. Reagan, *When Abortion Was a Crime: Women, Medicine, and the Law in the United States, 1867–1973* (Berkeley: University of California Press, 1997).

7. Courtni E. Molnar, "'Has the Millennium Yet Dawned?': A History of Attitudes toward Pregnant Workers in America," *Michigan Journal of Gender and Law* 12, no. 1 (2005): 163–87.

8. Mary Roth Walsh, *"Doctors Wanted: No Women Need Apply": Sexual Barriers in the Medical Profession, 1835–1975* (New Haven, CT: Yale University Press, 1977); Regina Markell Morantz-Sanchez, *Sympathy and Science: Women Physicians in American Medicine* (New York: Oxford University Press, 1985).

9. Barron H. Lerner, *The Breast Cancer Wars: Hope, Fear, and the Pursuit of a Cure in Twentieth-Century America* (New York: Oxford University Press, 2001); Ellen Leopold, *A Darker*

Ribbon: Breast Cancer, Women, and Their Doctors in the Twentieth Century (Boston: Beacon Press, 1999).

10. John Whyte and Lisa Capaldini, "Treating the Lesbian or Gay Patient," *Delaware Medical Journal* 52, no. 5 (May 1980): 271–80; Ronald Bayer, *Homosexuality and American Psychiatry: The Politics of Diagnosis* (1981; repr., Princeton, NJ: Princeton University Press, 1987).

11. Elizabeth Bucar and Finn Enke, "Unlikely Sex Change Capitals of the World: Trinidad, United States, and Tehran, Iran, as Twin Yardsticks of Homonormative Liberalism," *Feminist Studies* 37, no. 2 (Summer 2011): 301–28; Leslie Feinberg, "Trans Health Crisis: For Us It's Life or Death," *American Journal of Public Health* 91, no. 6 (June 2001): 897–900; Joanne J. Meyerowitz, *How Sex Changed: A History of Transsexuality in the United States* (Cambridge, MA: Harvard University Press, 2002); Charalampos Siotos, Paula M. Neira, Brandyn D. Lau, Jill P. Stone, James Page, Gedge D. Rosson, and Devin Coon, "Origins of Gender Affirmation Surgery: The History of the First Gender Identity Clinic in the United States at Johns Hopkins," *Annals of Plastic Surgery* 83, no. 2 (August 2019): 132–36.

12. Citizens Board of Inquiry into Health Services for Americans, *Heal Your Self*, 2nd ed. (Washington, DC: American Public Health Association, 1972), 127. See also Naomi Rogers, "'Caution: The AMA May Be Hazardous to Your Health': The Student Health Organizations (SHO) and American Medicine, 1965–1970," *Radical History Review* 2001, no. 80 (Spring 2001): 5–34.

13. Bonnie Lefkowitz, *Community Health Centers: A Movement and the People Who Made It Happen* (New Brunswick, NJ: Rutgers University Press, 2007); Alondra Nelson, *Body and Soul: The Black Panther Party and the Fight against Medical Discrimination* (Minneapolis: University of Minnesota Press, 2011).

14. Barbara Ehrenreich and Deirdre English, *Complaints and Disorders: The Sexual Politics of Sickness*, 2nd ed. (New York: Feminist Press, 2011), 159, quoted in Jennifer Nelson, *More Than Medicine: A History of the Feminist Women's Health Movement* (New York: New York University Press, 2015), 116.

15. Wendy Kline, *Bodies of Knowledge: Sexuality, Reproduction, and Women's Health in the Second Wave* (Chicago: University of Chicago Press, 2010), 4.

16. Susan M. Reverby, "Thinking through the Body and the Body Politic: Feminism, History, and Health-Care Policy in the United States," in *Women, Health, and Nation: Canada and the United States since 1945*, ed. Georgina Feldberg, Molly Ladd-Taylor, and Kathryn McPherson (Montreal: McGill-Queen's University Press, 2003), 411.

17. See, for example, Sandra Morgen, *Into Our Own Hands: The Women's Health Movement in the United States, 1969–1990* (New Brunswick, NJ: Rutgers University Press, 2002); Nelson, *More Than Medicine*; Nelson, *Women of Color*; Kluchin, *Fit to Be Tied*; Hannah Dudley-Shotwell, *Revolutionizing Women's Healthcare: The Feminist Self-Help Movement in America* (New Brunswick, NJ: Rutgers University Press, 2020); and Michelle Murphy, *Seizing the Means of Reproduction: Entanglements of Feminism, Health, and Technoscience* (Durham, NC: Duke University Press, 2012).

18. Helen Marieskind, "The Women's Health Movement," *International Journal of Health Sciences* 5, no. 2 (April 1975): 218.

19. Michelle Murphy uses the phrase *traveling technology* to describe menstrual extraction. See Murphy, *Seizing the Means*, 150–76.

20. Myra Marx Ferree and Patricia Yancey Martin, eds., *Feminist Organizations: Harvest of the New Women's Movement* (Philadelphia: Temple University Press, 1995), 4.

NOTES TO PAGES 8–10

21. Getting an exact count is difficult for a variety of reasons. At any point in time, it is un-clear exactly what should be considered a clinic and what should be considered feminist. One historian counted at least forty-two feminist clinics in nineteen states in 1975; using someone else's data, she counted fifteen in 2010. Daphne Spain, *Constructive Feminism: Women's Spaces and Women's Rights in the American City* (Ithaca, NY: Cornell University Press, 2016), 138.

22. Alice Echols, *Daring to Be Bad: Radical Feminism in America, 1967–1975* (Minneapo-lis: University of Minneapolis Press, 1989); Sara M. Evans, *Tidal Wave: How Women Changed America at Century's End* (New York: Free Press, 2003); Estelle B. Freedman, *No Turning Back: The History of Feminism and the Future of Women* (New York: Ballantine Books, 2002); Ruth Rosen, *The World Split Open: How the Modern Women's Movement Changed America* (New York: Viking, 2000). See also Finn Enke, *Finding the Movement: Sexuality, Contested Space, and Femi-nist Activism* (Durham, NC: Duke University Press, 2007); and Stephanie Gilmore, *Groundswell: Grassroots Feminist Activism in Postwar America* (New York: Routledge, 2013). Other histories of modern feminism appear in the chapters below.

23. Early women's rights movements also included advocates who focused on bodily autonomy and control. See, for example, Wendy L. Rouse, *Her Own Hero: The Origins of the Women's Self-Defense Movement* (New York: New York University Press, 2017); April R. Haynes, *Riotous Flesh: Women, Physiology, and the Solitary Vice in Nineteenth-Century America* (Chicago: University of Chicago Press, 2015); Katharina Vester, "Regime Change: Gender, Class, and the Invention of Dieting in Post-bellum America," *Journal of Social History* 44, no. 1 (Fall 2010): 39–70; and Judith Walzer Leavitt, "Birthing and Anesthesia: The Debate over Twilight Sleep," in *Mothers & Motherhood: Readings in American History*, ed. Rima D. Apple and Janet Golden (Columbus: Ohio State University Press, 1997), 242–58.

24. Jael Silliman, Marlene Gerber Fried, Loretta Ross, and Elena R. Gutiérrez, *Undivided Rights: Women of Color Organize for Reproductive Justice* (Cambridge, MA: South End Press, 2004); Nelson, *Women of Color*; Wendy Kline, *Coming Home: How Midwives Changed Birth* (New York: Oxford University Press, 2019); Schoen, *Choice and Coercion*; Kluchin, *Fit to Be Tied*.

25. Catherine O. Jacquet, *The Injustices of Rape: How Activists Responded to Sexual Violence, 1950–1980* (Chapel Hill: University of North Carolina Press, 2019); Danielle L. McGuire, *At the Dark End of the Street: Black Women, Rape, and Resistance—a New History of the Civil Rights Movement from Rosa Parks to the Rise of Black Power* (New York: Knopf, 2010); Susan Brown-miller, *Against Our Will: Men, Women and Rape* (New York: Simon and Schuster, 1975); Del Martin, *Battered Wives* (San Francisco: Glide Publications, 1976).

26. A representative from the Women's Community Health Center (WCHC) in Cambridge, Massachusetts, attended a meeting in 1979 where several feminist organizations considered a united statement on whether "transexuals" were welcome in "women's space." Several of the organizations refused to contribute to the statement on any side of the issue. As far as I could tell, the WCHC refused to articulate a position. Meeting notes, February 2, 1979, MC 512, box 3, folder 2, WCHC.

27. For a discussion of professional activism, see Lisa Levenstein, *They Didn't See Us Coming: The Hidden History of Feminism in the Nineties* (New York: Basic Books, 2020), 79–96.

28. Murphy, *Seizing the Means*; Kline, *Bodies of Knowledge*; Kathy Davis, *The Making of Our Bodies, Ourselves: How Feminism Travels across Borders* (Durham, NC: Duke University Press, 2007); Morgen, *Into Our Own Hands*; Nelson, *More Than Medicine*; Dudley-Shotwell, *Revolu-tionizing Women's Healthcare*.

29. With special thanks to Norman Bell, Carol Downer, Mary Lisbon, Val Leoffler, Loretta Mears, Kater Pollock, Joan Waitkevicz, and Linda Wilshusen.

30. Thanks to Teri McGinnis and Shauna Heckert, respectively.

Chapter One

1. Jean of Mountain Grove, "A Revolutionary Afternoon," *Women's Press*, July/August 1973, 18.

2. Donna J. Haraway, "The Virtual Speculum in the New World Order," *Feminist Review* 55, no. 1 (Spring 1997): 41. Michelle Murphy likewise criticized the rhetorical deployment of the power of seeing: "While appropriating anticolonial discourse, U.S. feminist self-help often remained insensible to the recapitulation of the rhetoric of domination at work in their calls to take possession of their flesh through a conquering gaze." Michelle Murphy, "Immodest Witnessing: The Epistemology of Vaginal Self-Examination in the U.S. Feminist Self-Help Movement," *Feminist Studies* 30, no. 1 (Spring 2004): 137.

3. In *Seizing the Means of Reproduction: Entanglements of Feminism, Health, and Technoscience* (Durham, NC: Duke University Press, 2012), Michelle Murphy focused on the embedded values of the tools and "protocols" of the feminist self-help gynecology movement as promoted by its California advocates. Hannah Dudley-Shotwell also examined feminist self-help, in *Revolutionizing Women's Healthcare: The Feminist Self-Help Movement in America* (New Brunswick, NJ: Rutgers University Press, 2020).

4. Nancy Tomes, *Remaking the American Patient: How Madison Avenue and Modern Medicine Turned Patients into Consumers* (Chapel Hill: University of North Carolina Press, 2016).

5. Merlin Chowkwanyun, "The New Left and Public Health: The Health Policy Advisory Center, Community Organizing, and the Big Business of Health, 1967–1975," *American Journal of Public Health* 101, no. 2 (February 2011): 238–49.

6. Citizens Board of Inquiry into Health Services for Americans, *Heal Your Self*, 2nd ed. (Washington, DC: American Public Health Association, 1972), 127. See also Theodore O. Cron, "A Patients' Revolt: Is It Possible?," *Hospital Progress* 51, no. 10 (October 1970): 69–71. The California Department of Health becomes the Department of Health Services in 1978; in 2007 it splits into the Department of Health Care Services and the Department of Public Health.

7. Ivan Illich, *Medical Nemesis: The Expropriation of Health* (London: Calder and Boyars: 1975), 11. See also Irving Kenneth Zola, "Medicine as an Institution of Social Control," *Sociological Review* 20, no. 4 (November 1972): 487–504.

8. See, for example, Fitzhugh Mullan, *White Coat, Clenched Fist: The Political Education of an American Physician* (New York: Macmillan, 1976); Thomas J. Ward Jr., *Out in the Rural: A Mississippi Health Center and Its War on Poverty* (New York: Oxford University Press, 2017); Naomi Rogers, "'Caution: The AMA May Be Hazardous to Your Health': The Student Health Organizations (SHO) and American Medicine, 1965–1970," *Radical History Review* 2001, no. 80 (Spring 2001): 5–34; David E. Smith, David J. Bentel, and Jerome L. Schwartz, eds., *The Free Clinic: A Community Approach to Health Care and Drug Abuse* (Beloit, WI: Stash Press, 1971); John Dittmer, *The Good Doctors: The Medical Committee for Human Rights and the Struggle for Social Justice in Health Care* (New York: Bloomsbury Press, 2009); and David Barton Smith, *The Power to Heal: Civil Rights, Medicare, and the Struggle to Transform America's Health Care System* (Nashville: Vanderbilt University Press, 2016).

9. For the "smart patient," see Marvin S. Belsky and Leonard Gross, *How to Choose and Use Your Doctor: The Smart Patient's Way to a Longer, Healthier Life* (New York: Arbor House,

1975), 101–29; for the "activated patient," see Keith W. Sehnert and Howard Eisenberg, *How to Be Your Own Doctor—Sometimes* (New York: Grosset and Dunlap, 1975), 1–2; for the "health consumer," see Arthur Levin, *Talk Back to Your Doctor: How to Demand (and Recognize) High-Quality Health Care* (Garden City, NY: Doubleday, 1975), 9. See also Arthur S. Freese, *Managing Your Doctor: How to Get the Best Possible Health Care* (New York: Stein and Day, 1975). For an early and more radical example of the genre, see Arthur Frank and Stuart Frank, *The People's Handbook of Medical Care* (New York: Vintage Books, 1972).

10. Frank and Frank, *People's Handbook of Medical Care*, 3.

11. Lowell S. Levin, Alfred H. Katz, and Erik Holst, *Self-Care: Lay Initiatives in Health* (New York: Prodist, 1976); and Belsky and Gross, *How to Choose Your Doctor*.

12. Belsky and Gross, *How to Choose Your Doctor*, 31.

13. Alfred H. Katz and Eugene I. Bender, *The Strength in Us: Self-Help Groups in the Modern World* (New York: New Viewpoints, 1976); Levin, Katz, and Holst, *Self-Care*, 31–47.

14. Keith W. Sehnert, "The Course for Activated Patients," in *Patient Education: An Inquiry into the State of the Art*, ed. Wendy D. Squyres (New York: Springer, 1980), 194.

15. Boston Women's Health Collective, *Women and Their Bodies: A Course* (Boston: Boston Women's Health Collective, 1970). For the history of *Our Bodies, Ourselves*, see Kathy Davis, *The Making of Our Bodies, Ourselves: How Feminism Travels across Borders* (Durham, NC: Duke University Press, 2007); and Wendy Kline, *Bodies of Knowledge: Sexuality, Reproduction, and Women's Health in the Second Wave* (Chicago: University of Chicago Press, 2010), 9–39.

16. See, for example, Sandra Morgen, *Into Our Own Hands: The Women's Health Movement in the United States, 1969–1990* (New Brunswick, NJ: Rutgers University Press, 2002), 22–26; Jennifer Nelson, *More Than Medicine: A History of the Feminist Women's Health Movement* (New York: New York University Press, 2015), 107–8; and Sheryl Burt Ruzek, *The Women's Health Movement: Feminist Alternatives to Medical Control* (New York: Praeger, 1978), 53–58.

17. Ninia Baehr, *Abortion without Apology: A Radical History for the 1990s* (Boston: South End Press, 1990), 7–20, 21.

18. Carol Downer, "No Stopping: From Pom-Poms to Saving Women's Bodies," *On the Issues Magazine*, October 17, 2011, https://www.womenshealthspecialists.org/health-alerts-for-women/no-stopping-from-pom-poms-to-saving-womens-bodies-by-carol-downer/.

19. Petrinovich and Downer eventually developed separate and perhaps rival approaches to women's reproductive autonomy. In April 1972, Petrinovich opened the Women's Clinic, allegedly the "first clinic run by women" in Los Angeles County. "Staffed by Volunteers: Clinic for Women Only Opens," *Los Angeles Times*, April 26, 1972; Francie Hornstein, letter to the editor, *Lesbian Tide*, July 1973, 20.

20. Baehr, *Abortion without Apology*, 22; Dudley-Shotwell, *Revolutionizing Women's Health-care*.

21. Carol Downer, "Through the Speculum," in *Test-Tube Women: What Future for Motherhood?*, ed. Rita Arditti, Renate Duelli Klein, and Shelley Minden (London: Pandora Press, 1984), 419.

22. Morgen notes that self-help advocates Lolly and Jeanne Hirsch were criticized for repeatedly lionizing Downer in the self-help periodical the *Monthly Extract*. They shrugged off the critique, proudly admitting that they were creating "women heroes for the 20th century." Morgen, *Into Our Own Hands*, 22–26. The original reads, "I hope to create women heroes for the twentieth century." Lolly [Hirsch], letter to Robin Christensen, *Monthly Extract*, January/February 1973, 4.

23. For a conversation on the contingent nature of "public" space in feminist institutions, see Finn Enke, *Finding the Movement: Sexuality, Contested Space, and Feminist Activism* (Durham, NC: Duke University Press, 2007), 177–216, esp. 180.

24. See, for example, "Women's Self-Help Clinic Comes to New Jersey," *NOW News, Central New Jersey Chapter*, November 1971, 19. According to one account, Downer and Rothman presented their "Learn In" to groups including the American Association of University Women, the Long Beach Women's Union, the Western Unitarian Ministers' conference, various NOW chapters in California and beyond, and the Western Psychological Association meeting. "Self-Help Clinics on the Move—and in the Media," *NOW News, Orange County Chapter*, May 1972, 5.

25. [Tallahassee] Feminist Women's Health Center, *Come to Self-Help Clinic*, [1977?], box 4, folder 69: FWHC; pamphlets, n.d., DFWHC; "The Self-Help Clinic Is Going on the Road," [November 1971?], box 61, folder: "Self-Help Tour," AFWHC.

26. For a sense of this slide show, see the color insert in Federation of Feminist Women's Health Centers, *A New View of a Woman's Body: A Fully Illustrated Guide* (New York: Touchstone Books, 1981).

27. For a description of a self-help demonstration at a NOW conference in Atlanta, Georgia, in June 1973, see Gena Corea, *The Hidden Malpractice: How American Medicine Treats Women as Patients and Professionals* (New York: William Morrow, 1977), 260–62.

28. Mary Heath and Ellen [Monahan], interview by the Salt Lake City Feminist Women's Health Center, August 16, 1975. This chapter relies in part on several interviews conducted in the 1970s by women associated with a Feminist Women's Health Center. The originals were in the Downer collection.

29. Anonymous, letter, *Monthly Extract*, August/September 1974, 15.

30. Anonymous, letter from Indiana, *Monthly Extract*, August/September 1975, 11.

31. Jeanne Hirsch, "The Third Eye," in *The Witch's Os*, ed. Millie Alleyn (Stamford, CT: New Moon, 1972), 31.

32. Heath and [Monahan], interview.

33. Laura K. Brown, "The Feminist Women's Health Center at Population Planners' Menstrual Regulation Conference," *Feminist Women's Health Center Report* (1974): 6; Lolly Hirsch, "Second Women-Controlled Women's Health Center Conference," *Monthly Extract*, December 1974/January 1975, 8; Laura Punnett, "The Politics of Menstrual Extraction," in *From Abortion to Reproductive Freedom: Transforming a Movement*, ed. Marlene Gerber Fried (Boston: South End Press, 1990), 107; Frances Hornstein, "An Interview on Women's Health Politics, Part I," *Quest*, Summer 1974, 27–36.

34. Lolly Hirsch, "Practicing Medicine without a License," *Monthly Extract*, July/August 1977, 3.

35. One hallmark of advanced self-help clinics was menstrual extraction. See chapter 3.

36. West Coast Sisters, "Self-Help Clinic," *Everywoman*, July 30, 1971, 6. Reprinted widely in periodicals and in stand-alone form. See, for example, West Coast Sisters, "Do It Yourself," *Great Speckled Bird*, September 13, 1971, 12.

37. Lorraine Rothman, "Self Help Clinic: Paramedic Politics," *NOW News, Central New Jersey Chapter*, March 1972, 8–9.

38. Ina Clausen and Jack Radey, letter to the editor, *People's World*, September 28, 1974, 6.

39. Miriam Frank, "Women's Health," *Fifth Estate*, April 28–May 11, 1973, 7. See also Corea, *Hidden Malpractice*, 261; Elizabeth Sommers, "Self-Help," in *Proceedings for the 1975 Conference*

on *Women and Health* (Boston: self-pub., 1975), 33; Linda Wilshusen, interview with the author, July 1, 2011; and Dudley-Shotwell, *Revolutionizing Women's Healthcare*, 25.

40. See Ruzek, *Women's Health Movement*, 53–54, 109–10.

41. Jody Peugh, interview with the author, September 30, 2011.

42. See Belsky and Gross, *How to Choose Your Doctor*; Freese, *Managing Your Doctor*; and Levin, *Talk Back to Your Doctor*.

43. Barbara Ehrenreich, "Feminism and the Cultural Revolution in Health," in *Proceedings for the 1975 Conference on Women and Health* (Boston: self-pub., 1975), 11. See also Barbara Ehrenreich and Deirdre English, *Complaints and Disorders: The Sexual Politics of Sickness* (New York: Feminist Press, 1973); Corea, *Hidden Malpractice*, 74–103; Ruzek, *Women's Health Movement*, 65–102; Jeanne [Hirsch], "Menstruation/Menstrual Extraction," *Monthly Extract*, January/February 1973, 3; Lolly [Hirsch], letter to Robin Christensen, *Monthly Extract*, January/February 1973, 5; and Alice Wolfson, "Caution: Health Care May Be Hazardous to Your Health," *Up from Under*, May/June 1970, 5–10.

44. [Federation of Feminist Women's Health Centers], "What This Book Is All About" (unpublished manuscript, n.d.), 6, Downer collection.

45. Elizabeth L. Campbell, "Why Self Health?," in *Circle One: A Woman's Beginning Guide to Self Health and Sexuality*, ed. Elizabeth L. Campbell and Vicki Ziegler, 2nd ed. (Colorado Springs, CO: Circle One, 1975), 4.

46. "Feminist Health: Reclaiming Your Body," *Maine Freewomen's Herald*, June/July 1974, 5. See also "Getting into Our Bodies," *Other Woman*, May 19, 1972, 15.

47. West Coast Sisters, "Self-Help Clinic," 6.

48. West Coast Sisters, *Self-Help Clinic Part II*. For the internal explanation of self-help, see, for example, West Coast Sisters, "Self-Help Clinic"; West Coast Sisters, *Self-Help Clinic Part II* (Los Angeles: Peace Press, 1971), in WHRC, reel 1-356; [Tallahassee] Feminist Women's Health Center, *Come to Self-Help Clinic*; and [Los Angeles] Feminist Women's Health Center, "Well Woman Health Care in Woman Controlled Clinics" (unpublished manuscript, 1976), Downer collection. *Self-Help Clinic Part II* has a mysterious publication history. According to a March 1972 NOW central New Jersey chapter newsletter, it was originally published in *Everywoman*. No evidence supports this. Instead, it was reprinted regularly with "Self-Help Clinic" in pamphlet form. For more on self-help gynecology, see Terri Kapsalis, *Public Privates: Performing Gynecology from Both Ends of the Speculum* (Durham, NC: Duke University Press, 1997), 161–82; Murphy, "Immodest Witnessing," 115–47; Murphy, *Seizing the Means*; and Dudley-Shotwell, *Revolutionizing Women's Healthcare*, 11–53.

49. Carol Downer and Ann Shalluck, interview, July 24, 1975, Downer collection.

50. Portland Women's Health Center, excerpts from *A Self-Help Manual for Women*, 1978, in *Self-Help*, National Women's Health Network Resource Guide 7 (Washington, DC: National Women's Health Network, 1980), 9. See also Elizabeth L. Campbell, "Women and Health Care: A Brief Chronicle," in *Circle One: A Woman's Beginning Guide to Self Health and Sexuality*, ed. Elizabeth L. Campbell and Vicki Ziegler, 2nd ed. (Colorado Springs, CO: Circle One, 1975), 4.

51. Pamela Parker Allen, "The Small Group Process," in *Dear Sisters: Dispatches from the Women's Liberation Movement*, ed. Rosalyn Baxandall and Linda Gordon (1969; repr., New York: Basic Books, 2000), 67–72; Janet Norman, "Consciousness-Raising: Self-Help in the Women's Movement," in Alfred H. Katz and Eugene I. Bender, *The Strength in Us: Self-Help Groups in the Modern World* (New York: New Viewpoints, 1976), 166–74.

52. By one source, there were "some 50 clinics" across the country by the end of 1972. I suspect this number is low. "Anne Arundel N.O.W. Sends Donation in Support of Women of Self-Help Clinic," *NOW News, Anne Arundel Chapter*, December 1972, 2.

53. A few examples from 1972 include Ruth and Cheryl, "Help Yourself," *Women's Liberation Newsletter* (San Francisco), May 1972, 9; "Self-Help: Off with the Sheet," *Mother Lode*, Spring 1972, 6–7; "Health Care: Low-Cost, Quality Care, the Right of All People," *Borrowed Times*, November 22, 1972, 14; "Self-Help," *Women's Voices* (Okinawa), [January 1972?], 11–12; Susan Williamson, "Lesbian Weekend," *Gay Liberator* (Detroit), March 1972, 7; "Women's Center Notes," *Joint Issue*, November 16, 1972, 3; and "Self-Help Clinics," *Chicago Seed*, February 1, 1972, 5.

54. This publication lasted into 1978.

55. B. Mitchell, "Self-Help: A Personal View," *WomenWise*, September 30, 1978, 2; West Coast Sisters, *How to Start a Self-Help Clinic* (Los Angeles: Self-Help Clinic One, 1971).

56. "Self-Knowledge—Our Bodies," *Women's Press* (Eugene, Oregon), December 1971, 3; "Women's Clinic," *Women's Press* (Eugene, Oregon), April 1972, 2. See also Judith Byrd, "Self-Help Clinic," *Women's Press* (Eugene, Oregon), April 1972, 6; Kay, "Women's Clinics—Eugene," *Women's Press*, May 1973, 12; "Feminist Health: Reclaiming Your Body," 5; and Frank, "Women's Health," 7.

57. "Self-Health: No More Shit," *Big Mama Rag*, July 1, 1973, 14.

58. Mitchell, "Self-Help," 2.

59. Miriam Frank, "German Self-Help," *Off Our Backs*, July/August 1977, 9.

60. Maud Anne Bracke, *Women and the Reinvention of the Political: Feminism in Italy, 1968–1983* (New York: Routledge, 2014), 106. For more about self-help in Europe, see "European Self-Help Conference," *Off Our Backs*, August/September 1980, 5. See also Christiane Ewert, "New Moon over Berlin?!," *Monthly Extract*, February/March 1976, 5–6.

61. Lorraine Rothman, "Self Help Clinics Start in New Zealand," *Her-Self*, April 1974, 22. A brief discussion of the New Zealand visit appeared as "Our Women Abroad," *Monthly Extract*, February/March 1974, 12.

62. See Hannah Grace Dudley Shotwell, "Empowering the Body: The Evolution of Self-Help in the Women's Health Movement" (PhD diss., University of North Carolina at Greensboro, 2016). For lesbian self-help groups, see "Coming Home: Feminist Self-Help Center," *Lansing Star*, April 15–28, 1976, 1, 9. See also Louise Corbett, "Getting Our Bodies Back: Menopausal Self-Help Groups," *WomenWise*, March 31, 1981, 2; and "Berkeley Women's Health Collective," *Monthly Extract*, September/October, 1976, 18.

63. Helen I. Marieskind, "Helping Oneself to Health," *Social Policy*, September/October 1976, 65; "Self Help: Off with the Sheet," 6–7.

64. West Coast Sisters, *How to Start a Self-Help Clinic, Level II* (Los Angeles: Self-Help Clinic One, 1971), box 62, folder: "Participatory Clinic," AFWHC.

65. Ruzek, *Women's Health Movement*, 188–92. Helen Marieskind disputes the characterization of self-help as largely middle class. Marieskind, "Helping Oneself to Health." This claim rankles the working-class activists in the movement. Shauna Heckert, for example, vociferously denied that she had ever been or ever aspired to be middle class. Shauna Heckert, interview with the author, October 13, 2006.

66. For a discussion of how self-exam and self-help clinics "shore[d] up the unmarked and normalized work of whiteness by unracing themselves," see Murphy, *Seizing the Means*, 41.

67. See Hirsch, "Second Women-Controlled Women's Health Center Conference," 4.

68. Sheryl Burt Ruzek, "Emergent Modes of Utilization: Gynecological Self-Help," in *Nurs-*

ing Dimensions, vol. 7, ed. Karren Kowalski (1977; repr., Wakefield, MA: Nursing Resources, 1979), 76.

69. Michelle Murphy, "Unsettling Care: Troubling Transnational Itineraries of Care in Feminist Health Practice," *Social Studies of Science* 45, no. 5 (October 2015): 720.

70. Ruzek, *Women's Health Movement*, 191. See also Angela Wilson, "Black Women's Health," *HealthRight*, Winter 1976–77, 1, 6.

71. See, for example, Jael Silliman, Marlene Gerber Fried, Loretta Ross, and Elena R. Gutiérrez, *Undivided Rights: Women of Color Organize for Reproductive Justice* (Cambridge, MA: South End Press, 2004), 65; Lyndie Brimstone, "Pat Parker: A Tribute," *Feminist Review* 34, no. 1 (Spring 1990): 4–7; Ruzek, *Women's Health Movement*, 191–92; Nelson, *More Than Medicine*, 158–66; and Enke, *Finding the Movement*, 197–216.

72. Julia Aihara, "Self-Help for Women," *Gidra*, April 1972, 8.

73. Luz Alvarez Martinez, interview by Loretta Ross, December 6–7, 2004, VFOHP, 36, https://www.smith.edu/libraries/libs/ssc/vof/transcripts/MartinezLuz.pdf.

74. Martinez, interview, 38.

75. Silliman et. al., *Undivided Rights*, 241–63.

76. Vicki Ziegler and Bonnie Poucel, interview, August 14, 1975, Downer collection.

77. Debra Brody, Sara Grusky, and Patricia Logan, "Self-Help Health," *Off Our Backs*, July 1982, 14, 17. See also Barbara Smith, ed., *Home Girls: A Black Feminist Anthology* (New York: Kitchen Table Press, 1983), xxxv–lii; and Silliman et al., *Undivided Rights*, 63.

78. Silliman et al., *Undivided Rights*, 56.

79. Corbett, "Getting Our Bodies Back," 2.

80. Jeanne [Hirsch], "Not Guilty, Not Guilty, Not Guilty," *Monthly Extract*, November/December 1972, 1–2.

81. For example, see Carol Downer to "Sisters," September 3, 1972, reel 1, WHRC. A probable 1971 version of the letterhead also refers to "Women's Choice Clinic."

82. Downer, "Through the Speculum," 420.

83. For more about the use of lay health workers, see chapters 2 and 4.

84. Rebecca M. Kluchin, "'Pregnant? Need Help? Call Jane': Service as Radical Action in the Abortion Underground in Chicago," in *Breaking the Wave: Women, Their Organizations, and Feminism, 1945–1985*, ed. Kathleen A. Laughlin and Jacqueline L. Castledine (New York: Routledge, 2011), 136–54; Laura Kaplan, *The Story of Jane: The Legendary Underground Feminist Abortion Service* (New York: Pantheon Books, 1995). See also Kelly Suzanne O'Donnell, "Reproducing Jane: Abortion Stories and Women's Political Histories," *Signs: Journal of Women in Culture and Society* 43, no. 1 (Autumn 2017): 77–96.

85. Chico Feminist Women's Health Center, "Participatory Clinic," n.d., Downer collection.

86. Quotations in [Los Angeles] Feminist Women's Health Center, "Well Woman Health Care in Woman Controlled Clinics." See also Ruzek, "Emergent Modes of Utilization," 73–77. For the use of participatory clinics beyond the FWHCs, see, for example, Santa Cruz Women's Health Collective, *The Self Help Clinic Booklet* (self-pub., n.d.), 11.

87. Judith A. Houck, "The Best Prescription for Women's Health: Feminist Approaches to Well-Woman Care," in *Prescribed: Writing, Filling, Using, and Abusing the Prescription in Modern America*, ed. Jeremy A. Greene and Elizabeth Siegel Watkins (Baltimore: Johns Hopkins University Press, 2012), 134–56.

88. According to Sandra Morgen's account of the Great Yogurt Conspiracy (GYC), police raided a self-help clinic. This is clearly the line that Downer and others among the FWHC toed.

It is not clear that this was true. For other historical treatments of the GYC, see Ruth Rosen, *The World Split Open: How the Modern Women's Movement Changed America* (New York: Viking, 2000), 177.

89. "Self-Examination on Trial," *Great Speckled Bird*, December 18, 1972, 7; Michael Seiler, "Feminists Run Afoul of the Law," *Los Angeles Times*, October 3, 1972. This account, which does not mention that yogurt was confiscated, was obviously based on a press release issued by the Feminist Women's Health Center. Feminist Women's Health Center, "Feminist Found Not Guilty of Practicing Medicine," December 6, 1972, in WHRC, reel 1-448–49.

90. Search warrant, Municipal Court of Los Angeles Judicial District, County of Los Angeles, State of California, September 20, 1971, 1, Downer collection. See also Corea, *Hidden Malpractice*, 262.

91. Stephanie Caruana, "Great Yogurt Conspiracy," *Off Our Backs*, January 1973, 7. The yogurt-as-lunch story was repeated in Deborah Rose, "Lookin' Around: How Women Are Regaining Control," *Second Wave*, March 1973, 26.

92. Helen Koblin, "Two Feminists Busted for 'Practicing Medicine,'" *Los Angeles Free Press*, September 29–October 9, 1972, 19.

93. Ellie, "Feminists Found 'Not Guilty' of Practicing Medicine," *Women's Press*, November 1972, 14–15.

94. Seiler, "Feminists Run Afoul," 1. See also "Self-Examination on Trial," 7.

95. John Urso, "Affidavit in Support of and Petition for Search Warrant," September 20, 1972, Women's Studies Archive, 4.

96. Seiler, "Feminists Run Afoul," 4. The affidavit in support of the search warrant alleges that Downer treated the infection with yogurt.

97. Seiler, 1.

98. Evelle J. Younger (California attorney general) and Louis C. Castro (deputy attorney general) to Michael R. Buggy (executive secretary, Board of Nursing Education and Nurse Registration), October 4, 1972, Downer collection.

99. Carol [Downer] and Alma to Laura and Friends of the Library, October 11, 1972, Downer collection.

100. Caruana, "Great Yogurt Conspiracy," 7. See also Seiler, "Feminists Run Afoul," 4; and "Feminist Rape," October 19, 1972, press release, Downer collection. This latter document suggests that because Wilson was "much more involved," she pled guilty and claims that Downer had the more "winable" [*sic*] case.

101. Seiler, "Feminists Run Afoul," 1.

102. "L.A. Cops Raid Women's Clinic," *Militant*, November 10, 1972, 11; Seiler, "Feminists Run Afoul," 4. See also "Feminist Health Center Director Acquitted," *Fifth Estate*, December 16, 1972–January 5, 1973, 8; Younger and Castro to Buggy, October 4, 1972; and [Downer] and Alma to Laura and Friends of the Library, October 11, 1972. Stephanie Caruana alleges that the state's case centered on an April 28, 1972, incident when Downer allegedly offered to provide an abortion or to fit an IUD on the state's undercover witness. Caruana then claims that Downer was not at the clinic on the day in question. It's unclear what to make of this story. April 28 was not listed in the affidavit in support of the search warrant. Caruana, "Great Yogurt Conspiracy," 7.

103. Jeanne Cordova, "Rape of 'Self-Help,'" *Lesbian Tide*, November 1972, 10. See also "Feminist Rape," n.d., and September 23, 1972, press releases, Women's Studies Archive.

104. Nancy D. Moser, October 18, 1972, Downer collection.

105. Lynn Bruner to Dr. Grennigan (Board of Medical Examiners) and J[oseph] Busch (dis-

trict attorney), n.d., Downer collection. See also affidavits from Lesley Salas, November 10, 1972; Sarah Sammons, November 11, 1972; Donna Davis, November 10, 1972, all from the Downer collection.

106. J. [Hirsch], "Not Guilty, Not Guilty," 2.

107. Barbara A. McGowan, "Heide, Wilma Scott," *American National Biography*, last modified February 2000, https://doi-org.ezproxy.library.wisc.edu/10.1093/anb/9780198606697.article .1500829.

108. Helen Koblin, "Feminist Benefit at Ash Grove," *Los Angeles Free Press*, December 1–10, 1972, 2.

109. Doug Shuit, "Jury Acquits Feminist in Yogurt Case," *Los Angeles Times*, December 6, 1972, B4.

110. "L.A. Cops Raid Women's Clinic," 11.

111. Jo Murray, "'Self-Help' Proponents to Speak at Tribunal," *Oakland Tribune*, October 27, 1972, 31.

112. "Feminist Health Center Director Acquitted," 8; Feminist Women's Health Center, "Feminist Found Not Guilty."

113. See, for example, Koblin, "Feminist Benefit at Ash Grove," 2. See also "Carol Downer Acquitted or 'The Yogurt Case,'" *NOW News, Pomona Valley Chapter*, December 1972, 1, 5.

114. "Self-Service Setback," *Time*, October 16, 1972, 74.

115. For numbers, see Jeanne Cordova, "Feminist Acquitted in 'Great Yogurt Conspiracy' Trial," *Lesbian Tide*, January 1973, 4, 15, 25; Shuit, "Jury Acquits Feminist," B4; and J. [Hirsch], "Not Guilty, Not Guilty," 1–2.

116. Note quoted in Cordova, "Feminist Acquitted," 4. Original from the Downer collection.

117. For Downer's comments, see Cordova, 4; and "Feminist Health Center Director Acquitted," 8.

118. Feminist Women's Health Center, "Feminist Found Not Guilty."

119. In 1974, three Santa Cruz, California, midwives were similarly "busted" for practicing medicine without a license. Like the Great Yogurt Conspiracy, this episode publicized home birth midwifery and generated conversations about the place of medicine and patient choice in childbirth practices. The Santa Cruz midwives ultimately lost their case. Wendy Kline, *Coming Home: How Midwives Changed Birth* (New York: Oxford University Press, 2019), 95–132.

120. See West Coast Sisters, "Self-Help Clinic," 6.

121. See, for example, West Coast Sisters, "Do It Yourself," 12.

122. See Peggy Grau, "Vaginal Politics," *Everywoman*, August 20, 1971, 16. The identity of Grau is not completely clear. At one point, the West Coast Sisters claimed that she was a fictitious front for a male abortionist. See chapter 3. Hannah Dudley-Shotwell notes that some members of the FWHC believed that "Peggy Grau" was merely a cover for Harvey Karman. Dudley-Shotwell, *Revolutionizing Women's Healthcare*, 32. Grau was likely one of the lay health workers who worked with Karman and John S. Gwynne.

123. See West Coast Sisters, "Do It Yourself," 12; and "Vaginal Politics: Self-Help Clinic," *Ain't I a Woman?*, November 19, 1971, 2. See also Peggy Grau, "Do-It-Yourself: Vaginal Examination," *Liberation News Service*, September 15, 1971, 2–3; and Peggy Grau, "Be Your Own Physician," *NOLA Express*, October 7, 1971, 10, which have the same text with different pictures.

124. "Self-Help Clinic Clarification," *Everywoman*, December 17, 1971, 17.

125. Peggy Grau, letter to readers, *Everywoman*, February 1972, 14. See also handout, "Self-Help Clinic: Vaginal Politics."

126. L. & M., "Iowa City," *Monthly Extract*, October/November 1972, 1.

127. L. & M., "Iowa City," 2.

128. Fran, Mae Dell, Margaret, and Tacie, "What Is 'Feminist' Health?," *Off Our Backs*, June 1974, 5.

129. Laura [Brown] and Barb [Hoke], interview by Lynn [Heidelberg], n.d., ca. 1974, Downer collection.

130. Levin, *Talk Back to Your Doctor*, 185.

131. Laura Tyner, "Another Look at Self Examination and Sacred Heart," *Women's Press*, October 1974, 21.

132. Barbara Monty, "Personal Action," *Second Wave*, March 1973, 27.

133. Jane Sussman, letter to the editor, *NOW News, Central New Jersey Chapter*, March 16, 1972, 10.

134. Maryann Barakso, *Governing NOW: Grassroots Activism in the National Organization for Women* (Ithaca, NY: Cornell University Press, 2004).

135. For Downer's take on feminist detractors, see [Federation of Feminist Women's Health Centers], "What This Book Is All About," 12.

136. Susan Reverby, "Our Bodies, Ourselves: Getting By with a Little Help from Our Friends," *University Review*, no. 28 (April 1973): 27.

137. Lorrien, "Remarks," in *Women's Sexuality Conference Proceedings*, ed. NOW (New York: NOW, 1974), 38. See also Stephen Grosz and Bruce McAuley, "*Self-Health* and *Healthcaring*," *Camera Obscura* 3, no. 1 (1981): 128–35.

138. Nora Ephron, "Women," *Esquire*, December 1972, 78.

139. Ellen Frankfort, "Vaginal Politics," *Village Voice*, November 25, 1971, 74.

140. Robin Cox, "An Interview with Kay Weiss," *Plexus*, June 1976, 6. Reverby made the same point in 1973, noting that the speculum might be a valuable weapon, but it was "no substitute for an army and a battle plan." Reverby, "Our Bodies, Ourselves," 27.

141. Stephanie Allan, "Some Horror Stories," *People's World*, September 14, 1974, 7. See a response in Clausen and Radey, letter to the editor, *People's World*, 6. For criticism of self-exam as an individual approach, see Rose, "Lookin' Around," 28; Elizabeth Fishel, "Women's Self-Help Movement: Or, Is Happiness Knowing Your Own Cervix?," *Ramparts*, November 1973, 29–31, 56–59; and Sharon Lieberman, "Women's Health: Professionalism Can Be Destructive," *Majority Report*, May 1975, 6.

Chapter Two

1. Kater Pollock, interview with the author, July 1, 2011; Robin Baker, interview with the author, July 1, 2011.

2. The word *clinic* was used several ways by feminist health activists. As we have already seen, a self-help clinic could refer to a course of study centered on self-discovery and shared insights. In this chapter, *clinic* refers to the provision of health services.

3. "The Medical Industrial Complex," *Health/PAC Bulletin*, November 1969, 1–2; Eli Ginzberg and Miriam Ostow, *Men, Money, and Medicine* (New York: Columbia University Press, 1969); Barbara Ehrenreich and John Ehrenreich, *The American Health Empire: Power, Profits, and Politics* (New York: Vintage Books, 1971); Marvin Henry Edwards, *Hazardous to Your Health: A New Look at the "Health Care Crisis" in America* (New Rochelle, NY: Arlington House, 1972).

4. Dispensaries, which provided outpatient care for the urban poor in the nineteenth and early twentieth centuries, were important precursors to some of the clinic experiments in the twentieth century. See, for example, Charles E. Rosenberg, "Social Class and Medical Care in Nineteenth-Century America: The Rise and Fall of the Dispensary," *Journal of the History of Medicine and Allied Sciences* 29, no. 1 (January 1974): 32–54; William Pencak, "Free Health Care for the Poor: The Philadelphia Dispensary," *Pennsylvania Magazine of History and Biography* 136, no. 1 (January 2012): 25–52; and Christopher Crenner, "Race and Medical Practice in Kansas City's Free Dispensary," *Bulletin of the History of Medicine* 82, no. 4 (Winter 2008): 820–47.

5. H. Jack Geiger, "Community Health Centers: Health Care as an Instrument of Social Change," in *Reforming Medicine: Lessons of the Last Quarter Century*, ed. Victor W. Sidel and Ruth Sidel (New York: Pantheon Books, 1984), 13, quoted in Jennifer Nelson, *More Than Medicine: A History of the Feminist Women's Health Movement* (New York: New York University Press, 2015), 23.

6. For a history of the MCHR and their work during Freedom Summer, see John Dittmer, *The Good Doctors: The Medical Committee for Human Rights and the Struggle for Social Justice in Health Care* (New York: Bloomsbury Press, 2009).

7. Nelson, *More Than Medicine,* 24–26. See also Bonnie Lefkowitz, *Community Health Centers: A Movement and the People Who Made It Happen* (New Brunswick, NJ: Rutgers University Press, 2007); Thomas J. Ward Jr., *Out in the Rural: A Mississippi Health Center and Its War on Poverty* (New York: Oxford University Press, 2016); and Jonathan Engel, *Poor People's Medicine: Medicaid and American Charity Care since 1965* (Durham, NC: Duke University Press, 2006).

8. Gregory L. Weiss, *Grassroots Medicine: The Story of America's Free Health Clinics* (Lanham, MD: Rowman & Littlefield, 2006), 28–33.

9. Weiss, *Grassroots Medicine*, 28–33.

10. "Free Clinics," *Health/PAC Bulletin*, October 1971, 1.

11. Weiss, *Grassroots Medicine*, 28–33.

12. See Weiss; Jerome L. Schwartz, "First National Survey of Free Medical Clinics, 1967–69," *HSMHA Health Reports* 86, no. 9 (September 1971): 775–87; and "Free Clinics," *Health/PAC Bulletin*, 1–16.

13. Alondra Nelson, *Body and Soul: The Black Panther Party and the Fight against Medical Discrimination* (Minneapolis: University of Minnesota Press, 2011), 79.

14. Nelson, *Body and Soul*, 75–114. See also Mary T. Bassett, "No Justice, No Health: The Black Panther Party's Fight for Health in Boston and Beyond," *Journal of African American Studies* 23, no. 4 (December 2019): 352–63.

15. "Free Clinics," 13.

16. The Berkeley Free Clinic adopted this motto as its own. It is unclear whether they originated it.

17. Niki A. Nibbe, "Beyond the Free Clinics Origin Myth: Reconsidering Free Clinics in the Context of 1960s and 1970s Social Movements and Radical Health Activism" (master's thesis, University of California, San Francisco, 2012), 41.

18. David E. Smith, Donald R. Wesson, and Rod Ciceri, "The National Free Clinic Movement: Historical Perspectives," *ADIT: Approaches to Drug Abuse and Youth*, October 2, 1973, 16.

19. Nibbe, "Beyond the Free Clinics Origin Myth," 21.

20. Nelson, *Body and Soul*, 96; "Gloria Arellanes," Chicana por mi Raza, Chicana por mi Raza Digital Memory Collective, last modified November 29, 2015, chicanapormiraza.org /chicanas/Gloria-arellanes.

21. "Women's Clinics," *Health/PAC Bulletin*, October 1971, 14. See also Kyla, "Free Clinic: Medical Center in Need of Improvement," *Quicksilver Times*, June 27, 1969, 4; "What Is a Free Clinic? Women in Imperial Beach," *Goodbye to All That* (San Diego), January/February 1973, 2–3; and "The Women's Clinic at Open Door," *Northwest Passage*, June 7–20, 1971, 12.

22. Smith, Wesson, and Ciceri, "The National Free Clinic Movement," 13.

23. H. Jack Geiger, "Hidden Professional Roles: The Physician as Reactionary, Reformer, Revolutionary," *Social Policy*, March/April 1971, 31, quoted in Robert J. Bazell, "Health Radicals: Crusade to Shift Medical Power to the People," *Science* 173, no. 3996 (August 6, 1971): 509.

24. Sandra Morgen, *Into Our Own Hands: The Women's Health Movement in the United States, 1969–1990* (New Brunswick, NJ: Rutgers University Press, 2002), 71.

25. For more about feminist clinics, see Wendy Simonds, *Abortion at Work: Ideology and Practice in a Feminist Clinic* (New Brunswick, NJ: Rutgers University Press, 1996); Johanna Schoen, *Abortion after Roe* (Chapel Hill: University of North Carolina Press, 2015); Nelson, *More Than Medicine*; and Hannah Dudley-Shotwell, *Revolutionizing Women's Healthcare: The Feminist Self-Help Movement in America* (New Brunswick, NJ: Rutgers University Press, 2020).

26. Julia McKinney Barfoot, "Free Health Care for Women by Women: The Berkeley Women's Health Collective," in *Getting Clear: Body Work for Women*, ed. Anne Kent Rush (New York: Random House, 1973), 89, 91.

27. "Berkeley Women's Clinic," *Everywoman*, June 18, 1971, 2.

28. "Berkeley Women's Clinic," 2; Barfoot, "Free Health Care," 95. For more on the BWHC, see Morgen, *Into Our Own Hands*, 79–85.

29. Barfoot, "Free Health Care," 95.

30. "Women's Clinics," 14. For a history of the Aradia Women's Health Center in Seattle, opened in April 1972, see Nelson, *More Than Medicine*, 91–122. Women's Health Clinic in Portland opened in June 1971. "Women's Clinic Opens," *Willamette Bridge*, June 24, 1971, 4; "The Women's Clinic at Open Door," 12; Wendy Kline, *Bodies of Knowledge: Sexuality, Reproduction, and Women's Health in the Second Wave* (Chicago: University of Chicago Press, 2010), 77–79.

31. Dudley-Shotwell, *Revolutionizing Women's Healthcare*, 38. For more on feminist clinics owned or managed by individual feminist women, see Schoen, *Abortion after Roe*, particularly as she describes the work of Susan Hill and Renee Chelian.

32. Dudley-Shotwell, *Revolutionizing Women's Healthcare*, 39–40; Morgen, *Into Our Own Hands*, 90–95; Schoen, *Abortion after Roe*, 41.

33. Joan McKinney, "New Clinic Offers a Choice to Women," *Oakland Tribune*, May 4, 1973, 33, 35.

34. Dudley-Shotwell, *Revolutionizing Women's Healthcare*, 38; Morgen, *Into Our Own Hands*, 71. See also Daphne Spain, "Appendix D: Feminist Health Centers in the United States, 1975," in *Constructive Feminism: Women's Spaces and Women's Rights in the American City* (Ithaca, NY: Cornell University Press, 2016), 201–2.

35. Kline, *Bodies of Knowledge*, 80.

36. Susan Reverby, "Alive and Well in Somerville, Mass." *HealthRight*, Winter 1975, 1.

37. Reverby, "Alive and Well," 1.

38. Dudley-Shotwell, *Revolutionizing Women's Healthcare*, 41.

39. G. William Domhoff, "History of Santa Cruz," *Who Rules America?* (blog), January 2009, https://whorulesamerica.ucsc.edu/santacruz/history.html. See also Richard Gendron and G. William Domhoff, *The Leftmost City: Power and Progressive Politics in Santa Cruz* (Boulder, CO: Westview Press, 2009).

40. Wendy Kline, *Coming Home: How Midwives Changed Birth* (New York: Oxford University Press, 2019), 95–132.

41. Kater Pollock, "Developing a Socialist-Feminist Model: The Growth of the Santa Cruz Women's Health Collective" (bachelor's thesis, University of California, Santa Cruz, 1978), 3.

42. Pollock, "Developing a Socialist-Feminist Model," 3.

43. Kline, *Coming Home*, 112–13; Pollock, "Developing a Socialist-Feminist Model," 6.

44. Quoted in Brian Pendleton, "The California Therapeutic Abortion Act: An Analysis," *Hastings Law Journal* 19, no. 1 (November 1967): 242–55.

45. Pollock, "Developing a Socialist-Feminist Model," 6. The hospital landscape in Santa Cruz was in flux during the last half of the twentieth century. The American Medical International Community Hospital, opened in 1959, was loosely affiliated with the Seventh Day Adventist Church via the Sundean Foundation. Dominican Santa Cruz Hospital opened in 1967. Santa Cruz County General Hospital opened in 1968, but it had discontinued most of its care by 1973. Thanks to Emma Wathen for this research.

46. Kline, *Coming Home*, 112.

47. "Self-Help," *NOW News, Santa Cruz Chapter*, July/August 1972, 5.

48. Pollock, "Developing a Socialist-Feminist Model," 6–8.

49. Dana Frank and Tinka Gordon, "The Santa Cruz Women's Health Collective: Collective Organization of Work," (unpublished manuscript, n.d., ca. 1981), Wilshusen collection.

50. "Our Editorial Policy," *Santa Cruz Women's Health Center Newsletter*, June 1978, 2.

51. Pollock, interview.

52. "Paper for New Members" (unpublished manuscript, May 1976), 2, Wilshusen collection.

53. Baker, interview.

54. Tinka Gordon, "Case Study: The Santa Cruz Women's Health Collective: The Collective Organization of Work" (unpublished document, n.d., ca. 1980), 3. This document is very similar to Frank and Gordon's unpublished manuscript, "Collective Organization of Work." The document authored by Gordon alone seems to predate the expanded version by Frank and Gordon.

55. Gordon, "Case Study," 3–4; "Santa Cruz Women's Health Project Position Paper" (unpublished document, n.d.), quoted in Kater Pollock, "Developing a Socialist-Feminist Model: The Growth of the Santa Cruz Women's Health Collective" (bachelor's thesis, University of California, Santa Cruz, 1978)," 11. See also "Collective Process: Meetings," *Santa Cruz Women's Health Center Newsletter*, June 1977, 4; and "Collective Process: Consensus," *Santa Cruz Women's Health Center Newsletter*, March 1978, 4.

56. Baker, interview.

57. Jody Peugh, interview with the author, September 30, 2011.

58. See, for example, David Priestland, *The Red Flag: A History of Communism* (New York: Grove Press, 2009), 144–45, 150, 246–47; and S. Tsirul, *The Practice of Bolshevik Self-Criticism: How the American Communist Party Carries Out Self-Criticism and Controls Fulfillment of Decisions* (New York: Central Committee, Communist Party USA, 1932).

59. "Collective Process: Meetings," 4. See also "Collective Process: C/SC," *Santa Cruz Women's Health Center Newsletter*, September 1977, 2; and "Collective Process: Strokes," *Santa Cruz Women's Health Center Newsletter*, December 1977, 3.

60. Peugh, interview.

61. Frank and Gordon, "Collective Organization of Work," 9.

62. "Paper for New Members," 5.

63. Radicalesbians, "The Woman-Identified Woman," in *Dear Sisters: Dispatches from the*

Women's Liberation Movement, ed. Rosalyn Baxandall and Linda Gordon (1970; repr., New York: Basic Books, 2000), 107–9.

64. "Santa Cruz Women's Health Project Position Paper," quoted in Kater Pollock, "Developing a Socialist-Feminist Model: The Growth of the Santa Cruz Women's Health Collective" (bachelor's thesis, University of California, Santa Cruz, 1978), 12.

65. "Santa Cruz Women's Health Collective New Members Orientation" (unpublished document, September 1975), 6, Wilshusen collection.

66. Pollock, "Developing a Socialist-Feminist Model," 16.

67. Pollock, 44.

68. Pollock, 44. The schisms defined by alliances with particular threads of feminism and their theoretical demands as described by Alice Echols do not seem to have been at play in the discussion of socialist feminism in Santa Cruz. Alice Echols, *Daring to Be Bad: Radical Feminism in America, 1967–1975* (Minneapolis: University of Minnesota Press, 1989).

69. Baker, interview; Colleen Douglas, interview with the author, September 11, 2011; Linda Wilshusen, interview with the author, July 1, 2011; Peugh, interview.

70. The Santa Cruz Women's Health Collective, "Position Paper of the Santa Cruz Women's Health Collective Concerning the Birth Center Arrests" (unpublished document, n.d., ca. March 1974), quoted in Kater Pollock, "Developing a Socialist-Feminist Model: The Growth of the Santa Cruz Women's Health Collective" (bachelor's thesis, University of California, Santa Cruz, 1978), 39–40.

71. Wilshusen, interview; Pollock, "Developing a Socialist-Feminist Model," 76.

72. Wilshusen, interview; Peugh, interview; Pollock, "Developing a Socialist-Feminist Model," 77.

73. Baker, interview. Several people contributed to the booklet itself, but Baker used her contribution for her thesis requirement.

74. Pollock, "Developing a Socialist-Feminist Model," 24.

75. Despite the SCWHC's resentment regarding the required board, it eventually proved quite useful: in 1982, the board stepped in and fired longtime employees to create a more diverse staff. See chapter 8.

76. Frank and Gordon, "Collective Organization of Work," 15.

77. In 1997, the Santa Cruz Women's Health Center bought this building. Vicki Winters, "A Clinic of One's Own: Santa Cruz Women's Health Center Buys Its Own Facility," *Mid-County Post* (Capitola, CA), January 20–February 2, 1998, 12.

78. Pollock, interview.

79. For a history of the "bust," see Kline, *Coming Home*, 95–132.

80. The Santa Cruz Women's Health Collective, "Position Paper Concerning the Birth Center Arrests," quoted in Pollock, "Developing a Socialist-Feminist Model," 40.

81. Pollock, 36.

82. Frank and Gordon, "Collective Organization of Work," 15.

83. Frank and Gordon, 16.

84. Frank and Gordon, 17.

85. Pollock, "Developing a Socialist-Feminist Model," 69–70; Pollock, interview.

86. Pollock, "Developing a Socialist-Feminist Model," 72.

87. Pollock, 72–73.

88. Pollock, 74.

89. Pollock, 90, 93.

90. "Women's Health Counseling Set at SC Center," *Santa Cruz Sentinel*, December 2, 1976, 11; "New Directions for the Health Collective," *Santa Cruz Women's Health Center Newsletter*, December 1976, 2. The clinic may have reopened briefly between January and March 1975, but it is not clear. See "Update on Our Clinics," *Santa Cruz Women's Health Center Newsletter*, March 1976, 3. By June 1978, Lloyd Benjamin had taken over the medical care, presumably under his license. "Women's Center Expands Service," *Santa Cruz Sentinel*, June 12, 1978, 22.

91. Pollock, "Developing a Socialist-Feminist Model," 61.

92. Pollock, 62–63.

93. Pollock, 50.

94. Pollock, 63.

95. Exactly what happened is unclear from the record.

96. "Update on Our Clinics," 3.

97. "Whatever Happened to Clinics? An Update from the Women's Health Collective" (unpublished manuscript, February 1976), Wilshusen collection.

98. These clinics included the Women's Choice abortion clinic in Oakland and the Choice Clinic in Los Gatos. Undated flyer for abortion services included in Pollock, "Developing a Socialist-Feminist Model," vi.

99. Gordon, "Case Study," 7; Frank and Gordon, "Collective Organization of Work," 18.

100. Baker, interview.

101. "Revenue Sharing Hearings," *Santa Cruz Women's Health Center Newsletter*, June 1976, 2.

102. Frank and Gordon, "Collective Organization of Work," 18.

103. Frank and Gordon, 18–19.

104. Wilshusen, interview.

105. Frank and Gordon, "Collective Organization of Work," 21–22.

106. *P.I.D.: Pelvic Inflammatory Disease*, 2nd ed. (Santa Cruz Women's Health Collective, 1978); *Herpes*, rev. ed. (Santa Cruz Women's Health Collective, 1977).

107. Frank and Gordon, "Collective Organization of Work," 18.

108. David O. Sears and Jack Citrin, *Tax Revolt: Something for Nothing in California*, enlarged ed. (Cambridge, MA: Harvard University Press, 1985).

109. Sue Reynolds, "Services in Danger," *Matrix*, August 1978, 1.

110. "Yes, We're Still Alive!," *Santa Cruz Women's Health Center Newsletter*, September 1978, 3.

111. "Womankind Health Services Expansion," *Santa Cruz Women's Health Center Newsletter*, March 1979, 4.

112. "Yes, We're Still Alive!," 3.

113. "Don't Recall Us, We'll Recall You," *Matrix*, September 1978, 3.

114. Judy Cassada, "Budget Blues," *Matrix*, September 1978, 5. See also "Budget Brief," *Santa Cruz Women's Health Center Newsletter*, September 1978, 4.

115. "Yes, We're Still Alive!," 3.

116. Wilshusen, interview.

117. Frank and Gordon, "Collective Organization of Work," 18.

118. For more about the changes in the SCWHC, see chapter 8.

119. The college was Humboldt State College, now Humboldt State University. Humboldt County, especially the southern region, has been called the "heartland of high-grade marijuana farming in California." David Samuels, "Dr. Kush: How Medical Marijuana Is Transforming the Pot Industry," *New Yorker*, July 28, 2008, 49.

120. Lorraine Carolan, interview with the author, January 5, 2010; Jan Rowen, interview with the author, December 3, 2009.

121. "Charges Refiled against Birth Center Operator," *Times Standard* (Eureka, CA), October 30, 1975, 5.

122. Edith Butler, *United Indian Health Services, Inc.: Celebrating 25 Years of Service to the American Indian Community, 1970–1995* (Trinidad, CA: United Indian Health Services, Inc., 1995); Edith Butler, *25 Years of Self Determination: A Commemorative History of the California Rural Indian Health Board, Inc.* (Sacramento: California Rural Indian Health Board, Inc., 1994). Butler credits the California Department of Public Health with this initiative. Because the Department of Public Health did not exist as such until 2007, the Department of Health probably led the project.

123. Butler, *United Indian Health Services*, 11–20; Paul D. Ward, "California Regional Medical Programs," *California Medicine* 118, no. 4 (April 1973): 88–90.

124. Butler, *United Indian Health Services*, 19–20. In 1971, UIHS joined the California Rural Indian Health Board. At least three of the people who worked at Northcountry Clinic also worked for UIHS: Nancy Henchell, Carol Ervin, and Bert Umland, a physician. Butler, 19–20.

125. Helen Sanderson, "Sign of the Times," *North Coast Journal*, September 14, 2006, http://www.northcoastjournal.com/091406/cover0914.html.

126. "Open Door Clinic Open Soon in Arcata; Varied Services," *Times Standard*, March 29, 1971, 16.

127. Sanderson, "Sign of the Times."

128. Paul Brisso, "Walkout Paralyzes Arcata's Open Door Clinic," *Times Standard*, October 19, 1973, 5.

129. Valerie Ohanian, "Being a Woman Doctor Is Sometimes Very Difficult," *Times Standard*, September 30, 1973, 5. This article suggests that Pennington, working through Open Door Clinic and working with Bill Fisher, delivered babies at women's homes, because women "absolutely refuse[d] to go to a hospital." See also Gena Pennington, interview with the author, October 9, 2006.

130. Suzanne Willow, interview with the author, December 30, 2009; Susan Riesel, interview with the author, July 6, 2011; Deborah Sweitzer, interview with the author, July 7, 2011.

131. Pennington, interview. See also Shulamith Firestone, *Dialectic of Sex* (New York: William and Morrow and Company, 1970).

132. Pennington, interview.

133. Pennington. There are some discrepancies about the years physicians started to work in the clinic and when Pennington started to work there. Although she may have begun as a volunteer, at some point, she became a paid part-time employee.

134. Patsy Ciardullo and Nevada Wagoner, "Title X Family Planning Program (1970–1977)," Embryo Project Encyclopedia, October 21, 2016, https://embryo.asu.edu/pages/title-x-family-planning-program-1970-1977.

135. Pennington, interview; Willow, interview.

136. Willow, interview. The broad strokes of this story were described in Judith A. Houck, "The Best Prescription for Women's Health: Feminist Approaches to Well-Woman Care," in *Prescribed: Writing, Filling, Using, and Abusing the Prescription in Modern America*, eds. Jeremy A. Greene and Elizabeth Siegel Watkins (Johns Hopkins University Press, 2012), 134–156.

137. National Advisory Commission on Health Manpower, *Report of the National Advisory Commission on Health Manpower* (Washington, DC: US Government Printing Office, 1967), 1:2.

138. Dick Howard and R. Douglas Roederer, *Health Manpower Licensing* (Lexington, KY: Council of State Governments, 1978), 2.

139. Howard and Roederer, *Health Manpower Licensing*, 15.

140. Richard M. Briggs, Barbara S. Schneidman, Eleanor N. Thorson, and Ronald D. Deisher, "Education and Integration of Midlevel Health-Care Practitioners in Obstetrics and Gynecology: Experience of a Training Program in Washington State," *American Journal of Obstetrics and Gynecology* 132, no. 1 (September 1, 1978): 68; Donald R. Ostergard, John E. Gunning, and John R. Marshall, "Training and Function of a Women's Health-Care Specialist, a Physician's Assistant, or Nurse Practitioner in Obstetrics and Gynecology," *American Journal of Obstetrics and Gynecology* 121, no. 8 (April 15, 1975): 1036.

141. Briggs et al., "Education and Integration of Midlevel Practitioners," 76.

142. Ostergard, Gunning, and Marshall, "Training and Function of a Specialist," 1030.

143. A similar program, the Gynecorps Training Program, was developed in 1972 by the Department of Obstetrics and Gynecology at the University of Washington School of Medicine. Briggs et al., "Education and Integration of Midlevel Practitioners," 68–77.

144. Richard M. Briggs, "The Use of Para-medical Personnel in Obstetrics and Gynecology," *Northwest Medical Journal* 1, no. 7 (July 1974): 13. Briggs describes programs in effect as of May 1, 1973, that trained "non-physician family planning specialists." Ibid.

145. Willow, interview.

146. These included Susan Anderson and Lorraine Carolan.

147. Henchell died in May 2006. Information about her part of the Women's Health Care Specialist programs comes primarily from author interviews with Carol Ervin and Suzanne Willow.

148. Norman Bell, handwritten notes for Open Door memoir (unpublished manuscript, n.d.), in the author's possession.

149. Willow, interview.

150. Willow, interview; Carol Ervin, interview with the author, October 16, 2006.

151. Ervin, interview. For reasons beyond the scope of this project, tensions grew within the governing board of the UIHS. Perhaps Henchell was caught up in those issues. "Court Injunction Halts Indian Health Services Election," *Times Standard*, July 13, 1973, 11.

152. Bell, handwritten notes. One source claimed that tensions over supplies also played a part in causing a rift between Bell and Pennington. Riesel, interview.

153. In some accounts it was Henchell and Ervin at the table.

154. Willow, interview; Felicia Oldfather, interview with the author, October 9, 2006.

155. "Announcing the Opening of North Country Clinic for Women and Children," *Times Standard*, December 8, 1976, 16. The Northcountry Clinic is also referred to as North Country Clinic; internal documents generally refer to it as Northcountry Clinic for Women and Children.

156. "Expanded Clinic Marks Progress," *Times Standard*, January 7, 1978; Bob Palomares, "North Country Clinic Becomes a Success Story," *Times Standard*, October 9, 1978.

157. Palomares, "North Country Clinic Becomes a Success Story."

158. Ervin, Henchell, Pennington, White, and Willow. Other women, including Beverley Allen (lab tech), Deborah Sweitzer (in the first class of WHCS trainees), and Edith Umland (physician), joined the clinic soon after its founding.

159. Pennington, interview.

160. "Expanded Clinic Marks Progress."

161. "Expanded Clinic Marks Progress."

162. Willow, interview.

163. Howard and Roederer, *Health Manpower Licensing*, 15, 22.

164. Lorraine Carolan, email message to author, February 25, 2010.

165. Office of Statewide Health Planning and Development, *Annual Report to the Legislature, State of California, and to the Healing Arts Licensing Boards*, November 1979, 17–18.

166. Briggs, "Use of Para-medical Personnel," 9–11; Evelyn T. Dravecky, "The Obstetric–Gynecologic Team: Focus on the Worker Member," *Clinical Obstetrics and Gynecology* 15, no. 2 (June 1972): 319–32.

167. Susan Riesel, interview with the author, October 10, 2006; Susan Anderson, interview with the author, July 27, 2006; Carolan, interview; Willow, interview.

Chapter Three

1. Ninia Baehr, *Abortion without Apology: A Radical History for the 1990s* (Boston: South End Press, 1990), 22.

2. For the most complete historical treatment of menstrual extraction to date, see Michelle Murphy, *Seizing the Means of Reproduction: Entanglements of Feminism, Health, and Techno-science* (Durham, NC: Duke University Press, 2012), 150–76; and Hannah Dudley-Shotwell, *Revolutionizing Women's Healthcare: The Feminist Self-Help Movement in America* (New Brunswick, NJ: Rutgers University Press, 2020), 20–35, 104–17.

3. In addition to Rothman and Downer, the founders of the Los Angeles FWHC included Julie Barton, Carol Broberg, Florence Ehring, Joyce Stanley, and Colleen Wilson. Elayne Heiman was involved in the early self-help clinics but may have left the project before the group called itself the Los Angeles FWHC. Carol Downer, Lorraine Rothman, and Eleanor Snow, "F.W.H.C. Response," *Off Our Backs*, August/September 1974, 17–18.

4. For early histories of abortion, see James C. Mohr, *Abortion in America: The Origins and Evolution of National Policy, 1800–1900* (Oxford: Oxford University Press, 1978); and Leslie J. Reagan, *When Abortion Was a Crime: Women, Medicine, and Law in the United States, 1867–1973* (Berkeley: University of California Press, 1997), esp. 11.

5. Rosalind Pollack Petchesky, *Abortion and Woman's Choice: The State, Sexuality, and Reproductive Freedom*, rev. ed. (Boston: Northeastern University Press, 1990), 111.

6. Thomas B. Littlewood, *The Politics of Population Control* (Notre Dame: University of Notre Dame Press, 1977), 55, quoted in Rosalind Pollack Petchesky, *Abortion and Woman's Choice: The State, Sexuality, and Reproductive Freedom*, rev. ed. (Boston: Northeastern University Press, 1990), 121. See also Emily Klancher Merchant, *Building the Population Bomb* (New York: Oxford University Press, 2021); and Donald T. Critchlow, *Intended Consequences: Birth Control, Abortion, and the Federal Government in Modern America* (New York: Oxford University Press, 1999).

7. Petchesky, *Abortion and Woman's Choice*, 123.

8. Reagan, *When Abortion Was a Crime*, 224. For a history of illegal abortion in California, see Alicia Gutierrez-Romine, *From Back Alley to the Border: Criminal Abortion in California, 1920–1969* (Lincoln: University of Nebraska Press, 2020). For more on the Army of Three, see Lawrence Lader, *Abortion II: Making the Revolution* (Boston: Beacon Press, 1973), 27–34.

9. See, for example, Lana Clarke Phelan and Patricia Maginnis, *The Abortion Handbook for Responsible Women* (North Hollywood: Contact Books, 1969).

10. Leslie J. Reagan, "Crossing the Border for Abortions: California Activists, Mexican Clinics, and the Creation of a Feminist Health Agency in the 1960s," *Feminist Studies* 26, no. 2 (Summer 2000): 323–48.

11. See, for example, Lucinda Cisler, "Unfinished Business: Birth Control and Women's Lib-

eration," in *Sisterhood Is Powerful: An Anthology of Writings from the Women's Liberation Movement*, ed. Robin Morgan (New York: Vintage Books, 1970), 277–78.

12. Richard Pérez-Peña, "'70 Abortion Law: New York Said Yes, Stunning the Nation," *New York Times*, April 9, 2000. For more on early abortion reform and legalization, see Johanna Schoen, *Abortion after Roe* (Chapel Hill: University of North Carolina Press, 2015), 9–11.

13. Leslie J. Reagan, *Dangerous Pregnancies: Mothers, Disabilities, and Abortion in Modern America* (Berkeley: University of California Press, 2010), esp. 139–79. See also Gutierrez-Romine, *From Back Alley to Border*, 179–80.

14. Lynn Lilliston, "New Law on Abortion Hailed as Health Aid," *Los Angeles Times*, June 20, 1967; Reagan, *When Abortion Was a Crime*, 166.

15. Lilliston, "New Law on Abortion"; Brian Pendleton, "The California Therapeutic Abortion Act: An Analysis," *Hastings Law Journal* 19, no. 1 (November 1967): 242–55; Lynn Lilliston, "Defects of Abortion Law Cited at Seminar," *Los Angeles Times*, May 30, 1968; Reagan, *When Abortion Was a Crime*, 166.

16. Lilliston, "Defects of Abortion Law."

17. Reagan, *When Abortion Was a Crime*, 167.

18. Lilliston, "Defects of Abortion Law."

19. "The Therapeutic Abortion Act," *Los Angeles Times*, April 24, 1967; Lilliston, "New Law on Abortion."

20. Lilliston, "New Law on Abortion"; Lynn Lilliston, "New Law Liberal in Intent, but Is It in Practice?," *Los Angeles Times*, March 1, 1970.

21. Keith Monroe, "How California's Abortion Law Isn't Working," *New York Times*, December 29, 1968.

22. People v. Belous, 71 Cal. 2d 954 (1969), quoted in Zad Leavy, "Living with the Therapeutic Abortion Act of 1967," *Clinical Obstetrics and Gynecology* 14, no. 4 (December 1971): 1156–57.

23. Nancy Briggs Reardan, "California's 1967 Therapeutic Abortion Act: Abridging a Fundamental Right to Abortion," *Pacific Law Journal* 2, no. 1 (January 1971): 186–203; quotation on 192. See also Gutierrez-Romine, *From Back Alley to Border*, 184–91.

24. Zad Leavy, "Living with the Therapeutic Abortion Act of 1967," *Clinical Obstetrics and Gynecology* 14, no. 4 (December 1971): 1155.

25. Gwen Gibson, "Liberalized Abortion Law: 4 Years Later," *Los Angeles Times*, November 21, 1971.

26. Barbara L., "Woman vs. Gynecology," *Women's Press*, May 1973, 2.

27. Bill Hazlett, "Young Doctor Puts State's Abortion Laws to the Test," *Los Angeles Times*, March 29, 1971; "Five Linked to Abortion Clinic Face Charges," *Los Angeles Times*, March 26, 1970.

28. "Court Ruling on Abortions," *Los Angeles Times*, November 28, 1972.

29. "Court Ruling on Abortions"; "Abortion Go-Ahead: State Court Voids Need for Panel OK, Decision Now Up to Woman and Physician," *Los Angeles Times*, November 22, 1972.

30. Schoen, *Abortion after Roe*, 10–12.

31. Schoen, 10–12.

32. Schoen, 38–45.

33. John Dart, "Abortion Decision Expected to Have Little Effect in California," *Los Angeles Times*, January 23, 1973.

34. Betty Liddick, "Effects of Supreme Court Abortion Ruling," *Los Angeles Times*, February 11, 1973.

35. Dart, "Decision Expected to Have Little Effect." See also Frances Hornstein, "The Woman-Controlled Abortion," in *Abortion in a Clinic Setting*, ed. Los Angeles Feminist Women's Health Center (Los Angeles: Feminist Women's Health Center, 1974), 6.

36. Dudley-Shotwell, *Revolutionizing Women's Healthcare*, 12–13.

37. Carol Downer, "No Stopping: From Pom-Poms to Saving Women's Bodies," *On the Issues Magazine*, October 17, 2011, https://www.womenshealthspecialists.org/health-alerts-for-women /no-stopping-from-pom-poms-to-saving-womens-bodies-by-carol-downer/.

38. For histories of Jane, see Laura Kaplan, *The Story of Jane: The Legendary Underground Feminist Abortion Service* (New York: Pantheon Books, 1995); Rebecca M. Kluchin, "'Pregnant? Need Help? Call Jane': Service as Radical Action in the Abortion Underground in Chicago," in *Breaking the Wave: Women, Their Organizations, and Feminism, 1945–1985*, ed. Kathleen A. Laughlin and Jacqueline Castledine (New York: Routledge, 2011): 136–54; and Kelly Suzanne O'Donnell, "Reproducing Jane: Abortion Stories and Women's Political Histories," *Signs: Journal of Women in Culture and Society* 43, no. 1 (Autumn 2017): 77–96.

39. For more about Koome, see Cassandra Tate, "Koome, Dr. Adriaan Frans (1929–1978)," *HistoryLink.org*, September 14, 2000, https://www.historylink.org/File/2642. For evidence that Koome did D&Cs, see Lorraine Rothman, "Medical Self-Help Clinic: Paramedical Politics," *NOW News, Central New Jersey Chapter*, March 1972, 4–5; originally presented at the Reproduction Workshop, NOW National Convention, Los Angeles, CA, September 5, 1971. See also Hornstein, "The Woman-Controlled Abortion," 5.

40. Rothman, "Medical Self-Help Clinic," 5.

41. Alan J. Margolis and Sadja Goldsmith, "Early Abortion without Cervical Dilation: Pump or Syringe Aspiration," *Journal of Reproductive Medicine* 9, no. 5 (November 1972): 237–40; *Feminist Manifesto: All You Ever Wanted to Know about Abortion (But Couldn't Find Out from Your Doctor)*, n.d., ca. 1971, FC, 3. Patricia Maginnis was the likely author.

42. Schoen, *Abortion after Roe*, 25–30.

43. Schoen, 28.

44. Dudley-Shotwell, *Revolutionizing Women's Healthcare*, 14–15; Murphy, *Seizing the Means*, 156–57.

45. For Russia, see "Menstrual Regulation—What Is It?," *Population Reports, Series F (Pregnancy Termination)*, no. 2 (April 1973): f11; for China, see "Harvey Karman: Another Vacuum Cleaner Salesman?," *Her-Self*, October/November 1973, 9, 21. See also Colette Price, "The Self-Help Clinic," *Woman's World*, March/May 1972, 4, 7; Murphy, *Seizing the Means*, 155–57; and Tanfer Emin Tunc, "Designs of Devices: The Vacuum Aspiration and American Abortion Technology," *Dynamis* 28 (2008): 353–76.

46. Lorraine Rothman, "Menstrual Extraction: Procedures," *Quest*, Summer 1978, 45.

47. Lorraine Rothman, "Speech by Lorraine Rothman," in *The Proceedings of the Menstrual Extraction Conference*, ed. Oakland Feminist Women's Health Center (Oakland: Oakland Feminist Women's Health Center, 1974), 12.

48. Rothman, "Speech," 12.

49. Feminist Women's Health Center (Oakland), "Menstrual Extraction: The Means to Responsibly Control Our Periods," n.d., WHRC, reel 1. See also Federation of Feminist Women's Health Centers, *A New View of a Woman's Body: A Fully Illustrated Guide* (New York: Touchstone Books, 1981), 121–27.

50. West Coast Sisters, "Self-Help Clinic," *Everywoman*, July 30, 1971, 6.

51. Products advertised as methods to bring on menstruation have been around since at

least the late nineteenth century. Lauren MacIvor Thompson, "Women Have Always Had Abortions," *New York Times*, December 13, 2019. See also Andrea Tone, "Contraceptive Consumers: Gender and the Political Economy of Birth Control in the 1930s," *Journal of Social History* 29, no. 3 (Spring 1996): 485–506.

52. West Coast Sisters, *Self-Help Clinic Part II* (Los Angeles: Peace Press, 1971), reel 1-356, WHRC. See also Tacie Dejanikus, "Menstrual Extraction," *Off Our Backs*, December 1972, 4–5.

53. Feminist Women's Health Center (Oakland), "Menstrual Extraction."

54. Laura Punnett, "Menstrual Extraction: Politics," *Quest*, Summer 1978, 48. See also "Advanced Self-Help Clinics," *NOW News, Central New Jersey Chapter*, March 1972, 9A.

55. Feminist Women's Health Center (Oakland), "Menstrual Extraction."

56. Carol Downer, "Covert Sex Discrimination against Women as Medical Patients" (80th Annual Convention of the American Psychological Association, Honolulu, HI, September 5, 1972), box 3, folder 23: "Feminism; Ideology, 1970–71," DFWHC.

57. Punnett, "Menstrual Extraction: Politics," 50.

58. Rothman, "Menstrual Extraction: Procedures," 44; Federation of Feminist Women's Health Centers, *A New View*, 121. See also Murphy, *Seizing the Means*, 150–54.

59. Rothman, "Speech," 12.

60. Dejanikus, "Menstrual Extraction," 4–5.

61. In *Seizing the Means of Reproduction*, Michelle Murphy described the importance of process ("arrangement, composition or *protocols* which actualized the elements in some ways, not others") to give actions and technologies particular meaning as "protocol feminism" (30). She referred directly to self-help as envisioned by the West Coast Sisters. Murphy, *Seizing the Means*, 25–67.

62. West Coast Sisters, *Self-Help Clinic Part II*.

63. West Coast Sisters.

64. Dejanikus, "Menstrual Extraction," 5.

65. Punnett, "Menstrual Extraction: Politics," 49.

66. Debra Law, "Speech by Debra Law," in *The Proceedings of the Menstrual Extraction Conference*, ed. The Oakland Feminist Women's Health Center (Oakland: Oakland Feminist Women's Health Center, 1974), 35. See also Murphy, *Seizing the Means*, 150–63.

67. Federation of Feminist Women's Health Centers, *A New View*, 123.

68. Rothman, "Menstrual Extraction: Procedures," 45.

69. Rothman, 46.

70. Barbara Hoke, "Letter: Another Look at Menstrual Extraction," *Daily Californian*, May 24, 1974, 7. The same language is used by Punnett, "Menstrual Extraction: Politics," 49.

71. Frances Hornstein and Rebecca Chalker, interview with the author, June 23, 2008. See also Carol Downer, interview with the author, June 26, 2008.

72. Big Pines meeting minutes, September 15, 1973, box 6, folder 26, DFWHC.

73. Janice Delaney, Mary Jane Lupton, and Emily Toth, *The Curse: A Cultural History of Menstruation* (New York: E. P. Dutton, 1976), 217.

74. Dejanikus, "Menstrual Extraction," 4–5. For more of the "tampering with nature" argument, see Evalyn S. Gendel, "It's Your Body, Not Your Doctor's," *Redbook*, March 1974, 170; and Barbara Seaman, *The Doctor's Case against the Pill* (New York: P. H. Wyden, 1969). For more about Barbara Seaman, see Kelly O'Donnell, "The Political Is Personal: Barbara Seaman and the History of the Women's Health Movement" (PhD diss., Yale University, 2015).

75. Ellen Frankfort, "Vaginal Politics," *Village Voice*, November 25, 1971, 74. See also Ellen

Frankfort, "Medicine, the Feminist Frontier," *New York Times*, March 3, 1973; Ellen Frankfort, "Man-Hating & Medicine," *Village Voice*, March 29, 1973, 9–11; and Ellen Frankfort, *Vaginal Politics* (New York: Quadrangle Books, 1972).

76. Dejanikus, "Menstrual Extraction," 5.

77. Laura Brown, presentation, n.d., box 2, folder 2–3: "Menstrual Extraction," DFWHC, 1. See also Feminist Women's Health Center (Oakland), "Menstrual Extraction"; and West Coast Sisters, *Self-Help Clinic Part II*. This latter publication stressed the need for safety as one of the reasons for using menstrual extraction in a group.

78. Ronald J. Pion, Alan J. Wabrek, and William B. Wilson, "Innovative Methods in Prevention of the Need for Abortions," *Clinical Obstetrics and Gynecology* 14, no. 4 (December 1971): 1313–16; Harvey Karman and Malcolm Potts, "Very Early Abortion Using Syringe as Vacuum Source," *Lancet* 299, no. 7759 (May 13, 1972): 1051–52; Margolis and Goldsmith, "Early Abortion without Cervical Dilation," 237–40; "Menstrual Regulation—What Is It?," f9–f21; William E. Brenner, David A. Edelman, and Elton Kessel, "Menstrual Regulation in the United States: A Preliminary Report," *Fertility and Sterility* 26, no. 3 (March 1975): 289–95.

79. Brenner, Edelman, and Kessel, "Menstrual Regulation in the United States," 289.

80. Milagros F. Atienza, Ronald T. Burkman, Theodore M. King, Lonnie S. Burnett, H. Lorrin Lau, Tim H. Parmley, and J. Donald Woodruff, "Menstrual Extraction," *American Journal of Obstetrics and Gynecology* 121, no. 4 (February 15, 1975): 490–95.

81. Pion, Wabrek, and Wilson, "Innovative Methods," 1313–16.

82. "Menstrual Regulation—What Is It?," f20.

83. Jane E. Hodgson, Roxanne Smith, and Daniella Milstein, "Menstrual Extraction: Putting It and All Its Synonyms into Proper Perspective as Pseudonyms," *JAMA* 228, no. 7 (May 13, 1974): 849.

84. Atienza et al., "Menstrual Extraction," 495.

85. Pion, Wabrek, and Wilson, "Innovative Methods," 1313–14.

86. "Menstrual Regulation—What Is It?," f18; Meyer, "Early Office Termination," 207.

87. Ralph W. Hale et al., "Office Termination of Pregnancy by 'Menstrual Aspiration,'" *American Journal of Obstetrics and Gynecology* 134, no. 2 (May 15, 1979): 216.

88. Gibson, "Liberalized Abortion Law."

89. Michael S. Goldstein, "Creating and Controlling a Medical Market: Abortion in Los Angeles after Liberalization," *Social Problems* 31, no. 5 (June 1984): 515.

90. Goldstein, "Creating and Controlling a Medical Market," 517.

91. Goldstein, 518. The term *abortion entrepreneur* is Goldstein's.

92. Goldstein, 518, 520, 523.

93. Goldstein, 523–25.

94. Lawrence Lader, *Abortion* (Boston: Beacon Press, 1966), 53, quoted in Johanna Schoen, *Abortion after Roe* (Chapel Hill: University of North Carolina Press, 2015), 4.

95. Doris Andrea Dirks and Patricia A. Relf, *To Offer Compassion: A History of the Clergy Consultation Service on Abortion* (Madison: University of Wisconsin Press, 2017); Arlene Carmen and Howard Moody, *Abortion Counseling and Social Change from Illegal Act to Medical Practice: The Story of the Clergy Consultation Service on Abortion* (Valley Forge, PA: Judson Press, 1973); Kaplan, *Story of Jane*; Schoen, *Abortion after Roe*, 4–5.

96. *Feminist Manifesto*, 2.

97. Nancy Banks, "The Truth about Abortion Referral," *Chicago Reader*, December 10,

1971, https://www.chicagoreader.com/chicago/the-truth-about-abortion-referral/Content?oid
=3006913. See also Anne Gardner, "Abortion Referrals," *Everywoman*, December 17, 1971, 13.

98. [West Coast Sisters], "Sisters," *Los Angeles Women's Liberation Newsletter*, November 1971, 6. See also Daphne Spain, *Constructive Feminism: Women's Spaces and Women's Rights in the American City* (Ithaca, NY: Cornell University Press, 2016), 123; and Liddick, "Effects of Supreme Court Ruling."

99. Debra Law, "The Woman-Controlled Abortion," in *Abortion in a Clinic Setting*, ed. Los Angeles Feminist Women's Health Center (Los Angeles: The Feminist Women's Health Center, 1974), 7.

100. "Helping Ourselves: The First Self-Help Clinic," in *Organizing Strategies in Women's Health: An Information and Action Handbook*, ed. Lakshmi Menon (Quezon City: Isis International, 1994), 59.

101. [West Coast Sisters], "Sisters," 6. See also Lorraine [Rothman], "W. L. Abortion Referral Service," *Women's Center Newsletter* (Los Angeles), June 1972, 3.

102. Spain, *Constructive Feminism*, 123.

103. Emily A. Champagne, "First Hand Report: Pregnancy Termination through the Feminist Women's Health Center," *NOW News, Berkeley Chapter*, May 1972, 7.

104. See, for example, Harry Nelson, "AMA Hits Commercialization of Abortion: Condemns Advertising by 'Mills,'" *Los Angeles Times*, September 22, 1970.

105. Schoen, *Abortion after Roe*, 45–59.

106. Carol Downer, "Through the Speculum," in *Test-Tube Women: What Future for Motherhood?*, ed. Rita Arditti, Renate Duelli Klein, and Shelley Minden (London: Pandora Press, 1984), 419; "Abortion Legalized: Supreme Court Ruling Opens Door for Feminist Abortion Clinic," *Sister*, February 1973, 5.

107. Feminist Women's Health Centers, "Synopsis of the Feminist Women's Health Centers' Development" (unpublished manuscript, n.d.), box 2, folder 2–3: "Menstrual Extraction," DF-WHC, 3. The Oakland FWHC opened in May 1973, and the Santa Ana FWHC opened in July 1973.

108. Fran Kaplan, "Owning Our Wellness: L.A. Feminist Women's Health Center: Services, Political Action," interview by Carolyn Keith, *Amazon: A Midwest Journal for Women*, June/July/August 1978, 24.

109. Barbara Hoke, interview with the author, March 19, 2008.

110. Carol Downer, "What Makes the Feminist Women's Health Center 'Feminist'?," *Feminist Women's Health Center Report*, 1974, 12.

111. Mary Heath, "How to Choose Your Abortionist," in *Abortion in a Clinic Setting*, ed. Los Angeles Feminist Women's Health Center (Los Angeles: The Feminist Women's Health Center, 1974), 26.

112. Law, "The Woman-Controlled Abortion," 8.

113. Schoen, *Abortion after Roe*, 45–49.

114. Law, "The Woman-Controlled Abortion," 8. The "physician as technician" model was widespread in feminist abortion clinics. Schoen, *Abortion after Roe*, 50.

115. Kaplan, "Owning Our Wellness," 21.

116. "Physician Training Program," n.d., MC 512, box 14, folder: "Los Angeles Feminist Women's Health Center, 1974–77," WCHC.

117. Carol Downer, "Abortion in a Women-Controlled Educational Setting Using Protocols

and Patient Participation as Quality Control Mechanisms," AB 1503 Grant Application, February 8, 1977, Downer collection.

118. National Advisory Commission on Health Manpower, *Report of the National Advisory Commission on Health Manpower* (Washington, DC: US Government Printing Office, 1967), 1:2.

119. Judith A. Houck, "The Best Prescription for Women's Health: Feminist Approaches to Well-Woman Care," in *Prescribed: Writing, Filling, Using, and Abusing the Prescription in Modern America*, ed. Jeremy A. Greene and Elizabeth Siegel Watkins (Baltimore: Johns Hopkins University Press, 2012), 134–56. See also Dana Gallagher, interview with the author, June 25, 2008.

120. Downer, "Abortion in a Women-Controlled Educational Setting."

121. "FWHC Proposes Laywomen Do Abortions," *Feminist Women's Health Center Report*, April 1977, 10–11.

122. Hope Blacker (Board of Medical Quality Assurance) to Wm. Gerber and Gene Feldman (members of the Division of Allied Health), February 27, 1977, Downer collection.

123. Carole Joffe, "The Politicization of Abortion and the Evolution of Abortion Counseling," *American Journal of Public Health* 103, no. 1 (January 2013): 57–65.

124. Joffe, "The Politicization of Abortion," 57–65.

125. Debra Law, "Counseling," in *Abortion in a Clinic Setting*, ed. Los Angeles Feminist Women's Health Center (Los Angeles: The Feminist Women's Health Center, 1974), 15.

126. Law, "The Woman-Controlled Abortion," 10.

127. Law, "Counseling," 15.

128. Kaplan, "Owning Our Wellness," 20–21. See also Law, "Counseling," 15–18; and Florence Ehring, "The Abortion Procedure," in *Abortion in a Clinic Setting*, ed. Los Angeles Feminist Women's Health Center (Los Angeles: The Feminist Women's Health Center, 1974), 20–22.

129. Carol Downer, interview with the author, March 28, 2007.

130. Feminist Women's Health Center of Detroit, "How to Pick Your Abortion Facility," *Her-Self*, July 1975, 8.

131. Heath, "How to Choose Your Abortionist," 26–27.

132. Lisa Cronin Wohl, "Would You Buy an Abortion from This Man? The Harvey Karman Controversy," *Ms. Magazine*, September 1975, 60–64, 113–20, 124; Elaine Woo, "Creator of Device for Safer Abortions," *Los Angeles Times*, May 18, 2008. Karman, who earned a bachelor's degree in theater and a master's degree in psychology, claimed to have a PhD in psychology from the International University in Geneva, Switzerland, likely a diploma mill.

133. Rothman, "Menstrual Extraction: Procedures," 44.

134. [Los Angeles] Feminist Women's Health Center, *Synopsis of the Activities of Harvey Karman*, n.d., box 2, folder 2–3: "Menstrual Extraction," DFWHC, 1.

135. Bella Stumbo, "Bangladesh War Toll: Mass Abortions," *Los Angeles Times*, March 31, 1972.

136. Murphy, *Seizing the Means*, 163–71.

137. "Women Seized in Cut-Rate Clinic: Nab 7 in Abortion Raid," *Chicago Daily News*, May 4, 1972.

138. Philadelphia Women's Health Collective, "The Philadelphia Story: Another Experiment on Women," *Her-Self*, February 1973, 15; Joan Sweeney, "Women Bused from Chicago: Philadelphia Says L.A. Man Performed Abortions for TV," *Los Angeles Times*, December 12, 1972.

139. Phyllis Ryan, "Karman Article in Error," *Her-Self*, April 1974, 2. Their suspicion of Gosnell's clinic was not misplaced. As of 2021, Gosnell was in prison, convicted of multiple counts of murder for deaths of women and possibly viable infants in his care. Katha Pollitt, "Dr. Kermit

Gosnell's Horror Show," *Nation*, January 27, 2011, https://www.thenation.com/article/archive/dr
-kermit-gosnells-horror-show/; Conor Friedersdorf, "Why Dr. Kermit Gosnell's Trial Should Be
a Front-Page Story," *Atlantic*, April 12, 2013, https://www.theatlantic.com/national/archive/2013
/04/why-dr-kermit-gosnells-trial-should-be-a-front-page-story/274944/.

140. Jan BenDor, "Supercoil Abortion, Karman Part 4," *Her-Self*, January 1974, 8.

141. Wohl, "Would You Buy an Abortion from This Man?," 114. See also Sweeney, "Women
Bused from Chicago"; and Joan Sweeney, "Man Accused of 11 Filmed Abortions to Fight Extradi-
tion," *Los Angeles Times*, December 13, 1972.

142. Ryan, "Karman Article in Error," 2.

143. "Dissension in Iowa City or Male Infiltration," *Monthly Extract*, October/November
1972, 3, in Philadelphia Women's Health Collective, "Philadelphia Story," 15.

144. BenDor, "Supercoil Abortion," 8.

145. Judith P. Bourne et al., "Medical Complications from Induced Abortion by the Super
Coil Method," *Health Services Report* 89, no. 1 (January/February 1974), 42.

146. Frances Chapman, "Supercoil Recoil: Karman Case Comes to Trial," *Off Our Backs*,
November 1973, 6.

147. [Los Angeles] Feminist Women's Health Center, *Synopsis of the Activities of Karman*,
3. For more about Karman's supercoil method, see Tanfer Emin Tunc, "Harvey Karman and
the Super Coil Fiasco: A Forgotten Episode in the History of American Abortion Technology,"
European Journal of Contraception and Reproductive Health Care 13, no. 1 (March 2008): 4–8.

148. See, for example, Linda Gordon, Helen Rodríguez Trías, and Bonnie Mass, "The Politics
of Population Control," in *Proceedings for the 1975 Conference on Women and Health* (Boston:
self-pub., 1975), 28–29.

149. Carol Downer, "Battle against Population Controllers Unite Radical Feminists and
People of Color," *Women's Health Movement Papers*, July 1980, 2. See also Lolly Hirsch, "Personal Response to the Journalists' Encounter on Population," *Monthly Extract*, August/Septem-
ber 1974, 4–11.

150. Helen Rodríguez Trías, "The Case of Puerto Rico," in *Proceedings for the 1975 Conference
on Women and Health* (Boston: self-pub., 1975), 28–29.

151. Linda Gordon, "History," in *Proceedings for the 1975 Conference on Women and Health*
(Boston: self-pub., 1975), 28. See also Laura Briggs, *Reproducing Empire: Race, Sex, Science, and
U.S. Imperialism in Puerto Rico* (Berkeley: University of California Press, 2003).

152. As Carole R. McCann points out, the IPPF was often an unwanted player in the population control community. Carole R. McCann, *Figuring the Population Bomb: Gender and De-
mography in the Mid-twentieth Century* (Seattle: University of Washington Press, 2017), 43–78.

153. Cynthia Pearson, "Women Beware: Planned Parenthood Is On the Move," *Big Mama
Rag*, December 1980, 8–9. See also "Feminist Women's Health Centers Meet Planned Parenthood Physicians," *Feminist Women's Health Center Report*, September 1975, 8–9.

154. Margolis and Goldsmith, "Early Abortion without Cervical Dilation," 240.

155. Jane E. Brody, "Physicians throughout the World Are Studying New, Simple Technique
for Terminating Pregnancies," *New York Times*, December 20, 1973. See also Clive Wood, "Menstrual Extraction: Some Statistics at Last," *British Journal of Sexual Medicine* 2, no. 4 (August
1975): 17.

156. Laura Brown, "Speech by Laura Brown," in *The Proceedings of the Menstrual Extraction
Conference*, ed. The Oakland Feminist Women's Health Center (Oakland: Oakland Feminist
Women's Health Center, 1974), 17; Farber, "Speech," 19.

157. Brody, "Physicians throughout the World."

158. Murphy, *Seizing the Means*, 169; Jack S. Hirsh, discussant, in Meyer, "Early Office Termination," 207.

159. Punnett, "Menstrual Extraction: Politics," 56–58; "Planned Parenthood World Population Washington Memo," *Monthly Extract*, February/March 1974, 12.

160. Pearson, "Women Beware," 8–9.

161. Planned Parenthood clinics composed 5 percent of the clinics listed on the 1982–83 National Abortion Federation roster. Schoen, *Abortion after Roe*, 20.

162. Jill Benderly, "Does Corporate Giant Fill Health Care Needs Like Feminist Clinics?," *New Directions for Women*, January/February 1990, 13, 16; Robert Speer, "Feminist Women's Health Center: Eight Years of Struggle and Success," *Chico News and Review*, February 3, 1983, 38. See also Schoen, *Abortion after Roe*, 20.

163. Downer, "Battle against Population Controllers," 2–3.

Chapter Four

1. Notes on June 9, 1994, Federation of Feminist Women's Health Centers conference call, June 17, 1994, Chico FWHC collection.

2. In 2023, the Feminist Abortion Network included thirteen abortion clinics. Feminist Abortion Network, accessed March 27, 2023, http://www.feministnetwork.org/.

3. The percentage of counties in California without an abortion provider increased from 19 percent in 1977 to 41 percent in 2000. The number of providers decreased from 583 in 1982 to 400 in 2000, a decline of 31 percent. Jacqueline Darroch Forrest, Ellen Sullivan, and Christopher Tietz, "Abortion in the United States, 1977–1978," *Family Planning Perspectives* 11, no. 6 (November/December 1979): 333; Stanley K. Henshaw, "Abortion Incidence and Services in the United States, 1995–1996," *Family Planning Practices* 30, no. 6 (November/December 1998): 267; Lawrence B. Finger and Stanley K. Henshaw, "Abortion Incidence and Services in the United States in 2000," *Perspectives on Sexual and Reproductive Health* 35, no. 1 (January/February 2003): 10.

4. For an analysis of how feminist health clinics changed over time in response to unrelenting opposition, see Sandra Morgen, *Into Our Own Hands: The Women's Health Movement in the United States, 1969–1990* (New Brunswick, NJ: Rutgers University Press, 2002), 110, 112. Other studies of change in the women's health movement include Ruth Simmons, Bonnie J. Kay, and Carol Regan, "Women's Health Groups: Alternatives to the Health Care System," *International Journal of Health Services* 14, no. 4 (1984): 619–34; Jan E. Thomas, "Everything about Us Is Feminist: The Significance of Ideology in Organizational Change," *Gender and Society* 13, no. 1 (February 1999): 101–19; Carol S. Weisman, *Women's Health Care: Activist Traditions and Institutional Change* (Baltimore: Johns Hopkins University Press, 1998), 10–98; Sheryl Burt Ruzek and Julie Becker, "The Women's Health Movement in the United States: From Grass-Roots Activism to Professional Agendas," *JAMWA* 54, no. 1 (Winter 1999): 4–8; and Susan M. Reverby, "Thinking through the Body and the Body Politic: Feminism, History, and Health-Care Policy in the United States," in *Women, Health, and Nation: Canada and the United States since 1945*, ed. Georgina Feldberg, Molly Ladd-Taylor, Alison Li, and Kathryn McPherson (Montreal: McGill-Queen's University Press, 2003), 404–20.

5. Douglas Shuit, "Bucolic Battleground: Tranquil Chico Is Caught in Bitter Political Crossfire," *Los Angeles Times*, April 28, 1985.

6. The reference to the "hippie-free-clinic" comes from Dido Hasper, Janice Turrini, Lor-

raine Rothman, and Lynne Randall, interview, September 9, 1975, Downer collection. The extant transcript, however, does not generally note who asked or answered any particular questions. Interviews later explicitly refute this characterization. Gayle Sweigert described it as a "neighborhood health clinic . . . with pretty good medical care"; Turrini called it a "family health center." Gayle Sweigert, interview with the author, March 18, 2008; Janice Turrini, interview with the author, October 15, 2006; Judy Rutherford and Betty Szudy, interview with the author, June 24, 2008.

7. Rutherford and Szudy, interview.

8. See People v. Belous, 71 Cal. 2d 954 (1969).

9. Hasper, Turrini, Rothman, and Randall, interview.

10. Hasper, Turrini, Rothman, and Randall.

11. Hasper, Turrini, Rothman, and Randall.

12. Hasper, Turrini, Rothman, and Randall.

13. The original nine founders were Dido Hasper, Helen Jones, Gayla Nicholson, Nancy Oakes, Judy Rutherford, Gayle Sweigert, Betty Szudy, Janice Turrini, and Diane. Before the clinic opened, Wendi Jones replaced Diane. Contradictory dates for the clinic's founding are given in "Chico Herstory," n.d., Chico FWHC collection, and Hasper, Turrini, Rothman, and Randall, interview.

14. Johanna Schoen, *Abortion after Roe* (Chapel Hill: University of North Carolina Press, 2015), 42.

15. According to Finn Enke, abortion provision was the lightning rod that led to the Detroit Feminist Women's Health Center's relocation after a neighborhood association used zoning rules to force it to move. Finn Enke, *Finding the Movement: Sexuality, Contested Space, and Feminist Activism* (Durham, NC: Duke University Press, 2007), 197–216.

16. Feminist entrepreneurs and businesswomen also entered the abortion marketplace in the 1970s. Johanna Schoen describes their struggles in *Abortion after Roe*.

17. Schoen, *Abortion after Roe*, 49–52. Schoen provides the history of the Emma Goldman Clinic in Iowa City in *Abortion after Roe*. For a history of feminist abortion provision in Chicago, see Wendy Kline, *Bodies of Knowledge: Sexuality, Reproduction, and Women's Health in the Second Wave* (Chicago: University of Chicago Press, 2010), 65–96; for Seattle, see Jennifer Nelson, *More Than Medicine: A History of the Feminist Women's Health Movement* (New York: New York University Press, 2015), 91–122; for Gainesville, see Evan Hart, "Building a More Inclusive Women's Health Movement: Byllye Avery and the Development of the National Black Women's Health Project, 1981–1990" (PhD diss., University of Cincinnati, 2012), 32–43; and chapter 7.

18. For a discussion of the politics of women-controlled health clinics, see [Los Angeles] Feminist Women's Health Center, "Well Woman Health Care in Woman Controlled Clinics" (unpublished manuscript, 1976), Downer collection.

19. Carol Downer, interview with the author, March 27, 2007. "Nice abortion clinics" provided competent care, but did not work for women's empowerment or challenge medical authority. See chapter 3.

20. Schoen, *Abortion after Roe*, 45–49.

21. Laura Kaplan, *The Story of Jane: The Legendary Underground Feminist Abortion Service* (New York: Pantheon Books, 1995); Kelly Suzanne O'Donnell, "Reproducing Jane: Abortion Stories and Women's Political Histories," *Signs: Journal of Women in Culture and Society* 43, no. 1 (Autumn 2017): 77–96.

22. "Founder. Visionary. Inspiration.," Women's Health Specialists of California, accessed

September 15, 2021, https://www.womenshealthspecialists.org/about/the-womens-movement/dido-hasper/; Rutherford and Szudy, interview; Sweigert, interview.

23. Betty Szudy, interview with the author, July 20, 2006; Turrini, interview.

24. Turrini, interview.

25. Hasper, Turrini, Rothman, and Randall, interview.

26. Kristen Olds, "A Woman-Controlled Clinic: The Chico Feminist Women's Health Care," *Wildcat*, February 27, 1975, 12. The Feminist Federal Credit Union was connected to the Detroit FWHC. Enke, *Finding the Movement*, 197–216.

27. Hasper, Turrini, Rothman, and Randall, interview.

28. Oddly, whether or not the Chico clinic was a collective, and when and if it stopped being a collective, is a matter of some dispute. For example, Dido Hasper claimed that the center stopped being a collective at one point. Dido Hasper, "Feminist Health Movement: Interview with Dido Hasper," by Gayle Kimball, in *Women's Culture in a New Era: A Feminist Revolution?*, ed. Gayle Kimball (Lanham, MD: Scarecrow Press, 2005), 223–29.

29. Szudy, interview.

30. Fran, Mae Dell, Margaret, and Tacie, "What Is 'Feminist' Health?," *Off Our Backs*, June 1974, 2–5; Carol Downer, Lorraine Rothman, and Eleanor Snow, "F.W.H.C. Response," *Off Our Backs*, August/September 1974, 17–18. See also Hannah Dudley-Shotwell, *Revolutionizing Women's Healthcare: The Feminist Self-Help Movement in America* (New Brunswick, NJ: Rutgers University Press, 2020), 45–49.

31. Frances Hornstein, "An Interview on Women's Health Politics, Part I," *Quest*, Summer 1974, 31–32. See also Joreen [Jo Freeman], "The Tyranny of Structurelessness," *Second Wave*, March 1972, 20–24, 42.

32. Hasper, Turrini, Rothman, and Randall, interview. For the criteria to become a director, see "Participation Criteria, Chico Feminist Women's Health Center," November 6, 1976, box 5, folder 42, DFWHC. Because of a policy of information sharing between FWHCs, this collection includes records from many FWHCs.

33. Hasper, Turrini, Rothman, and Randall, interview.

34. Olds, "A Woman-Controlled Clinic," 13.

35. Hasper, Turrini, Rothman, and Randall, interview.

36. Olds, "A Woman-Controlled Clinic," 12–13; Szudy quotation on 12.

37. Chico Feminist Women's Health Center, "Participatory Clinic," n.d., Downer collection.

38. [Los Angeles] Feminist Women's Health Center, *Well Woman Health Care*.

39. Staff meeting minutes, October 26, 1976, box 5, folder 42, DFWHC.

40. Gayle, "Referral Notes," March 1975, box 5, folder 46, DFWHC.

41. Laurie Clifton, "Hasper: Making a Difference in Women's Health," *Chico Enterprise-Record*, September 6, 1993.

42. For abortion as the economic base of a larger movement, see Paula Span, "Health: A New Era for Feminist Health Clinics," *New York Times*, November 23, 1980; and Shauna Heckert, interview with the author, June 21, 2007.

43. "Chico FWHC Clinic Statistics," February 15, 1975–December 31, 1979, "NORCAL Appeal" binder, Chico FWHC collection.

44. See chapter 3.

45. Staff meeting notes, September 21, 1976, box 5, folder 42, DFWHC.

46. Medical policy meeting notes, February 11, 1977, box 5, folder 42, DFWHC.

47. "Physician Training Program," n.d., MC 512, box 14, folder: "Los Angeles Feminist Women's Health Center, 1974–77," WCHC.

48. Olds, "A Woman-Controlled Clinic," 12. In 1982, representatives of the clinic continued to refer to the physicians as "technicians." Leslie Cagno, "A Matter of Choice," *Chico News and Review*, August 26, 1982.

49. Investigator notes, Employment Development Department Investigation, April 18, 1984, Chico FWHC collection, 64.

50. "Statement of Warren M. Hern, MD, before the NORCAL Review Board Concerning Malpractice Insurance Suspension Affecting the Chico Feminist Women's Health Center," March 10, 1980, "Physician Cover-Up" binder, Chico FWHC collection. Hern helped found the first freestanding nonprofit abortion clinic in Colorado. He continued in 2021 to be one of a handful of physicians to provide late-term abortions.

51. Hasper, Turrini, Rothman, and Randall, interview. Hanson's supervising physician was Carl Watson, one of the physicians who performed abortions at the clinic. Brenda Smith Hanson, interview with the author, March 19, 2008. For more about the role of the nurse practitioner at the clinic, see Judith A. Houck, "The Best Prescription for Women's Health: Feminist Approaches to Well-Woman Care," in *Prescribed: Writing, Filling, Using, and Abusing the Prescription in Modern America*, ed. Jeremy A. Greene and Elizabeth Siegel Watkins (Baltimore: Johns Hopkins University Press, 2012), 134–56.

52. Although the center often claimed that it was the only place in Northern California that offered abortions, at least two Chico ob-gyns occasionally performed abortions in the local hospital, and a third also offered abortion services at his office briefly between June 1977 and sometime in 1978. See Thomas Lorenz, deposition, June 20, 1980, "Physician Cover-Up" binder, Chico FWHC collection, 19.

53. [Anti-trust internal documents], "Background," January 22, 1981, Chico FWHC collection.

54. Hasper, Turrini, Rothman, and Randall, interview.

55. Sweigert, interview.

56. Judy Rutherford left in the fall or winter of 1976, feeling "spent" by all the service work in health care. "Directors' Notes," October 19, 1976, box 5, folder 42, DFWHC.

57. Turrini, interview; Szudy, interview.

58. Hilary Abramson, "Feminists vs. the State," *Sacramento Bee*, May 1, 1988, 8, citing a March 11, 1975, memo from the Butte-Glenn Medical Society directors' meeting.

59. Rebecca Chalker, "Chico Feminist Women's Health Center Files Second Major Antitrust Suit against OB/GYNS," *Health Activists' Digest* 3, no. 2 (Fall 1981), 42–45. Hans Freistadt, a semiretired ob-gyn in Oroville, twenty-six miles north of Chico, agreed to provide backup in December 1975. Hans Freistadt, contract, December 19, 1975, "NORCAL Appeal" binder, Chico FWHC collection.

60. Notes of conversation with Barry Furst and Chris Nelson-Watson, December 15, 1978, "Physician Cover-Up" binder, Chico FWHC collection.

61. Many of the facts in this case, including whether the hysterectomy was necessary, why Romano did not go to the hospital immediately, and whether Palmer was negligent, remain unresolved.

62. Audrey Pulis to Leonard and Lyde (attorneys at law), August 5, 1980, "Physician Cover-Up" binder, Chico FWHC collection.

63. D. Peter Harvey to Robert L. Bateman, February 28, 1980, "NORCAL Appeal" binder, Chico FWHC collection.

64. "Chronology," "Physician Cover-Up" binder, Chico FWHC collection.

65. News of this lawsuit was published widely in both mainstream and left-of-center periodicals. See, for example, Roger Aylworth, "$12 Million Conspiracy Suit Filed," *Chico Enterprise-Record,* January 22, 1981; Dale Vargas, "Doctors Named in Antitrust Suit," *Sacramento Bee,* January 23, 1981; Rebecca Chalker, "Clinic Sues Doctors," *Guardian,* February 25, 1981; "Women's Health Under Siege," *Revolutionary Worker,* February 27, 1981; and "California Center Sues Male MDs," *New Directions for Women,* March/April 1981, 10.

66. Kevin Jeys, "FWHC Files Massive Restraint of Trade, Conspiracy Suit," *Chico News and Review,* January 23, 1981; Chalker, "Chico Center Files Anti-trust Suit." See also Dudley-Shotwell, *Revolutionizing Women's Healthcare,* 59–62.

67. "Calls to Area Doctors Re: Abortion Referrals," "Physician Cover-Up" binder, Chico FWHC collection.

68. Notes of conversation with Furst and Nelson-Watson.

69. "Calls to Area Doctors Re: Abortion Referrals."

70. Notes of telephone conversation with Victor Mlotok, April 16, 1980, "Physician Cover-Up" binder, Chico FWHC collection. Shauna Heckert spoke to Mlotok on the phone while Dido Hasper took notes.

71. Notes of meeting with Richard MacDonald, Lisa Todd, and Jeannie Clayton, April 25, 1980, "Physician Cover-Up" binder, Chico FWHC collection.

72. Notes of conversation with Max Lee, Melanie, and Karen, April 15, 1980, "Physician Cover-Up" binder, Chico FWHC collection.

73. Kathy Funk, notes of conversation with Steven Pulverman, August 20, 1979, "Physician Cover-Up" binder, Chico FWHC collection.

74. Pulis to Leonard and Lyde.

75. Maureen Pierce, notes of conversation with Hans Freistadt and Shauna Heckert, August 6, 1979, "Physician Cover-Up" binder, Chico FWHC collection.

76. "Feminist Center, Physicians Settle Suit Out of Court," *Chico Enterprise-Record,* May 13, 1983. See also "Women's Clinic Wins Rights on Abortion, Settles Suit," *Oakland Tribune,* May 17, 1983; and Bee Metro Staff, "Feminist Health Center Wins Suit against Doctors, Hospital," *Sacramento Bee,* May 17, 1983.

77. See Morgen, *Into Our Own Hands,* 23–24; and chapter 1.

78. Ellen Peskin to Jacques Barzaghi (special assistant to the governor), March 23, 1978, "Briefing Notebook," Chico FWHC collection; Ellen Peskin to Jerome Lackner (Department of Health), March 25, 1978, "Briefing Notebook," Chico FWHC collection. The California FWHCs that were part of the federation were Chico, Los Angeles, Orange County, and San Diego.

79. See, for example, Mabel W. Daley (OFP) to Diane Hasper (Chico FWHC), December 16, 1975, "Briefing Notebook," Chico FWHC collection.

80. Barbara Aved (OFP) to Shauna Heckert (Chico FWHC), May 9, 1977, "Briefing Notebook," Chico FWHC collection.

81. Shauna Heckert and Diane Hasper (Chico FWHC) to Barbara Avid [*sic*] OFP, May 20, 1977, "Briefing Notebook," Chico FWHC collection.

82. Barbara Aved to Diane Hasper and Shauna Heckert, August 15, 1977, "Briefing Notebook," Chico FWHC collection.

83. See, for example, Dido Hasper to Thelma Fraziear (OFP), December 7, 1977; and Shauna Heckert to Dale Houghland (Office of Health Professions Development), February 23, 1978, both "Briefing Notebook," Chico FWHC collection.

84. Jerome A. Lackner to Ellen Peskin, March 29, 1978, "Briefing Notebook," Chico FWHC collection.

85. Dido Hasper to Thelma Fraziear, July 22, 1981, Chico FWHC collection, mentions this 1979 waiver.

86. See, for example, documentation of an investigation prompted by the lieutenant governor's office, "Mike Curb" file, Chico FWHC collection.

87. Josette Mondanaro and Lyn Headley to Philip Weiler (chief deputy director of the Department of Health Services), memorandum, May 15, 1979, Downer collection.

88. Report of phone call between Josette Mondanaro to Carol Downer, May 16, 1979, "Briefing Notebook," Chico FWHC collection; Mondanaro and Headley to Weiler, memorandum; Dido Hasper to Phil Weiler (Department of Health Services), June 21, 1979, "Briefing Notebook," Chico FWHC collection.

89. Dido Hasper to Beverlee Myers, July 12, 1979, "Briefing Notebook," Chico FWHC collection.

90. On and off for about a year between 1980 and 1981, Mike Curb was acting governor as Jerry Brown was frequently outside the state campaigning for president. Curb used this opportunity to further a conservative agenda.

91. Philip Weiler (Department of Health Services) to Jeannie Clayton, April 7, 1981, "Briefing Notebook," Chico FWHC collection.

92. A Planned Parenthood clinic moved into Humboldt County in 1980. Lynn Johnson, "Feminist Health Centers under Siege," *WIN*, March 1, 1981, 4–8.

93. Dido Hasper (Chico FWHC) to Barbara Aved (OFP), July 30, 1981, Chico FWHC collection.

94. Barbara Aved (OFP) to Thora DeLey, July 28, 1981, Chico FWHC collection; Thora DeLey (Chico FWHC) to Barbara Aved (OFP), August 14, 1981, Chico FWHC collection; Barbara Aved (OFP) to "Family Planning Providers," October 8, 1981, Chico FWHC collection.

95. See Webster v. Reproductive Health Services, 492 U.S. 490 (1989); and Planned Parenthood of Southeastern Pa. v. Casey, 505 U.S. 833 (1992).

96. Johanna Schoen's *Abortion after* Roe analyzes various tactics of antiabortion activists after 1973. For a look at antichoice tactics against abortion clinics, see 155–97. See also Wendy Simonds, *Abortion at Work: Ideology and Practice in a Feminist Clinic* (New Brunswick, NJ: Rutgers University Press, 1996), 103–33. For a history of the antichoice movement, see Dallas A. Blanchard, *The Anti-abortion Movement and the Rise of the Religious Right: From Polite to Fiery Protest* (New York: Twayne Publishers, 1994); James Risen and Judy L. Thomas, *Wrath of Angels: The American Abortion War* (New York: Basic Books, 1998); and Karissa Haugeberg, *Women against Abortion: Inside the Largest Moral Reform Movement of the Twentieth Century* (Urbana: University of Illinois Press, 2017).

97. Patricia Baird-Windle and Eleanor J. Bader, *Targets of Hatred: Anti-Abortion Terrorism* (New York: Palgrave, 2001), xviii; Cynthia Gorney, *Articles of Faith: A Frontline History of the Abortion Wars* (New York: Simon & Schuster, 1998), 521; James Risen and Judy L. Thomas, *Wrath of Angels: The American Abortion War* (New York: Basic Books, 1998), 340.

98. "Feminist Women's Health Center Summary of Anti-activity: Volunteer Logs," various

dates, 1993 ("baby-killer," November 9, 1993; "butcher," August 20, 1993), Chico FWHC collection; "Fire at Redding Abortion Clinic Probed," *Redding (CA) Record Searchlight,* October 2, 1989; Judi Lemos, "Blaze Guts Abortion Clinic," *Redding (CA) Record Searchlight,* July 12, 1990; "Arsonist Hits Women's Clinic," *Sacramento Bee,* June 7, 1992; Adrienne Packer, "Abortion Clinics Set Afire," *Redding (CA) Record Searchlight,* October 10, 1994.

99. Judi Lemos, "Abortion Foe Pleads Guilty," *Redding (CA) Record Searchlight,* October 20, 1993. See also "Abortion: Violence Raises Stakes at Clinics," *Sacramento Bee,* March 6, 1994.

100. Elaine Gray, "Stink Bomb Closes Chico Abortion Center," *Chico Enterprise-Record,* September 18, 1992.

101. Herbert A. Sample, "Court Spurns Plea of Abortion Foes," *Sacramento Bee,* November 28, 1995.

102. Carmen J. Lee, "Clinton Access Bill Signed," *Pittsburgh Post-Gazette,* May 27, 1994.

103. Cindy Pearson, "Self-Help Clinic Celebrates 25 Years," *Network News,* March/April 1996, 1–2, 4; Schoen, *Abortion after Roe,* 195; "Our Herstory," Women's Choice Clinic, accessed April 16, 2007, www.womenschoiceclinic.org/herstory.html.

104. Carol Downer, recorded public interview at Chico, CA, n.d., CD, Downer collection; Jill Benderly, "Does Corporate Giant Fill Health Care Needs Like Feminist Clinics?," *New Directions for Women,* January/February 1990, 13, 16. The San Diego FWHC was taken over by Planned Parenthood.

105. Heckert quotation in Robert Speer, "Feminist Women's Health Center: Eight Years of Struggle and Success," *Chico News and Review,* February 3, 1983, 39; all other quotations in Claudine Campbell, "Planned Parenthood: Year Old Clinic Will Offer Abortion Services," *Chico News and Review,* 1983, from clipping in Chico FWHC collection.

106. "Report on Planned Parenthood Competition, Competition in General, and Plans for the Future," *Economic Survival of Woman-Controlled Clinics: A Summit Meeting,* November 7–8, [1994?], Downer collection.

107. Benderly, "Does Corporate Giant Fill Needs?," 13.

108. Thora DeLey, interview with the author, October 12, 2006; Heckert, interview.

109. By October 2005, the truce had apparently expired, and the center issued the document "Call to Action: Understanding and Exposing Population Control: The Colonization of Women's Bodies," Chico FWHC collection.

110. For more about the history of Medicaid (and Medi-Cal) managed care, see Jonathan Engel, *Poor People's Medicine: Medicaid and American Charity Care since 1965* (Durham, NC: Duke University Press, 2006), 202–43.

111. Elizabeth C. Saviano and Margie Powers, *California's Safety-Net Clinics: A Primer* (Oakland: California HealthCare Foundation, 2005).

112. Andrew B. Bindman et al., "Medicaid Managed Care's Impact on Safety-Net Clinics in California," *Health Affairs* 19, no. 1 (January/February 2000): 194–202.

113. Federation of Feminist Women's Health Centers, "Health Care Reform: A Case for Single Payer Reimbursement for Abortion," February 1994, Chico FWHC collection.

114. Notes on June 9, 1994, Federation of FWHCs conference call.

115. Women's Health Specialists, "Annual Report 2003," Chico FWHC collection.

116. Notes on June 9, 1994, Federation of FWHCs conference call.

117. Chico Feminist Women's Health Center, "Herstory Timeline, 1971–1998" binder, Chico FWHC collection.

118. Heckert, interview.

Chapter Five

1. F[rances] Hornstein, *Lesbian Health Care* (1973; repr., Los Angeles: Feminist Women's Health Center, 1974), 1, 2.

2. Hornstein, *Lesbian Health Care*, 3.

3. Barbara Herbert, "'Nobody Knows What Lesbian Health Is, or What It Could Be': An Interview with Lesbian Health Activist and Doctor Barbara Herbert," interview by Louise Rice, *Gay Community News*, April 16–22, 1989, 9.

4. Henry L. Minton, "Community Empowerment and the Medicalization of Homosexuality: Constructing Sexual Identities in the 1930s," *Journal of the History of Sexuality* 6, no. 3 (January 1996): 435–58; Marcia M. Gallo, *Different Daughters: A History of the Daughters of Bilitis and the Rise of the Lesbian Rights Movement* (New York: Carroll & Graf, 2006); C. Todd White, *Pre-gay L.A.: A Social History of the Movement for Homosexual Rights* (Urbana: University of Illinois Press, 2009); Lillian Faderman, *The Gay Revolution: The Story of Struggle* (New York: Simon & Schuster, 2015).

5. Elizabeth A. Armstrong, *Forging Gay Identities: Organizing Sexuality in San Francisco, 1950–1994* (Chicago: University of Chicago Press, 2002); David Eisenbach, *Gay Power: An American Revolution* (New York: Carroll & Graf, 2006); Faderman, *The Gay Revolution*; Jeremiah J. Garretson, *The Path to Gay Rights: How Activism and Coming Out Changed Public Opinion* (New York: New York University Press, 2018). Surely people who might now identify as trans and not clearly gay or lesbian, including people who identified as "queens," were centrally involved in the gay liberation movement. See, for example, *Screaming Queens: The Riot at Compton's Cafeteria*, directed by Victor Silverman and Susan Stryker (2005; San Francisco: Frameline, 2006), streaming video, 56 minutes, https://www.youtube.com/watch?v=G-WASW9dRBU&ab_channel=KQEDArts.

6. Marc Stein, *City of Sisterly and Brotherly Loves: Lesbian and Gay Philadelphia, 1945–1972* (Philadelphia: Temple University Press, 2004), 350.

7. Del Martin, "If That's All There Is," *Ladder*, December/January 1970–1971, 4–5. See also Robin Morgan, "Goodbye to All That," in *Dear Sisters: Dispatches from the Women's Liberation Movement*, ed. Rosalyn Baxandall and Linda Gordon (1970; repr., New York: Basic Books, 2000), 53–57; and Faderman, *The Gay Revolution*, 227–32.

8. See Ellen Willis, "Letter to the Left," in *Dear Sisters: Dispatches from the Women's Liberation Movement*, ed. Rosalyn Baxandall and Linda Gordon (1969; repr., New York: Basic Books, 2000), 51. See also Alice Echols, *Daring to Be Bad: Radical Feminism in America, 1967–1975* (Minneapolis: University of Minnesota Press, 1989), 23–60. Some lesbian activists pushed back. Although not mentioning Martin by name, Gittings and coauthor Kay Tobin denounced lesbians who had a "supercharged response to sexism and male chauvinism," which led them to attack the "sexism of the handiest men around, the gay men in the movement." Barbara Gittings and Kay Tobin, "Lesbians and the Gay Movement," in *Our Right to Love: A Lesbian Resource Book*, ed. Ginny Vida (Englewood Cliffs, NJ: Prentice-Hall, 1978), 151.

9. Martin, "If That's All There Is," 5.

10. Radicalesbians, "The Woman-Identified-Woman," in *Dear Sisters: Dispatches from the Women's Liberation Movement*, ed. Rosalyn Baxandall and Linda Gordon (1970; repr., New York: Basic Books, 2000), 107–9. For the lesbian menace action, see Echols, *Daring to Be Bad*, 214–16; and Stephanie Gilmore and Elizabeth Kaminski, "A Part and Apart: Lesbian and Straight Feminist Activists Negotiate Identity in a Second-Wave Organization," *Journal of the History of Sexuality* 16, no. 1 (January 2007): 96–97.

11. See, for example, Arlene Stein, *Sex and Sensibility: Stories of a Lesbian Generation* (Berkeley: University of California Press, 1997), 1–23.

12. Finn Enke, *Finding the Movement: Sexuality, Contested Space, and Feminist Activism* (Durham, NC: Duke University Press, 2007); Keridwen N. Luis, *Herlands: Exploring the Women's Land Movement in the United States* (Minneapolis: University of Minnesota Press, 2018); Bonnie J. Morris, "'Anyone Can Be a Lesbian': The Women's Music Audience and Lesbian Politics," *Journal of Lesbian Studies* 5, no. 4 (2001): 91–120; Maria McGrath, "Living Feminist: The Liberation and Limits of Countercultural Business and Radical Lesbian Ethics at Bloodroot Restaurant," *The Sixties: A Journal of History, Politics and Culture* 9, no. 2 (2016): 189–217.

13. Stein, *Sex and Sensibility*, 13.

14. Stein, 20.

15. Ada Calhoun, *St. Marks Is Dead: The Many Lives of America's Hippest Street* (New York: W. W. Norton, 2016), 221–22; Franklin N. Judson, "Sexually Transmitted Disease in Gay Men," *Sexually Transmitted Diseases* 4, no. 2 (April/June 1977): 76.

16. Bert Hansen, "American Physicians' 'Discovery' of Homosexuals, 1880–1900: A New Diagnosis in a Changing Society," in *Sickness and Health in America*, ed. Judith Walzer Leavitt and Ronald L. Numbers, 3rd ed. (Madison, WI: University of Wisconsin Press, 1997), 13–31; Harry Oosterhuis, *Stepchildren of Nature: Krafft-Ebing, Psychiatry, and the Making of Sexual Identity* (Chicago: University of Chicago Press, 2000); Jennifer Terry, *An American Obsession: Science, Medicine, and Homosexuality in Modern Society* (Chicago: University of Chicago Press, 1999).

17. Annelise Orleck, "Lesbian Lives, Lesbian Rights, Lesbian Feminism," in *Rethinking American Women's Activism* (New York: Routledge, 2015), 180.

18. For a history of the efforts to remove homosexuality from the *DSM*, see Ronald Bayer, *Homosexuality and American Psychiatry: The Politics of Diagnosis* (1981; repr., Princeton, NJ: Princeton University Press, 1987).

19. Orleck, "Lesbian Lives, Lesbian Rights," 180; Bopper Deyton and Walter Lear, "A Brief History of the Gay/Lesbian Health Movement in the U.S.A.," in *The Sourcebook on Lesbian/Gay Health Care*, ed. Michael Shernoff and William A. Scott, 2nd ed. (Washington, DC: National Lesbian/Gay Health Foundation, 1988), 17–18.

20. "What's Happening with ALMA," *Lesbian Connection*, March 1975, 3.

21. John Whyte and Lisa Capaldini, "Treating the Lesbian or Gay Patient," *Delaware Medical Journal* 52, no. 5 (May 1980): 271–80. Gay People in Medicine, the precursor to LGPIM, was founded by Paul Paroski. John Whyte, email message to the author, April 15, 2020.

22. Deyton and Lear, "Brief History of the Gay/Lesbian Health Movement," 15, 18. By at least 1982, there were national and local groups of lesbian health providers, including Lesbians in Health Care in New York City. "Herstory of LIHC," *Lesbian Health News*, March 1982, Health 05760, LHA.

23. Judson, "Sexually Transmitted Disease in Gay Men," 76–78; David G. Ostrow et al., "Epidemiology of Gonorrhea Infection in Gay Men," *Journal of Homosexuality* 5, no. 3 (Spring 1980): 285–88. See also Katie Batza, "A Clinic Comes Out: Idealism, Pragmatism, and Gay Health Services in Boston, 1971–1985," in *Beyond the Politics of the Closet: Gay Rights and the American State Since the 1970s*, ed. Jonathan Bell (Philadelphia: University of Pennsylvania Press, 2020), 19–39; Katie Batza, *Before AIDS: Gay Health Politics in the 1970s* (Philadelphia: University of Pennsylvania Press, 2018), 233–65; Richard A. McKay, "Before HIV: Venereal Disease among Homosexually Active Men in England and North America," in *The Routledge History of Disease*, ed. Mark Jackson (New York: Routledge, 2017), 439–57; Michael Brown and Larry Knopp, "The

NOTES TO PAGES 155–158

Birth of the (Gay) Clinic," *Health & Place* 28 (July 2014): 99–108; and untitled grant proposal, National Alliance of Lesbian and Gay Health Clinics, n.d., ca. 1992.

24. In 1979, the clinic clarified its position, noting that while women would not be "discriminated against" if they sought STD screening or treatment, it did not have the staff or facilities to "comfortably accommodate women" who sought other gynecological services. Howard Brown noted that they welcomed ideas and volunteers to figure out how they could be more open to women, but programs for women did not develop for another decade. "Lesbian Health Issues Addressed," *Blazing Star*, November 1979, 3. For a history of gay health clinics, see Batza, *Before AIDS*.

25. Rona N. Affoumado to "Dear Friend," Winter 1988, MssCol 1483, box 3, folder: "Community Health Project (NYC)," IGIC.

26. In her history of the lesbian health movement, Risa Denenberg claims that many of the leaders of the women's health movement were lesbians. The proportion of lesbians in the movement seems to have varied significantly geographically. Risa Denenberg, "A History of the Lesbian Health Movement," in *The Lesbian Health Book: Caring for Ourselves*, ed. Jocelyn White and Marissa C. Martinez (Seattle: Seal Press, 1997), 3–22. See also Hannah Dudley-Shotwell, *Revolutionizing Women's Healthcare: The Feminist Self-Help Movement in America* (New Brunswick, NJ: Rutgers University Press, 2020), 52–53.

27. Dudley-Shotwell, *Revolutionizing Women's Healthcare*, 52. Women involved in the Santa Cruz Women's Health Center similarly describe sexual exploration. Kater Pollock, interview with the author, July 1, 2011.

28. Marion Banzhaf, interview by Sarah Schulman, April 18, 2007, ACT UP Oral History Project, 22, http://www.actuporalhistory.org/interviews/images/banzhaf.pdf.

29. "Emma Goldman Women's Free Clinic," *Workforce*, May 1974, 21–22.

30. Barbara Hoke, interview with the author, March 19, 2008.

31. Kathy Riley, "Self-Defense and Health Care," *Lavender Woman*, December 1974, 5.

32. "Is There Life after Abortions?," *Lesbian Connection*, November 1975, 12. See also "I Am a Lesbian Health Care Worker," n.d., box 5, folder 11: Lesbian Self-Help, DFWHC. On concerns regarding the heterosexist nature of the self-help movement, see Lolly Hirsch, "Second Women-Controlled Women's Health Center Conference," *Monthly Extract*, December 1974/January 1975, 5.

33. "Report of the Lesbian Working Group," in *Proceedings for the 1975 Conference on Women and Health* (Boston: self-pub., 1975), 50–51.

34. Sharon Lieberman, "Women's Health: Professionalism Can Be Destructive," *Majority Report*, May 1975, 6.

35. "Berkeley Women's Health Collective," *Monthly Extract*, September/October 1976, 18; Chicago Lesbian Liberation to Carol and Lorraine, letter, *Monthly Extract*, March/April 1973, 5. See also Carolyn Keith-Mueller, "Owning Our Wellness," *Amazon*, September/October, 1977, 6.

36. "Berkeley Women's Health Collective," 18. Lesbian activists outside the health movement also engaged with self-help. In September 1976, for example, the Atlanta Lesbian Feminist Alliance held a potluck dinner and a self-help clinic. "Self-Help Clinic," *ALFA Newsletter*, September 1976, 6.

37. "BACC Lesbian Clinic Opens," *Feminist Communications*, August 1978, 4; Atlanta Feminist Women's Health Center, *Lesbian Well-Woman Clinic*, n.d., ca. 1981, box 47, folder: "Lesbian Health Care Concerns," FWHCR; "Lesbian Health Services Beginning in February 1977," *Santa*

Cruz Women's Health Center Newsletter, March 1977, 5; Paula Klein, "Health Needs Assessment in a Lesbian Community," (unpublished manuscript, September 10, 1980), box 44, folder: "Lesbian Health Issues," EGC. A gynecology clinic was also offered at the Gay Community Health Services Center in Los Angeles, but I saw it mentioned only once, so it was likely short lived. See "Women's Clinic Opens," *Lesbian Tide*, February 1973, 21. See also the Philadelphia Lavender Health Coalition's Lesbian Clinic, mentioned in the February 27, 1981, minutes of the St. Marks Women's Health Collective, Mears collection.

38. Lesbian Health Committee meeting minutes, April 26, 1976, box 17, folder: "Lesbian Health Committee, 1976-1977," EGC.

39. Klein, "Health Needs Assessment in a Lesbian Community" The survey this report describes was circulated in 1976. [Permission to quote granted by the archive.]

40. Women's Community Health Center, annual report, August 1975, MC 512, box 1, folder 13, WCHC, 2; Women's Community Health Center, second annual report, 1976, MC 512, box 1, folder 13, WCHC, 2.

41. Women's Community Health Center, second annual report, 8. See also Women's Community Health Center, "Statement on Sexual Preference," n.d., box 6, folder 15, DFWHC.

42. Women's Community Health Center, "Fifth Anniversary Annual Report," 1979, MC 512, box 1, folder 13, WCHC, 3. The Women's Community Health Center closed in 1981.

43. See Boston Women's Health Collective, "Homosexuality," in *Women and Their Bodies: A Course* (Boston: Boston Women's Health Collective, 1970), 31-34; Boston Women's Health Course Collective, "Homosexuality," in *Our Bodies, Ourselves: A Course by and for Women* (Boston: New England Free Press, 1971), 19-21.

44. Boston Women's Health Book Collective, *Our Bodies, Ourselves: A Book by and for Women* (New York: Simon and Schuster, 1973), 56, quoted in Wendy Kline, *Bodies of Knowledge: Sexuality, Reproduction, and Women's Health in the Second Wave* (Chicago: University of Chicago Press, 2010), 37.

45. Boston Women's Health Book Collective, *Our Bodies, Ourselves*, 56.

46. Kline, *Bodies of Knowledge*, 38.

47. Radicalesbians Health Collective, "Lesbians and the Health Care System," mimeograph, 1971, Health 05760, LHA, 1, 15. This document was reprinted several times. See "Lesbians and the Health Care System," *Gay Alternative*, April 1973, 14-17; and "Lesbians and the Health Care System," in *Out of the Closets: Voices of Gay Liberation*, ed. Karla Jay and Allen Young, 20th anniversary ed. (New York: New York University Press, 1992), 122-41.

48. Radicalesbians Health Collective, "Lesbians and the Health Care System," 12, 14. In the early 1970s, no major American "mental health associations had enacted ethical codes disallowing sexual encounters" between therapists and clients. Lucas Richert, *Break On Through: Radical Psychiatry and the American Counterculture* (Cambridge, MA: MIT Press, 2019), 28-31, 29.

49. Radicalesbians Health Collective, "Lesbians and the Health Care System," 15. This set of demands was reiterated in Barb Terrien and Irene Nodel, "Lesbian Health Day Statement," *Her-Self*, November 1975, 14.

50. Kristi, "Lesbians & Alcoholism," *Lesbian Connection*, February 1975, 4. See also Kristi, "Lesbians & Alcoholism: Part II," *Lesbian Connection*, March 1975, 6-8; "Are You a Lesbian Alcoholic?," *Lesbian Connection*, December 1974, 18; Catherine, "An Address to Alcoholic Lesbians by a Drunken Dyke," *Lesbian Connection*, May 1975, 18-20; Jean Swallow, ed., *Out from Under: Sober Dykes and Our Friends* (San Francisco: Spinsters/Aunt Lute, 1983); Brenda Weathers, *Alcoholism and the Lesbian Community* (Washington, DC: Gay Council on Drinking Behavior, 1980);

and Audrey Borden, *The History of Gay People in Alcoholics Anonymous: From the Beginning* (New York: Haworth Press, 2007).

51. Patricia Robertson and Julius Schachter, "Failure to Identify Venereal Disease in a Lesbian Population," *Sexually Transmitted Diseases* 8, no. 2 (April–June 1981): 76. This claim is often repeated, but some survey data fails to support it. See, for example, n39.

52. "Lesbian Health Collective," *Pandora*, June 1975, 6.

53. "Lesbian Health Collective," 6.

54. "Creative Arts Shown at Gay Symposium," *Pandora*, April 1975, 11.

55. The Lesbian Health Collective (formerly known as the Lesbian Clinic) was advertised in *Lesbian Connection*, *Pandora*, and *Northwest Passage* between April 1974 and August 1976.

56. Francis X. Clines, "Village Youths Find Friend in Doctor," *New York Times*, July 13, 1970. St. Marks Community Clinic is sometimes seen in print as St. Mark's Clinic or St. Mark's Community Clinic, but the official letterhead from the era spells it without the apostrophe.

57. Calhoun, *St. Marks Is Dead*; James Nevius, "The Strange History of the East Village's Most Famous Street," *Curbed*, September 4, 2014, https://ny.curbed.com/2014/9/4/10052426/the-strange-history-of-the-east-villages-most-famous-street.

58. Leslie B. Tanner, "Sisterhood Is Medical at Free Clinic," *Majority Report*, April 1974, 10, 16.

59. Joan Waitkevicz, "Notes on a Lesbian Medical Clinic" (unpublished manuscript, 1975), Waitkevicz collection.

60. Joyce Hunter, "St. Mark's Clinic in Danger of Closing," *Gotham*, April 16, 1980, 5.

61. Peg Byron, "Lesbian Health Clinic Update," *WomaNews*, May 1980, 5.

62. Barbara Herbert, interview with the author, December 17, 2017. Herbert herself eventually left for medical school.

63. "CHP [Community Health Project] Update," March 23, 1989, TAM.162, box 3, folder: "Lesbian Issues," WHAM.

64. Patricia E. Stevens, "Lesbian Health Care Research: A Review of the Literature from 1970 to 1990," *Health Care for Women International* 13, no. 2 (1992): 91–120.

65. See, for example, Raphael S. Good, "The Gynecologist and the Lesbian," *Clinical Obstetrics and Gynecology* 19, no. 2 (June 1976): 473–82; and F. Edwin Kenyon, "Homosexuality in Gynaecological Practice," *Clinics in Obstetrics and Gynecology* 7, no. 2 (August 1980): 363–85.

66. Hornstein, *Lesbian Health Care*, 5–7.

67. Robertson and Schachter, "Failure to Identify Venereal Disease," 75–76.

68. Hornstein, *Lesbian Health Care*, 4, 5.

69. These groups included the Women's Community Health Center in Cambridge, Massachusetts, the Chico Feminist Women's Health Center, and the Emma Goldman Clinic for Women. Paula Klein and Suzanne Vilmain, *Self-Health for Lesbian Women* (Iowa City: Emma Goldman Clinic for Women, 1978), box 44, folder: "Lesbian Health Issues," EGC; Chico Lesbian Self-Help Group, *Health Care for Lesbians*, n.d., Feminism-International Lesbian Movement folder 05860, LHA; Lesbian Pamphlet Writing Group [of the Women's Community Health Center] to "Sisters," *Lesbian Tide*, November/December 1975, 29.

70. See "Report of the Lesbian Working Group," 51.

71. Mary O'Donnell, Kater Pollock, Val Leoffler, and Ziesel Saunders, *Lesbian Health Matters!* (Santa Cruz: Santa Cruz Women's Health Collective, 1979), 5.

72. O'Donnell et al., *Lesbian Health Matters!*, 45. For an overview of the state of lesbian health by mainstream and alternative publications, see Mary O'Donnell, "Lesbian Health Care: Issues and Literature," *Science for the People* 10, no. 3 (May/June 1978): 8–19.

73. Caitlin Ryan and Judith Bradford, "Conducting the National Lesbian Health Care Survey: First of Its Kind," *Journal of the Gay and Lesbian Medical Association* 3, no. 3 (September 1999): 91–97. See also Caitlin Ryan, "My Roots as an Activist," *Journal of Lesbian Studies* 5, no. 3 (2001): 141–49.

74. Caitlin Ryan and Judith Bradford, *The National Lesbian Health Care Survey: Final Report* (Washington, DC: National Lesbian and Gay Health Foundation, 1988), 1.

75. Ryan and Bradford, *NLHCS: Final Report*, preface.

76. Ryan and Bradford, 3.

77. Ryan and Bradford, "Conducting the National Lesbian Health Care Survey," 91. See also Deyton and Lear, "Brief History of the Gay/Lesbian Health Movement," 18.

78. Caitlin Ryan and Judith Bradford, "The National Lesbian Health Care Survey: An Overview," in in *The Sourcebook on Lesbian/Gay Health Care*, ed. Michael Shernoff and William A. Scott, 2nd ed. (Washington, DC: National Lesbian/Gay Health Foundation, 1988), 39. See also Ryan and Bradford, *NLHCS: Final Report*.

79. Ryan and Bradford, *NLHCS: Final Report*, 111.

80. See, for example, Susan Johnson, an ob-gyn resident at the University of Iowa medical school; Patricia Robertson, an ob-gyn resident at the University of California, San Francisco School of Medicine; and Lisa Capaldini, a medical student and internal medicine resident at the University of California, San Francisco School of Medicine.

81. Susan Johnson, interview with the author, October 7, 2013.

82. See, for example, Susan R. Johnson et al., "Factors Influencing Lesbian Gynecologic Care: A Preliminary Study," *American Journal of Obstetrics and Gynecology* 140, no. 1 (May 1981): 20–28; Susan R. Johnson, Elaine M. Smith, and Susan M. Guenther, "Comparison of Gynecologic Health Care Problems between Lesbians and Bisexual Women: A Survey of 2,345 Women," *Journal of Reproductive Medicine* 32, no. 11 (November 1987): 805–11; Robertson and Schachter, "Failure to Identify Venereal Disease," 75–76; and K. Degen and H. J. Waitkevicz, "Lesbian Health Issues," *British Journal of Sexual Medicine* 9 (May 1982): 40–47.

83. In Susan Johnson's 1981 study, for example, 95 percent of the participants were white and 52 percent reported some college education. Johnson et al., "Factors Influencing Lesbian Gynecologic Care," 21.

84. Ryan and Bradford, *NLHCS: Final Report*, 3.

85. Pat Maher, "Calling On Lesbian Health: An Interview with Pat Maher," by Barbara Turk, *WomaNews*, July/August 1984, 6.

86. For the political argument promoted by some lesbian separatists that lesbians shouldn't have children, see Elizabeth Alice Clement, "Debating the 'Man Child': Understanding the Politics of Motherhood through Debates in the US Lesbian Community, 1970–1990," *Journal of Women's History* 31, no. 4 (Winter 2019): 86–110.

87. Irene Toro Martinez and Barbara Butcher, interview with the author, November 2, 2017.

88. For children in women's space, see Clement, "Debating the 'Man Child,'" 86–110. For accounts of lesbian motherhood more generally, see Ellen Lewin, *Lesbian Mothers: Accounts of Gender in American Culture* (Ithaca, NY: Cornell University Press, 1993); and Daniel Winunwe Rivers, *Radical Relations: Lesbian Mothers, Gay Fathers, and Their Children in the United States since World War II* (Chapel Hill: University of North Carolina Press, 2013).

89. Katie Batza, "From Sperm Runners to Sperm Banks: Lesbians, Assisted Conception, and Challenging the Fertility Industry, 1971–1983," *Journal of Women's History* 28, no. 2 (Summer 2016): 89. See also Lewin, *Lesbian Mothers*.

NOTES TO PAGES 170–172

90. Kara Speltz, "In a Dragon's Mouth: Lesbian Motherhood," *Off Our Backs*, December 1979, 17; Liz Hjetness and Alice Fisher, "Lesbians Consider Motherhood," *Gay Community News*, March 31, 1979; "The Birthing Project," *Lyon-Martin Women's Health Services Newsletter Access*, Fall 1992, 4, 6.

91. In some states, adoptions by gay men and lesbians were prohibited outright. Other states failed to codify their prohibition in law, but lesbian and gay adoptions were nevertheless difficult or impossible. Adoption agencies frequently refused to work with single parents or same-sex couples. Laura Briggs, *Somebody's Children: The Politics of Transracial and Transnational Adoption* (New York: Duke University Press, 2012), 245, 252–3.

92. Susan R. Johnson, Elaine M. Smith, and Susan M. Guenther, "Parenting Desires among Bisexual Women and Lesbians," *Journal of Reproductive Medicine* 32, no. 3 (March 1987): 198.

93. See, for example, Laurel Galana, "Radical Reproduction: X without Y," in *The Lesbian Reader*, ed. Gina Covina and Laurel Galana (Oakland: Amazon Press, 1975), 122–37; and Mare, "Lesbian Health Issues," *Lesbian Connection*, September 1977, 12–13. See also Greta Rensenbrink, "Parthenogenesis and Lesbian Separatism: Regenerating Women's Community through Virgin Birth in the United States in the 1970s and 1980s," *Journal of the History of Sexuality* 19, no. 2 (May 2010): 288–316; and Klein and Vilmain, *Self-Health for Lesbian Women*.

94. Frances Chapman and Bernice, "A Conference Is Bringing Together," *Off Our Backs*, May/June 1975, 5.

95. Batza, "From Sperm Runners to Sperm Banks," 85.

96. As we now know, these donor networks sometimes included the physician himself. See, for example, Marlene Cimons, "Fertility Doctor's Case Raises Ethical Concerns," *Los Angeles Times*, February 13, 1992; and Jacqueline Mroz, "Their Mothers Chose Donor Sperm. The Doctors Used Their Own Sperm," *New York Times*, August 21, 2019, https://www.nytimes.com/2019/08/21/health/sperm-donors-fraud-doctors.html.

97. "Artificial Insemination—Do It Yourself," *Big Mama Rag*, April 1979, 11.

98. For a discussion of lesbians and assisted conception between 1971 and 1983, the period before sperm banks were open to lesbians, see Batza, "From Sperm Runners to Sperm Banks," 84–85.

99. Mary Wings, "Conception Comix," in *Dyke Shorts* (self-pub., 1978), reprinted in Mary O'Donnell, Kater Pollock, Val Leoffler, and Ziesel Saunders, *Lesbian Health Matters!* (Santa Cruz: Santa Cruz Women's Health Collective, 1979), 62.

100. Susan Stern, "Artificial Insemination for Lesbians: A Different Type of Baby Boom in S.F.," *Synapse*, December 6, 1979. See also Sara Matthiesen, *Reproduction Reconceived: Family Making and the Limits of Choice after* Roe v. Wade (Oakland: University of California Press, 2021), 42–43.

101. "Artificial Insemination—Do It Yourself," 11, 14; Sarah and Mary Anonymous [pseud.], *Woman Controlled Conception* (San Francisco: Womanshare Books, 1979), 1–11; O'Donnell et al., *Lesbian Health Matters!*, 49–57; Martha Heath, "Do It Yourself Artificial Insemination," *Lesbian Tide*, September/October 1978, 26–27; Marie Anoped, "Artificial Insemination for Lesbians," *Seattle Gay News*, March 2, 1979.

102. O'Donnell et al., *Lesbian Health Matters!*, 49.

103. Francie Hornstein, "Children by Donor Insemination: A New Choice for Lesbians," in *Test-Tube Women: What Future for Womanhood?*, ed. Rita Arditti, Renate Duelli Klein, and Shelley Minden (Boston: Pandora Press, 1984), 373–81. See also Batza, "Sperm Runners to Sperm Banks," 90.

104. By 1978, the Vermont Women's Health Center provided "artificial insemination . . . after a thorough medical screening and counseling." Vermont Women's Health Center [History], November 1978, MC 503, box 50, folder 10, BWHBC, 5.

105. Sarah and Mary Anonymous [pseud.], *Woman Controlled Conception*, 1–11. According to Rebecca Chalker, the sperm bank in Burbank willingly provided the sperm to the center. Rebecca Chalker, interview with the author, June 23, 2008.

106. For the history of sperm banks, see Cynthia R. Daniels and Janet Golden, "Procreative Compounds: Popular Eugenics, Artificial Insemination and the Rise of the American Sperm Banking Industry," *Journal of Social History* 38, no. 1 (Fall 2004): 5–27. See also Laura Mamo, *Queering Reproduction: Achieving Pregnancy in the Age of Technoscience* (Durham, NC: Duke University Press, 2007), 29; and Kara W. Swanson, *Banking on the Body: The Market in Blood, Milk, and Sperm in Modern America* (Cambridge, MA: Harvard University Press, 2014), 198–237.

107. Batza, "From Sperm Runners to Sperm Banks," 83.

108. Barbara Raboy, telephone interview by Katie Batza, September 16, 2013, cited at Batza, 91. See also "Feminists Open First Bay Area Sperm Bank," *Second Opinion: Coalition for the Medical Rights of Women*, December 1982/January 1983, 2. In 1988, the Sperm Bank of California split from the Oakland FWHC to create its own entity. "History," Sperm Bank of California (website), accessed July 10, 2019, https://www.thespermbankofca.org/content/history.

109. Batza, "From Sperm Runners to Sperm Banks," 91.

110. For Atlanta, see Judy Siff (director, Donor Insemination Services) to "Sisters," January 8, 1992, box 8, folder: "Feminist Women's Health Center," ALFA; and Maureen Downey, "New Conceptions: When Mom and Donor Make Three," *Atlanta Constitution*, March 1, 1990, 63.

111. See Gina Kolata, "Lesbian Partners Find the Means to Be Parents," *New York Times*, January 30, 1989. Other evidence of the gayby boom was the publication of several books on lesbian (and gay) parenthood. See Cheri Pies, *Considering Parenthood*, 2nd ed. (San Francisco: Spinsters, 1988); and Frederick W. Bozett, ed., *Gay and Lesbian Parents* (New York: Praeger, 1987).

112. Johnson, Smith, and Guenther, "Parenting Desires," 198–200.

113. Kathleen Baca, "Growing Pains," *San Francisco Bay Guardian*, June 26, 1991, quoted in John Morrison, "Twelve Percent," *Christopher Street*, April 13, 1992, 9. Although many sources document the rich lesbian contribution to the AIDS movement, at least one author denounced the image of women in general and lesbians in particular "lovingly helping" gay men—men who could not be counted on to reciprocate if the tables were turned—as a "complete fraud." See Morrison, "Twelve Percent," 9. Many sources point to lesbian leadership (often unacknowledged) in the fight against AIDS. See, for example, Amber L. Hollibaugh, "Lesbian Denial and Lesbian Leadership in the AIDS Epidemic: Bravery and Fear in the Construction of a Lesbian Geography of Risk (1999)," in *My Dangerous Desires: A Queer Girl Dreaming Her Way Home* (Durham, NC: Duke University Press, 2000), 204; Jennifer Brier, "Locating Lesbian and Feminist Responses to AIDS, 1982–1984," *Women's Studies Quarterly* 35, no. 1/2 (Spring/Summer 2007): 234–48; Ryan, "My Roots as an Activist," 141–49; Lisa Diedrich, "Doing Queer Love: Feminism, AIDS, and History," *Theoria*, no. 112 (April 2007): 25–50; and Anne-christine d'Adesky, "Lesbian Love and Activism," *Curve*, August/September 2017, 28–29.

114. Rebecca Chalker, "Lesbian Health Care," in *The Sourcebook on Lesbian/Gay Health Care*, ed. Fern H. Schwaber and Michael Shernoff (New York: National Gay Health Education Foundation, 1984), 92; Denise Kulp, "On Working with My Brothers: Why a Lesbian Does AIDS Work," *Off Our Backs*, August/September 1988, 22.

115. Maxine Wolfe, "AIDS and Politics: Transformation of Our Movement," in *Women, AIDS,*

and Activism, ed. ACT UP/New York Women and AIDS Book Group (Boston: South End Press, 1990), 233.

116. Banzhaf, interview. See also Sarah Schulman, "Becoming an Angry Mob in the Best Sense: Lesbians Respond to AIDS Hysteria (1985)," in *My American History: Lesbian and Gay Life during the Reagan and Bush Years*, 2nd ed. (New York City: Routledge, 2019), 123–24. For more about lesbian involvement in AIDS work as a stand against homophobia, see Rose Appleman and Linda Kahn, "Lesbians Face AIDS on Several Fronts," *New Directions for Women*, May/June 1989, 12; and Brier, "Locating Responses to AIDS."

117. See Brier, "Locating Responses to AIDS," 235–36.

118. Zoe Leonard, "Lesbians in the AIDS Crisis," in *Women, AIDS, and Activism*, ed. ACT UP/New York Women and AIDS Book Group (Boston: South End Press, 1990), 117.

119. ACT UP/New York Women and AIDS Book Group, ed., *Women, AIDS, and Activism* (Boston: South End Press, 1990); Cindy Patton, *Sex and Germs: The Politics of AIDS* (Boston: South End Press, 1985); Nancy E. Stoller, "Lesbian Involvement in the AIDS Epidemic: Changing Roles and Generational Difference," *Women Resisting AIDS: Feminist Strategies of Empowerment*, eds. Beth E. Schneider and Nancy E. Stoller (Philadelphia: Temple University Press, 1995), 270–85; Hollibaugh, "Lesbian Denial and Lesbian Leadership," 210–14.

120. D'Adesky, "Lesbian Love and Activism," 28–29. Marj Plumb, a central player in lesbian and AIDS organizing, argues just the opposite, claiming that HIV/AIDS work brought an analysis of race and class into the lesbian health movement. Marj Plumb, Susan Rochman, and Jocelyn White, "From the Margins to the Mainstream: Lesbian Health Public Policy Advocacy," *Journal of the American Medical Women's Association* 54, no. 1 (Winter 1999): 21.

121. See, for example, Faith Guinchard, "AIDS: The Impact on Women's Lives," *WomenWise*, September 30, 1986, 6–7, 9.

122. Sarah Schulman, "The Denial of AIDS and the Construction of a Fake Life (1992)," in *My American History: Lesbian and Gay Life during the Reagan and Bush Years*, 2nd ed. (New York City: Routledge, 2019), 238.

123. Karla Jay, "Ties That Bind: Friendship between Lesbians and Gay Men," *Harvard Gay & Lesbian Review* 4, no. 1 (Winter 1997): 9; Caitlin Ryan, "Lesbians Working in AIDS: An Overview of Our History and Our Experience," in *The Sourcebook on Lesbian/Gay Health Care*, ed. Michael Shernoff and William A. Scott, 2nd ed. (Washington, DC: National Lesbian/Gay Health Foundation, 1988), 200–201. See also Deborah Bergman, "Has AIDS Finally Bonded Lesbians and Gay Men?," *Advocate*, December 18, 1990, 106.

124. Sarah Schulman, "Whatever Happened to Lesbian Activism? (1991)," in *My American History: Lesbian and Gay Life during the Reagan and Bush Years*, 2nd ed. (New York City: Routledge, 2019), 216.

125. Jay, "Ties That Bind," 9.

126. Diane Richardson, *Women and AIDS* (New York: Routledge, 1989), 90.

127. Bergman, "Has AIDS Finally Bonded Lesbians and Gay Men?," 106.

128. Laura Giges, "AIDS: A Woman's Issue," *WomenWise*, December 31, 1985, 3.

129. Susan Y. Chu et al., "Epidemiology of Reported Cases of AIDS in Lesbians, United States 1980–89," *American Journal of Public Health* 80, no. 11 (November 1990): 1380–81.

130. Jackie Winnow, "Lesbians Working on AIDS: Assessing the Impact on Health Care for Women," *Outlook*, Summer 1989, 10.

131. Winnow, "Lesbians Working on AIDS," 12–13; Sonia Johnson, *Wildfire: Igniting the She/Volution* (Albuquerque: Wildfire Books, 1989), 189–91.

132. Michael Shernoff and William A. Scott, introduction to *The Sourcebook on Lesbian/Gay Health Care*, ed. Michael Shernoff and William A. Scott, 2nd ed. (Washington, DC: National Lesbian/Gay Health Foundation, 1988), 10. For language of delay, see also Plumb, Rochman, and White, "From the Margins to the Mainstream," 22. For raising the alleged neglect of lesbians by gay men, see Kulp, "On Working with My Brothers," 22; and Leonard, "Lesbians in the AIDS Crisis," 117.

133. Beth Elliott, "Does Lesbian Sex Transmit AIDS? Get Real!," *Off Our Backs*, November 1991, 6.

134. Giges, "AIDS: A Woman's Issue," 3. See also June Thomas, "Lesbian/Gay Health Conference," *Off Our Backs*, May 1986, 1.

135. Risa Denenberg, "What the Numbers Mean," in *Women, AIDS, and Activism*, ed. ACT UP/New York Women and AIDS Book Group (Boston: South End Press, 1990), 3.

136. Gayle Green, "In This Together," review of *The Invisible Epidemic: The Story of Women and AIDS*, by Gena Corea, *Nation*, February 22, 1993, 239. See also Christie Jansky, "Focus on Women and AIDS," *Gay Community News*, March 25, 1991, 8.

137. Chu et al., "Epidemiology of Reported Cases," 1381.

138. Mary Bednarz et al., "Lesbians Living with AIDS Talk about Sex," *New York City Lesbian Health Fair*, May 3, 1997, 57.

139. Amber L. Hollibaugh, "Transmission, Transmission, Where's the Transmission? (1994)," in *My Dangerous Desires: A Queer Girl Dreaming Her Way Home* (Durham, NC: Duke University Press, 2000), 195.

140. Lesli Gaynor, "The Damned Sex Debate: Are Lesbians at Risk of Getting AIDS?," *Herizons*, Winter 1993, 16–20.

141. S. Y. Chu, T. A. Hammett, and J. W. Buehler, "Update: Epidemiology of Reported Cases of AIDS in Women Who Report Sex Only with Other Women, 1980–1991," *AIDS* 6, no. 5 (1992): 519. Indeed, as late as 2014, the Centers for Disease Control (CDC) reported no confirmed cases of HIV transmission from woman-to-woman sexual contact, although the researchers conceded that a scant few (less than five) were possible and one case was "likely." A. Deol and A. Heath-Toby, *HIV Risk for Lesbians, Bisexuals & Other Women Who Have Sex with Women* (New York: Women's Institute at Gay Men's Health Crisis, 2009); A. Prilfool, "Shocking Finding," *Off Our Backs*, May 1987, 15; Shirley K. Chan, Lupita R. Thornton, Karen J. Chronister, Jeffrey Meyer, Marcia Wolverton, Cynthia K. Johnson, Raouf R. Arafat, M. Patricia Joyce, William M. Switzer, Walid Heneine, Anupama Shankar, Timothy Granade, S. Michele Owen, Patrick Sprinkle, and Vickie Sullivan, "Likely Female-to-Female Sexual Transmission of HIV—Texas, 2012," *Morbidity and Mortality Weekly Report* 63, no. 10 (March 14, 2014): 209–12.

142. Lena Einhorn, "New Data on Lesbians and AIDS," *Off Our Backs*, April 1989, 10.

143. See, for example, Hollibaugh, "Lesbian Denial and Lesbian Leadership," 203–18.

144. See, for example, Amber L. Hollibaugh, "Lesbianism Is Not a Condom," in *My Dangerous Desires: A Queer Girl Dreaming Her Way Home* (Durham, NC: Duke University Press, 2000), 188.

145. Elliott, "Does Lesbian Sex Transmit AIDS?," 6.

146. Stoller, "Lesbian Involvement," 278–79. See also *Lesbians Address AIDS* (San Francisco: Women's AIDS Project, 1986).

147. See, for example, *Lesbians Address AIDS*. The language of *safe* and *safer sex* is noteworthy within a context where woman-to-woman sexual transmission of HIV was itself con-

tested. Lesbian activists referred to both *safe* and *safer sex*, with *safer sex* being slightly more common. I use it here unless the context warrants the use of *safe sex*.

148. Cindy Patton, "Mapping: Lesbians, AIDS and Sexuality: An Interview with Cindy Patton," by Sue O'Sullivan, *Feminist Review* 34 (Spring 1990): 120.

149. Herbert, "'Nobody Knows What Lesbian Health Is,'" 9.

150. "Lesbians: Low-Risk Identity, High-Risk Behavior," *WomenWise*, July 31, 1991, 5.

151. Einhorn, "New Data on Lesbians and AIDS," 10.

152. Gaynor, "The Damned Sex Debate," 16–20. See also Nancy Solomon, "Risky Business: Should Lesbians Practice Safer Sex?," *Outlook*, Spring 1992, 47–52.

153. Bednarz et al., "Lesbians Living with AIDS," 59–61.

154. Elizabeth Walber, editor's note to "Lesbians Living with AIDS Talk about Sex," *New York City Lesbian Health Fair*, May 3, 1997, 58.

155. Quotations: "hysterical": Patton, "Mapping," 120; "AIDS envy": Stoller, "Lesbian Involvement," 285; and Leonard, "Lesbians in the AIDS Crisis," 113, quoting Darrell Yates Rist, "The Deadly Costs of an Obsession," *Nation*, February 13, 1989, 181; "urban legend . . .": Elliott, "Does Lesbian Sex Transmit AIDS?," 6. For the argument that a focus on safer-sex methods might discourage lesbian sex, see Laurie Sherman, "Lesbians and AIDS: What Are the Risks?," *Gay Community News*, May 7–13, 1989, 3.

156. Hollibaugh, "Lesbianism Is Not a Condom," 187–91. Barbara Herbert explained in 1986, "We don't know how many lesbians use drugs, and it is generally one of the 'areas of silence' in the community." Thomas, "Lesbian/Gay Health Conference," 1.

157. Hollibaugh, "Lesbianism Is Not a Condom," 189.

158. Hollibaugh, 190. See also Appleman and Kahn, "Lesbians Face AIDS," 12.

159. Thomas, "Lesbian/Gay Health Conference," 1. See also Chyrell D. Bellamy, "Lesbians and HIV—What's the Connection?," *New York City Lesbian Health Fair*, April 3, 1993, 15.

160. Hollibaugh, "Transmission, Transmission," 194.

161. Hollibaugh, "Lesbian Denial and Lesbian Leadership," 207.

162. Hollibaugh, 210.

163. Whitman-Walker launched its Lesbian Health Program and its Lesbian Services Program in 1990. Whitman-Walker Health, "Lesbian Services Program, Meeting the Health Needs of Women," *Whitman-Walker Health*, August 5, 2018, https://www.whitman-walker.org/blogs-and-stories/40-stories-lesbian-services-program. See also Masha Gessen, "New York Lesbians Demand AIDS Care from GMHC," *The Advocate*, April 9, 1991, 55.

164. Lynn Warshafsky, *Lesbian Health Needs Assessment* (Los Angeles: Los Angeles Gay and Lesbian Community Services Center, 1992); Michigan Organization for Human Rights, *Michigan Lesbian Health Survey* (Lansing: Michigan Organization for Human Rights, 1991).

165. See, for example, Cuca Hepburn and Bonnie Gutierrez, *Alive & Well: A Lesbian Health Guide* (Freedom, CA: Crossing Press, 1988); Jocelyn White and Marissa C. Martinez, eds., *The Lesbian Health Book: Caring for Ourselves* (Seattle: Seal Press, 1997); Phyllis Noerager Stern, ed., *Lesbian Health: What Are the Issues?* (Washington, DC: Taylor & Francis, 1993); and Christy M. Ponticelli, *Gateways to Improving Lesbian Health and Health Care: Opening Doors* (New York: Haworth Press, 1998).

166. The Mautner Project for Lesbians with Cancer, founded in 1990, is the most important of these private ventures. In 2013, the Mautner Project, which had abandoned its exclusive focus on cancer and had expanded its mission to include bisexual and transgender individuals, merged

with Whitman-Walker Health in Washington, DC. *Mautner Project for Lesbians with Cancer*, n.d., ca. 1998, MC 683, box 7, folder 9: "Mission Statement, History, 1990–1997," RMP. See also the Lesbian Community Cancer Project, founded in 1990 in Chicago. It eventually became part of Howard Brown Health Center.

167. New York City, for example, established the Office of Gay and Lesbian Health Concerns in 1983 to cope with the flood of requests for information about AIDS. In 1984, the office created the Lesbian Health Project (LHP). The LHP claimed to be the first "government" project focused on the health needs of lesbians and bisexual women. Yvette C. Burton to "Sisters," December 23, 1992, TAM.162, box 4, folder: "Lesbian Health Project: City of New York Department of Health," WHAM.

168. Andrea L. Solarz, ed., *Lesbian Health: Current Assessment and Directions for the Future* (Washington, DC: National Academy Press, 1999), viii.

169. Mairead Sullivan argues that this publication "marks a significant attempt to consolidate the lesbian as a biopolitical category." Mairead Sullivan, "A Crisis Emerges: Lesbian Health between Breast Cancer and HIV/AIDS," *Journal of Lesbian Studies* 22, no. 2 (2018): 220.

170. Solarz, *Lesbian Health*, 64.

171. Solarz, 66.

172. Solarz, 98, 73.

173. "APHA Policy Statement 9819: The Need for Public Health Research on Gender Identity and Sexual Orientation," *American Journal of Public Health* 89, no. 3 (March 1999): 444–45.

174. See *American Journal of Public Health* 91, no. 6 (June 2001).

175. Allison L. Diamant, Cheryl Wold, Karen Spritzer, and Lillian Gelberg, "Health Behaviors, Health Status, and Access to and Use of Health Care: A Population-Based Study of Lesbian, Bisexual, and Heterosexual Women," *Archives of Family Medicine* 9, no. 10 (November 2000): 1043–51.

176. Solarz, *Lesbian Health*, 97–114.

177. M. B. Kennedy et al., "Assessing HIV Risk among Women Who Have Sex with Women: Scientific and Communication Issues," *Journal of the American Medical Women's Association* 50, no. 3–4 (May–August 1995): 103–7.

178. Greta R. Bauer and Jennifer A. Jairam, "Are Lesbians Really Women Who Have Sex with Women (WSW)? Methodological Concerns in Measuring Sexual Orientation in Health Research," *Women & Health* 48, no. 4 (2008): 385.

179. Rebecca M. Young and Ilan H. Meyer, "The Trouble with 'MSM' and 'WSW': Erasure of the Sexual-Minority Person in Public Health Discourse," *American Journal of Public Health* 95, no. 7 (July 2005): 1144–49.

Chapter Six

1. Seth Hemmelgarn, "Lyon-Martin on Life Support," *Bay Area Reporter*, January 27, 2011, https://www.ebar.com/news///241304; Lyon-Martin Health Services, "Lyon-Martin Health Services Announces Plan to Close Clinic," Facebook, January 25, 2011, https://www.facebook.com/notes/lyon-martin-health-services/lyon-martin-health-services-announces-plan-to-close-clinic/179282982107463/; "Health Clinic Falls Down," *Bay Area Reporter*, January 28, 2011, https://www.ebar.com/opinion/editorial/235213.

2. By March 16, 2011, community fundraising provided $339,000. Seth Hemmelgarn, "Clinic Reduces Amount of Money It's Seeking," *Bay Area Reporter*, March 16, 2011, https://www.ebar.com/news///241440.

3. Linda Nicholson, *Identity before Identity Politics* (Cambridge: Cambridge University Press, 2008), 2. For the critique of sexism in the New Left and its relationship to the rise of women's liberation, see Alice Echols, *Daring to Be Bad: Radical Feminism in America, 1967–1975* (Minneapolis: University of Minnesota Press, 1989).

4. Combahee River Collective, "A Black Feminist Statement," in *The Second Wave: A Reader in Feminist Theory*, ed. Linda Nicholson (New York: Routledge, 1997), 65.

5. Jeffrey Escoffier, *American Homo: Community and Perversity* (Berkeley: University of California Press, 1998), 190–201, quotation on 191.

6. Kimberle Crenshaw, "Mapping the Margins: Intersectionality, Identity Politics, and Violence against Women of Color," *Stanford Law Review* 43, no. 6 (July 1991): 1241–99, quotation on 1242; Shane Phelan, *Identity Politics: Lesbian Feminism and the Limits of Community* (Philadelphia: Temple University Press, 1989); Arlene Stein, "Seventies Questions for Nineties Women," in *Identity Politics in the Women's Movement*, ed. Barbara Ryan (New York: New York University Press, 2001), 227–41.

7. Martha E. Gimenez, "With a Little Class: A Critique of Identity Politics," *Ethnicities* 6, no. 3 (September 2006): 423–39; "Identity Politics," special issue, *Historical Materialism* 26, no. 2 (July 2018); Keeanga-Yamahtta Taylor, *From #BlackLivesMatter to Black Liberation* (Chicago: Haymarket Books, 2016); Adolph Reed Jr., "The Limits of 'Anti-racism,'" *Left Business Observer*, no. 121 (September 2009), https://www.leftbusinessobserver.com/Antiracism.html.

8. Joshua Gamson, "Messages of Exclusion: Gender, Movements, and Symbolic Boundaries," in *Identity Politics in the Women's Movement*, ed. Barbara Ryan (New York: New York University Press, 2001), 211–26, esp. 212.

9. Jeffrey Escoffier, "Culture Wars and Identity Politics: The Religious Right and the Cultural Politics of Homosexuality," in *Radical Democracy: Identity, Citizenship, and the State*, ed. David Trend (New York: Routledge, 1996): 165–78.

10. L. A. Kauffman, "The Anti-politics of Identity," in *Identity Politics in the Women's Movement*, ed. Barbara Ryan (New York: New York University Press, 2001), 30.

11. Raphael S. Good's "The Gynecologist and the Lesbian" was a notable exception, but it mostly describes and decries the lack of research on lesbian health. See Raphael S. Good, "The Gynecologist and the Lesbian," *Clinical Obstetrics and Gynecology* 19, no. 2 (June 1976): 473–82.

12. Patricia Robertson, unpublished interview by Kea Hedberg, July 19, 1994, LMHS collection. See also Patricia Robertson, interview with the author, October 17, 2006.

13. Benedict Anderson famously created the idea of the imagined community in his 1983 discussion of nationalism, *Imagined Communities: Reflections on the Origin and Spread of Nationalism* (London: Verso Editions, 1983). The idea has been used extensively outside this original context, including to analyze LGBTQ communities. See, for example, Charlotte Ross, "Imagined Communities: Initiative around LGBTQ Ageing in Italy," *Modern Italy* 17, no. 4 (November 2012): 449–64.

14. Alana Schilling, interview with the author, December 5, 2006.

15. See "How We Started," n.d., LMHS collection; and "History of Lyon-Martin Health Services," n.d., LMHS collection.

16. Patricia Robertson and Julius Schachter, "Failure to Identify Venereal Disease in a Lesbian Population," *Sexually Transmitted Diseases* 8, no. 2 (April–June 1981): 75.

17. Robertson and Schachter, "Failure to Identify Venereal Disease," 75.

18. Robertson and Schachter, 76.

340

19. Bay Area Physicians for Human Rights, "Perception of Health Issues by Sexual Minority Consumers," in *Lesbian Health Care: Information, Research, and Reports*, ed. Lyon-Martin Women's Health Services, n.d., quoted in Sherron Mills, "Overview: The Lesbian Patient and the Health Care System" (unpublished manuscript, November 1982), LMHS collection. The BAPHR was one of the first gay physicians' organization; Robertson was one of its founders.

20. Women's Alternative Health Services Articles of Incorporation, May 12, 1979, LMHS collection. See also Schilling, interview; and Sherron Mills, interview with the author, December 6, 2006. Although these three women signed the articles of incorporation and appear in most of the internally created histories of the clinic, women who might also deserve the designation of "founder" include Eileen Teitle, a nurse practitioner, and Lesley Anderson, an orthopedic medicine resident and Robertson's then partner. Lesley Anderson, interview with the author, December 6, 2006; Mary Ann Swissler, "The Lyon-Martin Clinic and the Rise of Lesbian Health," *Bay Area Reporter*, April 4, 1996, 49; "History of Lyon-Martin Health Services."

21. After its initial founding, Robertson had little to do with the clinic. Indeed, by 1981, she was living in Southern California. Still, after she returned to San Francisco in 1987, she frequently offered her home for organizing meetings and fundraisers. Robertson, interview. Schilling and Mills retained closer ties to the clinic, Mills serving on the board for several years. Schilling, interview; Mills, interview.

22. Although incorporated as Women's Alternative Health Services, the clinic did business as Lyon-Martin Women's Health Services. Martin and Lyon remained stalwart supporters of the clinic, but they had no formal connection to it. "Birth of Lyon Martin Women's Health Services," n.d., LMHS collection.

23. Marcia M. Gallo, *Different Daughters: A History of the Daughters of Bilitis and the Rise of the Lesbian Rights Movement* (New York: Carroll & Graf, 2006). See also Del Martin, *Battered Wives* (San Francisco: Glide Publications, 1976).

24. For histories of the San Francisco gay communities, see Nan Alamilla Boyd, *Wide Open Town: A History of Queer San Francisco to 1965* (Berkeley: University of California Press, 2003); John D'Emilio, "Gay Politics and Community in San Francisco Since World War II," in *Hidden from History: Reclaiming the Gay and Lesbian Past*, ed. Martin Duberman, Martha Vicinus, and George Chauncey Jr. (New York: Meridian, 1990), 456–73; and Gallo, *Different Daughters*. For gay migration, especially to San Francisco, see also Kath Weston, "Get Thee to a Big City: Sexual Imaginary and the Great Gay Migration," *GLQ* 2, no. 3 (June 1995): 253–277; and Elizabeth A. Armstrong, *Forging Gay Identities: Organizing Sexuality in San Francisco, 1950–1994* (Chicago: University of Chicago Press, 2002), 117–19.

25. Schilling, interview.

26. Lyon-Martin Women's Health Services mission statement, January 9, 1988, LMHS collection.

27. Bopper Deyton and Walter Lear, "A Brief History of the Gay/Lesbian Health Movement in the U.S.A.," in *The Sourcebook on Lesbian/Gay Health Care*, ed. Michael Shernoff and William A. Scott, 2nd ed. (Washington, DC: National Lesbian/Gay Health Foundation, 1988), 15, 18. For the history of the gay health movement, see also Katie Batza, *Before AIDS: Gay Health Politics in the 1970s* (Philadelphia: University of Pennsylvania Press, 2018).

28. Robertson, interview by Hedberg; Schilling, interview.

29. The lesbian focus of the clinic was more explicit after 1980, as described in chapter 5.

30. Advertisements for this clinic appeared in *Pandora*, *Lesbian Connection*, and *Northwest Passage*. Last mention of it appears in *Northwest Passage*, July 19–August 8, 1976, 27.

31. Lesbian Health Committee meeting minutes, April 26, 1976, box 17, folder: "Lesbian Health Committee, 1976–1977," EGC.

32. For a history of gay health clinics before the AIDS epidemic, see Batza, *Before AIDS*; and Thomas Martorelli, *For People, Not for Profit: A History of Fenway Health's First Forty Years* (Bloomington, IN: AuthorHouse, 2012).

33. Armstrong, *Forging Gay Identities*, 142–43.

34. *Gayellow Pages, West Coast Edition* (New York: Renaissance House, 1979), 31, 46.

35. Partial draft of unpublished Lyon-Martin history, n.d., LMHS collection.

36. Schilling, interview.

37. Marj Plumb, "One for the History Books," *Lyon-Martin Women's Health Services: The Clinic Line*, Winter 1999, 1–2.

38. "Client Insurance Use," n.d., LMHS collection.

39. "Staff Retreat," n.d., ca. 1987, LMHS collection; "Utilization of Office Space and Resources," n.d., ca. November 1987, LMHS collection.

40. Summary of February 1987 BACW Survey of Lyon-Martin Women's Health Services, September 1987, LMHS collection.

41. A sense of the BACW can be found in its newsletter, *Uncommon Voices*, published between 1982 and 1996. In addition to high-end social events (galas, cruises), it sponsored workshops for "corporate" women on entrepreneurship, wealth management, professional networking, real estate, and insurance, among other topics.

42. "Lyon-Martin Board-Staff Planning Work Session," January 9, 1988, LMHS collection.

43. Lyon-Martin mission statement.

44. On increased political clout of the lesbian and gay community in San Francisco, see Armstrong, *Forging Gay Identities*; and Jeremiah J. Garretson, *The Path to Gay Rights: How Activism and Coming Out Changed Public Opinion* (New York: New York University Press, 2018), 82–86, 96–121.

45. Marj Plumb, interview with the author, December 5, 2006.

46. See handwritten focus group notes, n.d., ca. 1990, LMHS collection.

47. "Lyon-Martin Women's Health Services Strategic Plan," May 22, 1990, LMHS collection.

48. "Lyon-Martin Strategic Plan."

49. *Lyon-Martin Women's Health Services 1992 Multi-cultural Report*, March 1992, LMHS collection, 7, 2.

50. See, for example, *Lyon-Martin Women's Health Services Access Newsletter*, Spring 1992.

51. John M. Luce, "A Strange New Disease in San Francisco: A Brief History of the City and Its Response to the HIV/AIDS Epidemic," *AnnalsATS* 10, no. 2 (April 2013): 143–47. See also Guenter Risse, "Caring for the Incurable: AIDS at San Francisco General Hospital," in *Mending Bodies, Saving Souls: A History of Hospitals* (New York: Oxford University Press, 1999), 619–73.

52. Risse, "Caring for the Incurable," 650–51.

53. In 1988, most statistics looked at AIDS diagnoses, but many HIV-positive women were diagnosed with AIDS-related complex (ARC) rather than AIDS.

54. The data used to confirm the statistics in this paragraph came from NCHHSTP AtlasPlus and the AIDS Public Information Dataset U.S. Surveillance from CDC WONDER. "NCHHSTP Atlas Plus," Centers for Disease Control and Prevention, accessed September 28, 2022, https://www.cdc.gov/nchhstp/atlas/index.htm; and Centers for Disease Control and Prevention, "AIDS Public Information Data Set (APIDS) US Surveillance Data for 1981–2002," accessed September 28, 2022, https://wonder.cdc.gov/aidspublic.html. Thanks to Emma Wathen for this analysis.

55. Lea Sanchez, "You Have to Know Street Talk," in *AIDS: The Women*, ed. Ines Rieder and Patricia Ruppelt (San Francisco: Cleis Press, 1988), 151–54.

56. J. H., "Just Getting By," in *AIDS: The Women*, ed. Ines Rieder and Patricia Ruppelt (San Francisco: Cleis Press, 1988), 80.

57. D. R., "My Kids Keep Me Going," in *AIDS: The Women*, ed. Ines Rieder and Patricia Ruppelt (San Francisco: Cleis Press, 1988), 96.

58. J. H., "Just Getting By," 78.

59. For more about the CARE Act, see Patricia D. Siplon, "Washington's Response to the AIDS Epidemic: The Ryan White CARE Act," *Policy Studies Journal* 27, no. 4 (November 1999): 796–808.

60. Lyon-Martin Women's Health Services, "Background and Agency Description," n.d., ca. 1989, LMHS collection. See also *Brothers for Sisters Campaign*, pamphlet, n.d., LMHS collection, 5, which claims that Lyon-Martin created "the nation's first safe sex kit for women in 1986."

61. Fran Miller to "Friends," n.d., ca. 1986, LMHS collection; Kim Corsaro, "Women Taking Care of Women," *Coming Up!*, July 1987, LMHS collection.

62. [Rita Shimmin], "Woman-to-Woman," *Lyon-Martin Women's Health Services Newsletter Access*, Spring 1992, 1.

63. Nancy Boutilier, "Lyon-Martin's Women's HIV Group: 'A Lot of Support—and the Right Kind,'" *Bay Area Reporter*, March 11, 1993, 20–21. See also "Lyon-Martin Clients with HIV: Showing Up for Their Lives," *Lyon-Martin Women's Health Services Newsletter Access*, Summer 1993, 1–2.

64. "Lesbians/Bisexual Women HIV Prevention Project," *Lyon-Martin Women's Health Services Newsletter Access*, Fall 1992, 6; Lani Ka'ahumanu, email message to author, July 1, 2021.

65. Plumb, interview. See also flyer, August 1991, LMHS collection.

66. In 1992, 33 percent of the clinic's clientele were women of color; 85 percent of clients had incomes below 200 percent of the poverty level. State of California Health and Welfare Agency, *Annual Utilization Report of Primary Care Clinics*, 1992, https://data.chhs.ca.gov/dataset/pre-2012-primary-care-clinic-utilization-data.

67. Plumb, interview. Kaiser Permanente was founded in the late 1930s in Oakland, California, to provide health care for the workers of Kaiser Industries. By the 1970s, it was widely recognized as the leading model of a prepaid, comprehensive program of health care, covering prevention, primary care, and hospitalization. Rickey Hendricks, *A Model for National Health Care: The History of Kaiser Permanente* (New Brunswick, NJ: Rutgers University Press, 1993).

68. Steven Seidman, "Identity and Politics in a 'Postmodern' Gay Culture: Some Historical and Conceptual Notes," in *Fear of a Queer Planet: Queer Politics and Social Theory*, ed. Michael Warner (Minneapolis: University of Minnesota Press, 1993), 127–32.

69. Plumb, interview.

70. L. Dymond Austin to Dee Mosbacher (president, Board of Directors), January 24, 1992, LMHS collection.

71. Nancy Puttkammer and Deborah Workman, "Lyon-Martin Women's Clinic Process Evaluation Plan," May 6, 1994, LMHS collection, 5.

72. Plumb, interview. Shimmin does not recall saying this.

73. Plumb. See also Brandy Sebron-Kelley (program coordinator, Voices and Choices) to Marj Plumb, June 28, 1993; Marj Plumb to Brandy Sebron-Kelley, July 1, 1993; Brandy Sebron-Kelley to Marj Plumb, July 15, 1993; and Brandy Sebron-Kelley to Marj Plumb, n.d., all from LMHS collection.

74. "Lyon-Martin Women's Health Services Long Term Fiscal Planning, Organizational Plan, January 1990 to January 1993" (draft, March 30, 1990), LMHS collection, 1. See also "Finance Report," July 1993, LMHS collection, which indicated expenses and income above $1 million with a deficit at about $100,000.

75. Plumb, interview.

76. Deborah Riggins (July 1993–December 1994); Terry Greenblatt (Spring 1995–July 1995); Donna Canali (September 1995–October 1998); Rita Shimmin (January 1999–March 1999); Marj Plumb (May 1999–January 2000); Jane Stafford (February 2000–May 2000); and Carol Newkirk (June 2000–May 2001).

77. See, for example, "Clinic Client Survey," 1994, LMHS collection.

78. Seven percent identified as transgender and another 15 percent identified as bisexual. 1999 HIV Client overview, May 24, 2000, Board of Directors meeting materials, LMHS collection.

79. Tamara Ooms, interview with the author, July 27, 2009.

80. Naomi Prochovnick, interview with the author, July 29, 2009.

81. Rose Quinones, interview with the author, March 22, 2011.

82. Beth Rittenhouse, interview with the author, March 22, 2011.

83. Nevertheless, many lesbians played important roles as caretakers for gay men with AIDS and as AIDS activists. See chapter 5.

84. Prochovnick, interview.

85. "Lesbian Mixed Doubles Tennis Tournament," *Lyon-Martin Women's Health Services Access*, Fall 1992, 3.

86. Rita Shimmin, interview with the author, July 28, 2009.

87. Plumb, interview.

88. Marj Plumb, "State of the Agency Presentation," n.d., ca. March 1999, LMHS collection.

89. Staff of Lyon-Martin Women's Health Services to Tina Ahn (board president), March 1, 1999, LMHS collection; staff of Lyon-Martin Women's Health Services to management staff and Board of Directors, March 24, 1999, LMHS collection; staff statement to Board of Directors, n.d., ca. March 17, 1999, LMHS collection. See also Elaine Herscher, "Lesbian Clinic On the Brink: S.F.'s Pioneering Lyon-Martin Facility Struggles to Survive as Many Wonder If It Should Stay Alive," *San Francisco Chronicle*, August 3, 1999.

90. Plumb, "State of the Agency Presentation."

91. Plumb, interview.

92. "90-Day Stability and Recovery Plan," version 2, April 7, 1999, LMHS collection.

93. Plumb, "State of the Agency Presentation."

94. Plumb.

95. Lyon-Martin Women's Health Center, "Summary of Staff Interviews," June 9, 1999, LMHS collection.

96. Marj Plumb and Tina Ahn to "Friend," June 4, 1999, LMHS collection.

97. "Staff Presentation Notes," n.d., ca. February or March 2000, LMHS collection.

98. See, for example, "Lesbian Outreach Work in Progress" documents, n.d., LMHS collection.

99. Doretha Williams-Flournoy, interview with the author, January 6, 2010.

100. Prochovnick, interview.

101. Alexandra L. Woodruff, "Lyon-Martin Health Clinic On the Mend," *Bay Area Reporter*, December 7, 2005, https://www.ebar.com/news///236577. Ostensibly, the walkout was a staff

protest against the policies of Doretha Williams-Flournoy, the clinic's first African American permanent executive director, and the board's lax oversight of Williams-Flournoy.

102. Centers for Disease Control, *Issue Brief: HIV and Transgender Communities*, April 2019, https://www.cdc.gov/hiv/pdf/policies/cdc-hiv-transgender-brief.pdf.

103. Prochovnick, interview. See also Rittenhouse, interview.

104. Willi McFarland, Erin C. Wilson, and Henry F. Raymond, "HIV Prevalence, Sexual Partners, Sexual Behavior and HIV Acquisition Risk among Trans Men, San Francisco, 2014," *AIDS and Behavior* 21, no. 12 (December 2017): 3346–52.

105. W. O. Bockting, B. E. Robinson, and B. R. S. Rosser, "Transgender HIV Prevention: A Qualitative Needs Assessment," *AIDS Care* 10, no. 4 (August 1998): 505–25.

106. Leslie Feinberg, "Trans Health Crisis: For Us It's Life or Death," *American Journal of Public Health* 91, no. 6 (June 2001): 897–900; Kim D. Jaffee, Deirdre A. Shires, and Daphna Stroumsa, "Discrimination and Delayed Health Care among Transgender Women and Men: Implications for Improving Medical Education and Health Care Delivery," *Medical Care* 54, no. 11 (November 2016): 1010–16.

107. *Transgender Tuesdays: A Clinic in the Tenderloin*, directed by Mark Freeman and Nathaniel Walters-Koh (San Francisco: Healing Tales Productions, 2012), https://www.youtube.com/watch?v=g_-2qLW2O7Y.

108. Prochovnick, interview.

109. Susan Stryker, *Transgender History* (Berkeley: Seal Press, 2008), 41–43; San Francisco Human Rights Commission, "Appendix M: San Francisco Human Rights Commission Announces Findings and Recommendations on Discrimination against Transgendered People," in *Proceedings from the Third International Conference on Transgender Law and Employment Policy*, ed. Phyllis Randolph Frye (Houston: ICTLEP, Inc., 1994), Digital Transgender Archive; Human Rights Commission, City and County of San Francisco, "Compliance Guidelines to Prohibit Gender Identity Discrimination," effective December 10, 2003, accessed February 12, 2019, https://sf-hrc.org/compliance-guidelines-prohibit-gender-identity-discrimination.

110. Jean Chin and Terry Greenblatt (LMWHS) to Larry Brinkman (Human Rights Commission), July 6, 1995, LMHS collection.

111. Edwin M. Lee (director, Human Rights Commission Dispute Resolution) to Donna Canali (LMWHS), June 20, 1996, LMHS collection.

112. Donna Canali (LMWHS) to Larry Brinkman (HRC), July 11, 1996, LMHS collection.

113. Jim Peterson (LAI Insurance Agents and Brokers) to Donna [Canali] (LMWHS), August 15, 1996, LMHS collection.

114. LMWHS Board of Directors meeting minutes, May 30, 2001, LMHS collection.

115. LMWHS Board of Directors meeting minutes, April 25, 2001, LMHS collection.

116. Quinones, interview; Prochovnick, interview.

117. Quinones, interview.

118. Finn Enke, "Collective Memory and the Transfeminist 1970s: Toward a Less Plausible History," *Transgender Studies Quarterly* 5, no. 1 (February 2018): 9–29; Cristan Williams, "Radical Inclusion: Recounting the Trans Inclusive History of Radical Feminism," *Transgender Studies Quarterly* 3, no. 1–2 (May 2016): 254–58; Emma Heaney, "Women-Identified Women: Trans Women in 1970s Lesbian Feminist Organizing," *Transgender Studies Quarterly* 3, no. 1–2 (May 2016): 137–45. See also Christoph Hanssmann, "Passing Torches? Feminist Inquiries and Trans-Health Politics and Practices," *Transgender Studies Quarterly* 3, no. 1–2 (May 2016): 120–

36; and Aaron H. Devor and Nicholas Matte, "One Inc. and Reed Erickson: The Uneasy Collaboration of Gay and Trans Activism, 1964–2003," *GLQ* 10, no. 2 (April 2004): 179–209.

119. Janice G. Raymond, *The Transsexual Empire: The Making of the She-Male* (Boston: Beacon Press, 1979), xx, 103–4.

120. Gamson, "Messages of Exclusion," 211–26; Susanne Sreedhar and Michael Hand, "The Ethics of Exclusion: Gender and Politics at the Michigan Womyn's Music Festival," in *Trans/forming Feminisms: Trans-feminist Voices Speak Out*, ed. Krista Scott-Dixon (Toronto: Sumach Press, 2006), 161–69.

121. Armstrong, *Forging Gay Identities*, 180.

122. Seidman, "Identity and Politics," 133, quoted in Armstrong, 182.

123. Armstrong, 182–83.

124. Stryker, *Transgender History*, 134–37. For more about trans activism in San Francisco before Queer Nation, see Elliot Blackstone, "MTF Transgender Activism in the Tenderloin and Beyond, 1965–1975: Commentary and Interview with Elliot Blackstone," by members of the Gay and Lesbian Historical Society of Northern California, *GLQ* 4, no. 2 (April 1998): 349–72.

125. Stryker, *Transgender History*, 136–37. See also K. L. Broad, "GLB + T?: Gender/Sexuality Movements and Transgender Collective Identity (De)Constructions," *International Journal of Sexuality and Gender Studies* 7, no. 4 (October 2002): 241–64.

126. Dawn Harbatkin, interview with the author, January 5, 2011. For the generational shift, see also Armstrong, *Forging Gay Identities*, 183.

127. "Mission," *Lyon-Martin Women's Health Services Quarterly Newsletter*, May 2003, 1. It's unclear when this mission statement was adopted. The proposed mission statement developed at a June 6–8, 2002, retreat read: "Lyon-Martin provides culturally-sensitive healthcare to women who have inequitable access to quality healthcare because of their sexual or gender identity, regardless of their ability to pay." Lyon-Martin Women's Health Services, *Strategic Planning Retreat Summary Report Draft*, June 8–9, 2002, LMHS collection.

128. Heather Cassell, "Lyon-Martin Drops 'Women' from Name," *Bay Area Reporter*, June 20, 2007, https://www.ebar.com/news///238033.

129. LMHS Board of Directors meeting minutes, April 25, 2007, LMHS collection.

130. Cassell, "Lyon-Martin Drops 'Women' from Name." See also "What's in a Name?," *Bay Area Reporter*, June 19, 2007, https://www.ebar.com/opinion/editorial/235028.

131. Pike Long, interview with the author, March 23, 2011.

132. According to fundraising appeals on the "Save Lyon-Martin" Facebook page, they had raised $501,001 by April 30, 2011. Save Lyon-Martin, "Thank you. Lyon-Martin's doors are still open because of you!," Facebook, May 4, 2011, https://www.facebook.com/notes/264221261616915/.

133. Save Lyon-Martin, "An Open Letter to the Lyon-Martin Community," Facebook, August 1, 2011, https://www.facebook.com/notes/3256760354372625/. Emphasis in the original.

134. Victoria Colliver, "Lyon-Martin Health Services Taking New Patients," *SFGate*, September 1, 2011, https://www.sfgate.com/news/article/Lyon-Martin-Health-Services-taking-new-patients-2311634.php.

135. HealthRIGHT 360 is now a group of several primary care and specialty clinics dedicated to the health needs of people in need, in San Francisco and beyond. HealthRIGHT 360, *Impact Report 2016*, https://www.healthright360.org/sites/default/files/HR360_2016_AnnualReport_TallWeb_02.png.

136. The Women's Community Clinic was founded in 1999 in the aftermath of the 1999

closure of the Women's Needs Clinic, a member of Haight Ashbury Free Clinics, Inc. The Lee Woodward Counseling Center for Women provides outpatient substance abuse and mental health treatment for women.

137. In March 2022, the clinic, now named Lyon-Martin Community Health, severed its relationship with HealthRIGHT 360 in its most recent effort to stay afloat. At that moment, it promoted itself as a trans-staffed and -led organization. Eric Burkett, "Lyon-Martin Center Breaks from HealthRIGHT 360, Changes Name," *Bay Area Reporter*, March 23, 2022, https:// www.ebar.com/story.php?ch=news&sc=news&id=314083.

Chapter Seven

1. We first met Martinez in chapter 1. She founded the National Latina Health Organization in 1986. In 1997 she became a cofounder of SisterSong Women of Color Reproductive Health Collective. Jael Silliman et al., *Undivided Rights: Women of Color Organize for Reproductive Justice* (Cambridge, MA: South End Press, 2004), 241–63.

2. Felicia Ward, interview with the author, September 17, 2017. This was a group interview that included Carol Granison, Rita Shimmin, Mandolin Kadera-Redmond, and Yvette Aldama. Irene Toro Martinez, a project assistant, was also in the room. Martinez's friend was likely Zakiya Somburu.

3. Ward, interview.

4. Ward.

5. Ward.

6. "Felicia Janet Ward" (autobiographical note), in *Black & Female: What Is the Reality? Black Women's Voices, Experiences, and Leadership*, ed. Be Present, Inc., n.d., 23, https://www .bepresent.org/images/stories/Black%20Women's%20Voices,%20Experiences,%20Leadership _2013.pdf.

7. Ward, interview.

8. According to the conference program, its official name was the First National Conference on Black Women's Health Issues. "First National Conference on Black Women's Health Issues," 1983, box 1, folder 7, AAOC. Estimates of the number of attendees vary from seventeen hundred to two thousand, well exceeding the organizers' expectations. Silliman et al., *Undivided Rights*, 70; Byllye Y. Avery, interview by Loretta Ross, July 21–22, 2005, VFOHP, 27, https://www.smith .edu/libraries/libs/ssc/vof/transcripts/Avery.pdf.

9. As this chapter will tell, Byllye Avery founded the Gainesville Women's Health Center; African American poet Pat Parker was a director of the Oakland FWHC; Brenda Joyner was a director of the Tallahassee FWHC; Loretta Mears worked at St. Marks Clinic; Rita Shimmin led the HIV/AIDS programs at Lyon-Martin; and Felicia Ward also worked at Lyon-Martin.

10. Other women of color created identity-specific health organizations a bit later. The National Latina Health Organization was founded in 1986; the National Asian Women's Health Organization was founded in 1993. Silliman et al., *Undivided Rights*, 241–63, 197–213.

11. Evan Hart, "Building a More Inclusive Women's Health Movement: Byllye Avery and the Development of the National Black Women's Health Project, 1981–1990" (PhD diss., University of Cincinnati, 2012), 28–29. On Byllye Avery's early health activism and the founding of the NBWHP, see also Hannah Dudley-Shotwell, *Revolutionizing Women's Healthcare: The Feminist Self-Help Movement in America* (New Brunswick, NJ: Rutgers University Press, 2020), 83–94.

12. Hart, "Building a More Inclusive Movement," 30.

13. Hart, 31–32.

14. Avery, interview, 16. See also Betty Freidan, *The Feminine Mystique* (New York: Dell, 1963).

15. See Beverly Jones and Judith Brown, *Toward a Female Liberation Movement* (Boston: New England Free Press, 1968), Roz Payne Sixties Archive, https://rozsixties.unl.edu/items/show/686. Casey Hayden and Mary King's "Sex and Caste" (1965), written from within the civil rights movement, was an early statement of the need for a movement focused on women's liberation. Rosalyn Baxandall and Linda Gordon, eds., *Dear Sisters: Dispatches from the Women's Liberation Movement* (1970; repr., New York: Basic Books, 2000), 21–22.

16. Avery, interview, 14–15.

17. Avery, 18.

18. Avery, interview, 16; Hart, "Building a More Inclusive Movement," 38.

19. Avery, interview, 17.

20. Avery, 17. For more about Black women and abortion, see Byllye Avery, "A Question of Survival/a Conspiracy of Silence: Abortion and Black Women's Health," in *From Abortion to Reproductive Freedom: Transforming a Movement*, ed. Marlene Gerber Fried (Boston: South End Press, 1990), 75–81; Beverly Smith, "Choosing Ourselves: Black Women and Abortion," in Fried, *From Abortion to Reproductive Freedom*, 83–86; and Loretta Ross, "Raising Our Voices," in Fried, *From Abortion to Reproductive Freedom*, 139–43.

21. Avery, interview, 20–24.

22. Lolly Hirsch, "Second Women-Controlled Women's Health Center Conference," *Monthly Extract*, December 1974/January 1975, 7.

23. Avery, interview, 18.

24. Avery, 18–20.

25. Hart, "Building a More Inclusive Movement," 52–54.

26. Hart, 54.

27. Hart, 56–58.

28. Barbara Smith, ed., introduction to *Home Girls: A Black Feminist Anthology* (New Brunswick, NJ: Rutgers University Press, 2000), xxxi, xxxv. Reproductive rights organizing by women of color was already robust in the 1970s. Jennifer Nelson, *Women of Color and the Reproductive Rights Movement* (New York: New York University Press, 2003); Silliman et al., *Undivided Rights*.

29. Stephanie Gilmore, *Groundswell: Grassroots Feminist Activism in Postwar America* (New York: Routledge, 2013).

30. Avery, interview, 26.

31. Avery, 26.

32. Silliman et al., *Undivided Rights*, 68.

33. Hart, "Building a More Inclusive Movement," 93.

34. Hart, 90–93.

35. Hart, 90–105.

36. Dennis Tourish and Pauline Irving, "Group Influence and the Psychology of Cultism within Re-evaluation Counselling: A Critique," *Counselling Psychology Quarterly* 8, no. 1 (March 1995): 35–50, quoted in Evan Hart, "Building a More Inclusive Women's Health Movement: Byllye Avery and the Development of the National Black Women's Health Project, 1981–1990" (PhD diss., University of Cincinnati, 2012), 100.

37. Silliman et al., *Undivided Rights*, 69.

38. Hart, "Building a More Inclusive Movement," 107, 108.

39. Hart, 111–12.

40. Beverly Smith, "Looking at the Total Picture: A Conversation with Health Activist Beverly Smith," by Andrea Lewis, in *The Black Women's Health Book: Speaking for Ourselves*, ed. Evelyn C. White, rev. ed. (Seattle: Seal Press, 1994), 180. See also Audre Lorde's famous articulation of the tensions between Black women forged in rampant anti-Black racism in "Eye to Eye: Black Women, Hatred, and Anger," in *Sister Outsider: Essays and Speeches* (Berkeley: Crossing Press, 1984), 145–75.

41. Byllye Y. Avery, "Breathing Life into Ourselves: The Evolution of the National Black Women's Health Project," in *The Black Women's Health Book: Speaking for Ourselves*, ed. Evelyn C. White, rev. ed. (Seattle: Seal Press, 1994), 4–10. See also Audre Lorde, "The Transformation of Silence into Language and Action," in *Available Means: An Anthology of Women's Rhetoric(s)*, ed. Joy Ritchie and Kate Ronald (Pittsburgh: University of Pittsburgh Press, 2001), 302–5; and Evelynn M. Hammonds, "Toward a Genealogy of Black Female Sexuality: The Problematic of Silence," in *Feminist Theory and the Body*, ed. Janet Price and Margrit Shildrick (New York: Routledge, 1999), 93–104.

42. Silliman et al., *Undivided Rights*, 69. Allen referred to her work as "Self-Help" and the National Black Women's Health Project referred to the community groups based on Black and Female as "Self-Help Groups." It is impossible, in, some instances, to distinguished officially sponsored Self-Help Groups from other self-help groups. I adopt "self-help" as the default.

43. Avery, interview, 26.

44. Shay Youngblood, "Self-Help Groups: Taking Charge and Taking Care," *Network News: Newsletter of the National Women's Health Network*, May/June 1983, 8.

45. Youngblood, "Self-Help Groups," 8.

46. Youngblood, 8.

47. Byllye Avery, "Who Does the Work of Public Health?," *American Journal of Public Health*, 92, no. 4 (April 2002), 570–75; Youngblood, "Self-Help Groups," 8.

48. Youngblood, 8.

49. Youngblood, 8–9.

50. Hart, "Building a More Inclusive Movement," 65.

51. H. Tia Juana Malone, "Reflections on Our Decade," *Vital Signs*, July–September 1994, 34.

52. "2,000 Black Women at Health Conference," *Upfront*, Fall 1983, 1.

53. Dudley-Shotwell, *Revolutionizing Women's Healthcare*, 88.

54. "2,000 Black Women at Conference," 1.

55. Malone, "Reflections on Our Decade," 34–35; Dázon Dixon Diallo, interview by Loretta Ross, April 4, 2009, VFOHP. In 1992, the organization changed its name to SisterLove, Inc. See "Biographical Notes," SisterLove records, Sophia Smith Collection of Women's History.

56. Malone, "Reflections on Our Decade," 34.

57. "Sharon Gary-Smith" (autobiographical note), in *Black & Female, What Is the Reality? Black Women's Voices, Experiences, and Leadership*, ed. Be Present, Inc., n.d., 7, https://www.bepresent.org/images/stories/Black%20Women's%20Voices,%20Experiences,%20Leadership_2013.pdf.

58. Malone, "Reflections on Our Decade," 67.

59. Black Women's Health Project, *First National Conference*, 8–25.

60. Silliman et al., *Undivided Rights*, 69.

61. Black Women's Health Project, *First National Conference*, 10, 16.

62. "2,000 Black Women," *Upfront*, 1, 3.

63. Ward, interview.

64. Silliman et al., *Undivided Rights*, 70.

65. Silliman et al., 70; Ward, interview. See also Be Present, Inc., ed., *Black & Female: What Is the Reality? Black Women's Voices, Experiences, and Leadership*, n.d., https://www.bepresent.org/images/stories/Black%20Women's%20Voices,%20Experiences,%20Leadership_2013.pdf.

66. Byllye Avery, "Toward Independence: NBWHP Update," *National Black Women's Health Project News*, July 1984, 2.

67. Lillie Allen, interview by Loretta Ross, February/March 2003, Ross papers, https://media.smith.edu/departments/ssc/ross/audio/ross-db2606a.mp3; Silliman et al., *Undivided Rights*, 70.

68. National Black Women's Health Project, *Self-Help Manual*, n.d., BWHIR, 9.

69. "Sharon Gary-Smith," 8.

70. Sharon Gary-Smith, "Self-Help: Our Past, Present and Future," *Vital Signs*, February 1989, 6.

71. See National Black Women's Health Project, *Self-Help Manual*, n.d., BWHIR.

72. National Black Women's Health Project, *Self-Help Manual*, 2-3.

73. Loretta Ross, interview by Joyce Follet, December 2, 2004, VFOHP, 204, https://www.smith.edu/libraries/libs/ssc/vof/transcripts/Ross.pdf.

74. Ross, interview, 209-10.

75. Susan L. Smith, *Sick and Tired of Being Sick and Tired: Black Women's Health Activism in America, 1890-1950* (Philadelphia: University of Pennsylvania Press, 1995), 74-75. See also Vanessa Northington Gamble, *Making a Place for Ourselves: The Black Hospital Movement, 1920-1945* (New York: Oxford University Press, 1995); Alondra Nelson, *Body and Soul: The Black Panther Party and the Fight against Medical Discrimination* (Minneapolis: University of Minnesota Press, 2011); and Madeleine Ware, Cara Delay, and Beth Sundstrom, "Abortion and Black Women's Health Networks in South Carolina, 1940-70," *Gender & History* 32, no. 3 (October 2020): 637-56.

76. Eleanor Hinton-Hoytt, "I'm Sick and Tired of Being Sick and Tired!," *Network News: Newsletter of the National Women's Health Network*, May/June 1983, 11.

77. National Black Women's Health Project, *Self-Help Manual*, 3. See also Youngblood, "Self-Help Groups," 8.

78. Ross, interview, 206; Silliman et al., *Undivided Rights*, 72.

79. Gary-Smith, "Self-Help," 6.

80. Silliman et al., *Undivided Rights*, 72.

81. Silliman et al., 72.

82. Hart, "Building a More Inclusive Movement," 209; Avery, interview, 45.

83. Ross, interview, 215-16; Silliman et al., *Undivided Rights*, 76.

84. Silliman et al., *Undivided Rights*, 76.

85. Hart, "Building a More Inclusive Movement," 211.

86. Hart, 212-13.

87. Byllye Avery, "The Next Step," *Vital Signs*, Summer 1991, 2.

88. Silliman et al., *Undivided Rights*, 77.

89. Carol Fox, "Parenting: Free Lectures and Weekend Workshops at UCSF," in University of California, San Francisco, *UCSF News* (San Francisco: University of California, San Francisco, 1988). See also Ward, interview.

90. Ward, interview.

91. Ward. One of these groups met monthly at Lyon-Martin Women's Health Services.

92. Carol Granison, interview with the author, September 17, 2017.

93. Granison, interview.

94. Mandolin Kadera-Redmond, interview with the author, September 17, 2017.

95. Kadera-Redmond, interview.

96. Kadera-Redmond.

97. Kadera-Redmond.

98. Rita Shimmin, interview with the author, September 17, 2017.

99. "Rita Shimmin" (autobiographical note), in *Black & Female: What Is the Reality? Black Women's Voices, Experiences, and Leadership*, ed. Be Present, Inc., n.d., 20.

100. Carolyn R. Shaffer and Kristin Anundsen, *Creating Community Anywhere: Finding Support and Connection in a Fragmented World* (New York: Jeremy P. Tarcher/Perigee Books, 1993), 81, 84.

101. Yvette Aldama, interview with the author, September 17, 2017.

102. Aldama, interview.

103. Roland G. Fryer Jr. et al., "Measuring Crack Cocaine and Its Impact," *Economic Inquiry* 51, no. 3 (July 2013): 1651–81; Robert E. Fullilove et al., "Risk of Sexually Transmitted Disease among Black Adolescent Crack Users in Oakland and San Francisco, Calif," *JAMA* 263, no. 6 (February 9, 1990): 851–55; Donald Sutton and Ralph F. Baker, *Oakland Crack Task Force: A Portrait of Community Mobilization* (Washington, DC: ERIC Clearinghouse, 1990); Michelle Alexander, *New Jim Crow: Mass Incarceration in the Age of Colorblindness* (New York: New Press, 2010)

104. Granison, interview.

105. Ward, interview.

106. Rachel L. Bagby, *Divine Daughters: Liberating the Power and Passion of Women's Voices* (San Francisco: HarperSanFrancisco, 1999), 98.

107. Bagby, *Divine Daughters*, 100.

108. Bagby, 103–4.

109. Aldama and Ward, interview.

110. Shaffer and Anundsen, *Creating Community Anywhere*, 84.

111. Ward, interview.

112. Ward.

113. Felicia Ward, email message to author, September 18, 2017.

114. Debra Brody, Sara Grusky, and Patricia Logan, "Self-Help Health," *Off Our Backs*, July 1982, 14, 17. See also Smith, *Home Girls*, xxxvi–lii; and Silliman et al., *Undivided Rights*, 63.

115. Silliman et al., *Undivided Rights*, 56.

116. Anne M. Valk, *Radical Sisters: Second-Wave Feminism and Black Liberation in Washington, D.C.* (Urbana: University of Illinois Press, 2008), 2.

117. Valk, *Radical Sisters*, 158–80.

118. Valk, 112.

119. Valk, 131.

120. Marion Banzhaf, interview with the author, October 13, 2022.

121. Mary Lisbon, interview with the author, May 31, 2018. This was a group interview that included Lisbon, Linda Leaks, and Ajowa Ifateyo. Irene Toro Martinez, a project assistant, was also in the room.

122. "You are cordially invited," undated flyer, Lisbon collection.

123. "Why a 'Black Women's Only' Program," undated flyer, Lisbon collection.

124. "Why a 'Black Women's Only' Program."

125. Attendance at meetings ranged from a low of four members to a high of twenty. The women who attended the initial meeting included Rosa Bowens (later Brunson Bowens), Monica Brown, Ajowa Ifateyo, Faida Lampley, Mary Lisbon, Doris A. Long, Sandra Marshall, Phyllis Meyers, Robin Roberts, Audrey Sartin, and Faye Williams.

126. "BWSHC Organizing Meeting Agenda," April 25, 1982, and draft agenda, both from Lisbon collection.

127. Rosa M. Brunson, "A New Direction in Black Women's Health," *Upfront*, Fall 1983, 11.

128. Faye Williams to "Sisters," July 7, 1982, Lisbon collection.

129. "BWSHC Meeting Agenda," September 26, 1982, Lisbon collection.

130. Lisbon, interview.

131. Ajowa Ifateyo, interview with the author, May 31, 2018.

132. Lisbon, interview.

133. Miscellaneous BWSHC agendas and meeting notes, Lisbon collection.

134. BWSHC meeting minutes, November 21, 1982, Lisbon collection.

135. "BWSHC Organizing Meeting Agenda."

136. Pre-reading for the meeting included chapters from *A New View of a Woman's Body* on the clitoris and reproductive anatomy. BWSHC meeting agenda, October 17, 1982, Lisbon collection.

137. BWSHC meeting minutes, October 31, 1982, Lisbon collection; Lisbon and Ifateyo, interview.

138. BWSHC meeting minutes, November 21, 1982, Lisbon collection.

139. Linda Leaks, "Can Feminism Liberate Black Women?," *Upfront*, Fall 1983, 5.

140. For more about the DC Rape Crisis Center and the role of Black women within it, see Valk, *Radical Sisters*, 158–80. See also Ross, interview.

141. "2000 Black Women at Health Conference," *Upfront: A Black Women's Newspaper*, 3. Ross has suggested that the DC BWSHC became an affiliate of the NBWHP (Ross, interview, 206), but no meeting minutes of the BWSHC after the June 1983 conference suggest a connection with the larger organization. Ross has also suggested that she was a member of this group (Ross, interview, 206), but she never appears on a membership list, nor did she attend any meeting. Still, she was friendly with the women. There was a DC group affiliated with the NBWHP, headed by Nkenge Touré. Perhaps Ross was a member of this group. Dudley-Shotwell, relying on Ross, repeats this claim. See Dudley-Shotwell, *Revolutionizing Women's Healthcare*, 90–91.

142. For references to Williams's mental health crisis, see Ross, interview, and BWSHC materials, Lisbon collection.

143. Comments from members of BWSHC, July 31, 1983, Lisbon collection.

144. "Black Women's Self-Help Collective Statement of Purpose," n.d., ca. 1983, Lisbon collection. This document is undated, but it was clearly affirmed between October 9 and November 20, 1983.

145. "BWSHC Statement of Purpose."

146. "BWSHC Statement of Purpose."

147. "BWSHC Statement of Purpose."

148. "BWSHC Statement of Purpose."

149. BWSHC meeting notes, December 4, 1983, Lisbon collection.

150. BWSHC meeting minutes, January 29, 1984, Lisbon collection.

151. Ajowa Ifateyo to "Sisters of the BWSHC," December 6, 1983, Lisbon collection.

152. BWSHC agenda, December 18, 1983 [misdated as 1984], Lisbon collection.

153. BWSHC meeting minutes, December 18, 1983, Lisbon collection. They did take up the issue on January 29, 1984.

154. Lauren [Austin] and Audrey [Sartin] to "Sisters [of the BWSHC]," n.d., Lisbon collection; BWSHC Meeting Minutes, December 18, 1984, Lisbon collection.

155. Irene Phillips to Black Women's Self-Help Collective, July 9, 1984, Lisbon collection.

156. [Austin] and [Sartin] to "Sisters," n.d.

157. [Austin] and [Sartin] to "Sisters," n.d.

158. Faye Williams to "Sisters of the BWSHC," November 26, 1984, suggests that an agenda had been set into January 1985.

159. Rosa Brunson to the women of the Black Women's Self-Help Collective, October 5, 1984, Lisbon collection.

160. "Felicia Janet Ward," 23.

Chapter Eight

1. LG [Laura Giges], "The Challenge of Change," *Santa Cruz Women's Health Center Newsletter*, March 1982, 1–2. This version of the article was attributed to LG; a later version (*Matrix*, July 1982, 1, 8) was attributed to Giges.

2. Giges, "Challenge of Change," 2.

3. Byllye Avery was a notable exception.

4. See, for example, the definition of *feminism* established by the Rising Sun Feminist Health Alliance, "Feminism," MC 503, box 50, folder 6: "RSFHA: Mailing and Related, Most about July 1979 Conference, October 13, 1979," BWHBC.

5. Wendy Simonds, *Abortion at Work: Ideology and Practice in a Feminist Clinic* (New Brunswick, NJ: Rutgers University Press, 1996).

6. Benita Roth, *Separate Roads to Feminism: Black, Chicana, and White Feminist Movements in America's Second Wave* (New York: Cambridge University Press, 2004), 7, 8; Finn Enke, "Collective Memory and the Transfeminist 1970s: Toward a Less Plausible History," *Transgender Studies Quarterly* 5, no. 1 (February 2018): 9–29. See also Kimberly Springer, *Living for the Revolution: Black Feminist Organizations, 1968–1980* (Durham, NC: Duke University Press, 2005), 28.

7. See Winifred Breines, *The Trouble between Us: An Uneasy History of White and Black Women in the Feminist Movement* (New York: Oxford University Press, 2006), 19–49. See also Jo Freeman, "On the Origins of Social Movements," in *Social Movements of the Sixties and Seventies*, ed. Jo Freeman (New York: Longman, 1983), 8–30.

8. Breines, *The Trouble between Us*, 105–6.

9. See, for example, the 1975 national socialist feminist conference in Yellow Springs, Ohio, in 1975, a conference attended by some of the women in the SCWHC. Breines, 153.

10. Breines, 51–78.

11. Robyn C. Spencer, *The Revolution Has Come: Black Power, Gender, and the Black Panther Party in Oakland* (Durham, NC: Duke University Press, 2016); Ashley D. Farmer, *Remaking Black Power: How Black Women Transformed an Era* (Chapel Hill: University of North Carolina Press, 2017); Bettye Collier-Thomas and V. P. Franklin, eds., *Sisters in the Struggle: African American Women in the Civil Rights–Black Power Movement* (New York: New York University Press, 2001).

12. Springer, *Living for the Revolution*, 29.

13. Roth, *Separate Roads to Feminism*, 79.

14. Springer, *Living for the Revolution*; Keeanga-Yamahtta Taylor, ed., *How We Get Free: Black Feminism and the Combahee River Collective* (Chicago: Haymarket Books, 2017).

15. Breines, *The Trouble between Us*, 117. See also Anne M. Valk, *Radical Sisters: Second-Wave Feminism and Black Liberation in Washington, D.C.* (Urbana: University of Illinois Press, 2008); Springer, *Living for the Revolution*; and Finn Enke, *Finding the Movement: Sexuality, Contested Space, and Feminist Activism* (Durham, NC: Duke University Press, 2007).

16. Roth, *Separate Roads to Feminism*, 129–77. See also Alma M. Garcia, "The Development of Chicana Feminist Discourse, 1970–1980," *Gender & Society* 3, no. 2 (June 1989): 217–38; Marisela R. Chávez, "'We Have a Long, Beautiful History': Chicana Feminist Trajectories and Legacies," in *No Permanent Waves: Recasting Histories of U.S. Feminism*, ed. Nancy A. Hewitt (New Brunswick, NJ: Rutgers University Press, 2010), 77–97; and Lilia Fernandez, "The Limits of Nationalism: Women's Activism and the Founding of Mujeres Latinas en Acción," in *Brown in the Windy City: Mexicans and Puerto Ricans in Postwar Chicago* (Chicago: University of Chicago Press, 2012), 239–61.

17. Breines, *The Trouble between Us*, 168.

18. Breines, 167–68.

19. Breines, 168.

20. Valk, *Radical Sisters*, 10.

21. Valk, 84–109, quotation on 96.

22. Rebecca M. Kluchin, *Fit to Be Tied: Sterilization and Reproductive Rights in America, 1950–1980* (New Brunswick, NJ: Rutgers University Press, 2009), 198–203.

23. Jennifer Nelson, *Women of Color and the Reproductive Rights Movement* (New York: New York University Press, 2003), 136.

24. Nelson, *Women of Color*, 133–77. See also Kluchin, *Fit to Be Tied*, 196–213.

25. Jael Silliman et al., *Undivided Rights: Women of Color Organize for Reproductive Justice* (Cambridge, MA: South End Press, 2004), 32–34.

26. Nelson, *Women of Color*, 169–70.

27. Karen Starr (Concord Feminist Health Center) to "folks," August 5, 1985, MC 503, box 51, folder 9: "RSFHA: R2N2: Letter and Reports about November 1984 Conference and Racism, Found Loose, 1984–1985," BWHBC. Some might date the collapse to November 11, 1984, when the Women of Color Task Force withdrew from the network.

28. Kluchin, *Fit to Be Tied*, 184–85.

29. Nelson, *Women of Color*, 85–111. See also Silliman et al., *Undivided Rights*.

30. "Racism and Women's Health Movement" discussion notes, n.d., MC 503, box 50, folder 6: "RSFHA: Mailing and Related, Most about July 1979 Conference," October 13, 1979, BWHBC.

31. Jennifer Nelson, *More Than Medicine: A History of the Feminist Women's Health Movement* (New York: New York University Press, 2015), 96, 93.

32. Nelson, *More Than Medicine*, 91–122, esp. 115. On page 116, Nelson identifies these founders as Theresa Saludo, Sarah Sakuma, Shelley Yapp, and Janet Krause. Although the use of *Third World* to refer to countries of the Global South is now widely considered inappropriate, reflecting a Cold War hierarchy of national worth, in the 1960s and '70s, many organizations of Indigenous, Black, and other people of color frequently adopted the term. At the time, it signaled the common oppression of people of color in the US and elsewhere and the shared struggle for liberation. The term *Global South* also has its detractors.

33. Enke, *Finding the Movement*, 212–13. FWHCs in cities and neighborhoods with large

communities of color, including Oakland, California, and Tallahassee, Florida, attracted diverse staffs and clienteles. Carol Downer, interview with the author, June 26, 2008.

34. Unpublished 1977 BWHC document, quoted in Sandra Morgen, *Into Our Own Hands: The Women's Health Movement in the United States, 1969–1990* (New Brunswick, NJ: Rutgers University Press, 2002), 79–85.

35. Katherine Freeburg, "Health Clinic Open for Women of Color," *Plexus*, February 1983, 7.

36. St. Marks Women's Health Collective meeting minutes, March 28, 1980, Mears collection.

37. Handwritten notes, n.d., Waitkevicz collection.

38. Loretta Mears, interview with the author, January 11, 2018.

39. The April 11, 1980, meeting minutes of the St. Marks Womyn's Health Collective note the establishment of twice monthly meetings on racism. St. Marks Women's Health Collective meeting minutes, April 11, 1980, Waitkevicz collection. Sometimes the minute taker used this alternative spelling.

40. St. Marks Women's Health Collective meeting minutes, May 30, 1980, Waitkevicz collection.

41. St. Marks Women's Health Collective meeting minutes, June 20, 1980, Waitkevicz collection.

42. The May 30, 1980, meeting minutes note the unanimous decision to continue the meetings despite the "poor attendance." St. Marks Women's Health Collective meeting minutes, May 30, 1980.

43. St. Marks Women's Health Collective meeting minutes, July 25, 1980, Waitkevicz collection.

44. St. Marks WHC meeting minutes, July 25, 1980.

45. St. Marks Women's Health Collective meeting minutes, October 24, 1980, Waitkevicz collection.

46. St. Marks WHC meeting minutes, May 30, 1980.

47. St. Marks WHC meeting minutes, October 24, 1980.

48. St. Marks Women's Health Collective meeting minutes, November 23, 1980, Waitkevicz collection.

49. St. Marks Women's Health Collective meeting minutes, April 24, 1981, Waitkevicz collection.

50. "Statement of Philosophy and Function of St. Mark's Women's Health Collective Inc.," n.d., ca. summer 1985, Waitkevicz collection.

51. Agenda for October 4 workshop, September 27, 1983, Waitkevicz collection; agenda for Clinic CR workshop, April 12, 1986, Waitkevicz collection.

52. St. Marks Women's Health Collective ultimately closed in April 1995 because it could not attract enough volunteers to keep it open. "To All Members and Patients of the St. Mark's Women's Health Collective," *Sappho's Isle*, April 1995, 5.

53. The SCWHC, an organization, ran the Santa Cruz Women's Health Center. One of the projects of the health center was a health clinic.

54. Ciel Benedetto, interview with the author, September 30, 2011; Ciel Benedetto, interview by Irene Reti, in *Ciel Benedetto: A History of the Santa Cruz Women's Health Center, 1985–2000*, ed. Irene Reti and Randall Jerrell (Santa Cruz: Regional History Project, 2000), https://escholarship.org/uc/item/6bb2z21w.

55. In the 1970 census, less than 10 percent of the residents of Santa Cruz County identified as Hispanic; in 1980, the percentage had grown to 21. By 2010, 32 percent of the residents of Santa

Cruz County identified as Hispanic according to US census data. The term *Hispanic* reflects the language of the census.

56. Reyes did not disclose a racial or ethnic identity to me in our interview beyond identifying as a woman of color. Indeed, she commented on her ability to "blend in" because "people don't know what I am, what my background is." Jane Reyes, interview with the author, September 30, 2011.

57. Reyes, interview. According to membership records, Reyes joined in the fall of 1976 but may have taken a leave right away. She was listed as a member (not on leave) in the fall of 1977. "WHC Membership by Date," n.d., Wilshusen materials. Her own account of this is slightly different. See, for example, Jacquelyn Marie, "Jane Reyes," *Hotflash: Newsletter of the Santa Cruz Women's Health Center*, Spring 2000, 3.

58. Reyes, interview.

59. Reyes.

60. Reyes.

61. "Santa Cruz Women's Health Project Position Paper," quoted in Kater Pollock, "Developing a Socialist-Feminist Model: The Growth of the Santa Cruz Women's Health Collective" (bachelor's thesis, University of California, Santa Cruz, 1978), 11.

62. Giges, "Challenge of Change," 1.

63. JP [Jody Peugh], "Collective Process: Training and Integration," *Santa Cruz Women's Health Center Newsletter*, December 1978, 3.

64. Jody Peugh, interview with the author, September 30, 2011.

65. Peugh, interview.

66. Reyes, interview.

67. Giges, "Challenge of Change," 1.

68. Giges, 1.

69. CH [Carol Haber], "Beach Flats: The Community Comes Together," *Santa Cruz Women's Health Center Newsletter*, June 1983, 3. The phrase *bicultural/bilingual* likely highlighted their intention to hire Latina counselors as opposed to white women who spoke Spanish. It is not entirely clear whether the BOP predated the hire of Zayas and Saavedra. Zayas's name can be found both as RosaMaria Zayas and as Rosa Maria Zayas. I believe the former is correct.

70. JK [Jo Kenny], "Health Shorts," *Santa Cruz Women's Health Center Newsletter*, December 1981, 4.

71. Inger Giffin, "Laura Giges," *Hotflash: Newsletter of the Santa Cruz Women's Health Center*, Spring 2000, 4.

72. Marilyn Marzell, interview with the author, June 30, 2011. See also Kater Pollock, interview with the author, July 1, 2011. Pollock blamed "white guilt" and the willingness of one individual to exploit it for situations like these. Ibid.

73. Marzell, interview.

74. Giffin, "Laura Giges," 4.

75. Giges, "Challenge of Change," 8.

76. Pollock, interview.

77. Zayas did not remain long with the SCWHC; there is no trace of her in association with the clinic after 1983. She became executive director of the Community United in Response to AIDS/SIDA (CURAS) in San Francisco sometime after April 1991. By October 1992, because of "widespread fiscal and management problems," Zayas had been fired and the Department of Public Health had withdrawn its funding. In the press coverage of the problems at the organiza-

tion, Zayas was described as a "dictatorial leader who intimidates employees." David O'Connor, "City's Biggest Hispanic AIDS Service Provider Defunded," *Bay Area Reporter*, October 29, 1992, 33; David O'Connor, "Chaos at CURAS: Community United against AIDS Isn't," *Bay Area Reporter*, September 10, 1992, 4.

78. Giges, "Challenge of Change," 8.

79. Peugh, interview.

80. Laurie Slothower, "Taking It to the Streets: Health Counselors Figure: If They Can't Come to Us, We'll Go to Them," *Santa Cruz Sentinel*, August 15, 1982.

81. Morgen, *Into Our Own Hands*, 83–84.

82. Marilyn Marzell, "Reaching for Diversity," *Hotflash: Newsletter of the Santa Cruz Women's Health Center*, Spring 2000, 1.

83. Giges, "Challenge of Change," 8.

84. Giges, 8.

85. Marzell, interview; Reyes, interview; Benedetto, interview with the author.

86. Reyes, interview; Marzell, interview; Benedetto, interview by Reti, 40.

87. Marzell, interview.

88. Peugh, interview; Marzell, interview.

89. Pollock, interview.

90. Reyes, interview.

91. Barbara Garcia, "Barbara Garcia," interview by Ciel Benedetto, *Hotflash: Newsletter of the Santa Cruz Women's Health Center*, Spring 2000, 5.

92. Kenny, "Health Shorts," 4.

93. Rosamaria Zayas and Martha Ways to Ms. Foundation, quoted in Boston Women's Health Book Collective, *The New Our Bodies, Ourselves* (New York: Simon & Schuster, 1984), 603. This source lists the BOP as Laura Giges, Marilyn Marzell, Jody Peugh, Carmella Saavedra, Hermalinda Saavedra, Lucy Trujillo, Martha Ways, and Rosamaria Zayas. Zayas's name was styled as "Rosamaria" in this source.

94. MW [Martha Ways] and DA [Deborah Abbott], "Have Van, Will Travel," *Santa Cruz Women's Health Center Newsletter*, March 1982, 3.

95. Zayas and Ways to Ms. Foundation, 603.

96. Ways and Abbott, "Have Van, Will Travel," 3.

97. Slothower, "Taking It to the Streets." Salud Para La Gente, originally known as La Clinica, was founded in 1979 to provide health care to the children of farmworkers. It eventually developed into a full-service health clinic. Some women from the SCWHC volunteered at La Clinica. LP [Laura Partch], "La Clinica: A Positive Approach," *Santa Cruz Women's Health Center Newsletter*, September 1980, 2; MB [Mary Bush], "Migrant Health Care," *Santa Cruz Women's Health Center Newsletter*, Spring 1985, 2–3.

98. Slothower, "Taking It to the Streets"; and Ways and Abbott, "Have Van, Will Travel," 3. This early medical clinic may refer to the Mobile Health Unit. Some evidence suggests that the clinic within the La Familia building did not open until 1984. See LG [Laura Giges], "SCWHC–Eight Days a Week," *Santa Cruz Women's Health Center Newsletter*, December 1983, 3.

99. Ways and Abbott, "Have Van, Will Travel," 3.

100. Haber, "Beach Flats," 3.

101. In June 1983, the SCWHC requested $21,000 from city revenue funds to continue to fund the outreach program. Rosamaria Zayas and Martha Ways, "Cuts into Lives," *Matrix*, June 1983, 2.

102. Haber, "Beach Flats," 3; Giges, "SCWHC–Eight Days a Week," 3.

103. "La Familia Crisis Intervention Center Opens in Beach Flats," *Santa Cruz Sentinel*, July 18, 1983. See also Boston Women's Health Book Collective, *The New Our Bodies, Ourselves: Updated and Expanded for the '90s* (New York: Simon & Schuster, 1992), 707.

104. Giges, "SCWHC–Eight Days a Week," 3.

105. See "Santa Cruz Women's Health Center History/Timeline," in *Ciel Benedetto: A History of the Santa Cruz Women's Health Center, 1985–2000*, ed. Irene Reti and Randall Jerrell, 111.

106. Benedetto, interview with the author.

107. Irene Reti and Randall Jerrell, eds., *Ciel Benedetto: A History of the Santa Cruz Women's Health Center, 1985–2000*, 25.

108. Reti and Jerrell, *Ciel Benedetto*, 26, 41, 23–25; Benedetto, interview with the author.

109. Reti and Jerrell, 41.

110. Reti and Jerrell, 45–47.

111. Peugh, interview.

112. Reyes, interview.

113. Benedetto, interview with the author.

114. Marzell, interview.

115. Bernice Johnson Reagon, "Coalition Politics: Turning the Century," in *Home Girls: A Black Feminist Anthology*, ed. Barbara Smith (New Brunswick, NJ: Rutgers University Press, 2000), 349.

Conclusion

1. Soumya Karlamangla, "Male Doctors Are Disappearing from Gynecology. Not Everybody Is Thrilled about It," *Los Angeles Times*, March 7, 2018; orwh.od.nih.gov; Kathleen Sebelius, "Attention All Women: Trump Is Coming for Your Health Care," *New York Times*, July 13, 2020.

2. Jan E. Thomas and Mary K. Zimmerman, "Feminism and Profit in American Hospitals: The Corporate Construction of Women's Health Centers," *Gender and Society* 21, no. 3 (June 2007): 359–83.

3. Deirdre Cooper Owens and Sharla Fett, "Black Maternal and Infant Health: Historical Legacies of Slavery," *American Journal of Public Health* 109, no. 10 (October 2019): 1343.

4. Sheryl Gay Stolberg, "Biden Rule Would Strengthen Health Protections for Gay and Transgender People," *New York Times*, July 22, 2022.

5. Johanna Schoen, *Abortion after Roe* (Durham, NC; University of North Carolina Press, 2015), 219–37.

6. Felicia Ward, interview with the author, September 18, 2017.

Index

Page numbers in italics refer to figures.

Abbott, Deborah, 275

abortion, *89*; access, 2–3, 12, 13, 52, 56–57, 61, 69, 72, 88–93, 99, 119–26, 142–46, 151, 223, 256–58, 266, 285; activism and activists, 19, 93, 112–13; advocacy, 57, 90, 104; aspiration, 93–95, 109, 132; in California, 87–93; in Chicago, 321n17; community support for, 118; complications, 69, 137, 256; continual threats to, 13; counseling, 46, 57, 70–71, 110–12, 132, 260; deaths from, 3; as demystified, 94; do-it-yourself kits in Third World, 113; as economic base of larger movement, 322n42; education about, 37; entrepreneurs, 105, 316n91; as exploitation, 112–19; federal funds prohibited for, 117; feminist, health clinics, 322n42; feminist, history of, 321n17; feminist, politics of, 12–13, 86–119; feminist, providing, 108–12, 283; and fertility control, 131, 149; and free choice, 90; histories of, 87–88, 312n4; humane, 88; infection, post-, 137; late-term, 323n50; legal, 2, 12, 88–91, 105–10, 119, 122–23, 126; legislation, 12, 19, 52, 57, 88–93, 117, 123, 142, 256–57, 313n12; male physicians limiting access to, 3; marketplace, 68, 90–93, 105–9, 112, 118–19, 321n16; medical, 69; medical hostility to, 69; and menstrual regulation, 104; in Mexico, 88, 126; mills, 106–7; misuse of as instrument of birth control, preventing, 90; need and demand for more readily available, 87–88; need for services, 13; nontraumatic, 107; possible alternatives to, 111; practice shaped, 105–8; practitioners, 113–14; providers, 13, 19, 52–53, 69, 88, 92–95, 106–14, 118, 125, 132–33, 137, 143, 260, 320n3, 321n17; and quality care, 107; quasi-legal, market for, 91–92; referral services, 9, 34, 53, 70, 87, 105–7, 114, 266; reform, 88, 90, 113, 313n12; rights, 88, 118, 156, 175–76, 256–57; safe and affordable, 6, 12, 88, 105, 119, 122, 126, 262; second trimester restrictions, 92; self-, 30, 88; and self-help, 46, 69; social and personal meaning of, 12; and the state, 87–93; supercoil method, 114–15, 319n47; therapeutic, 2, 57, 87, 89–94, 106, 256; in Third World, 113; as tool of exploitation and control, 13; and transportation, 114; as unavailable, 2; underground, 53, 113, 256–57; unsafe, prosecuted, 114; vacuum aspiration, 93–95, 109, 132; woman-centered provision, 13; women's conflicted feelings about, 111–12; and women's empowerment, 321n19; and women's health clinics, 13; and women's health movement, 12; and women's right to control their reproduction, 88. *See also* abortion, illegal; abortion centers and clinics; abortion politics; antiabortion movement; menstrual extraction

abortion, illegal: in California, 91–92, 312n8; clinics, 20, 86, 94; complications of, 256; feminist health activist providers, 282–83; and legislation, 90; market for, 91–92; practitioners, 95, 106, 113; and self-help politics, 93–94; in states, 88; underground, 53, 113, 256–57; women of color deaths from, 2–3

Abortion after Roe (Schoen), 306n31, 313n12, 317n114, 321nn16–17, 325n96

abortion centers and clinics, 13, 34, 37, 58, 72, 118–20, 144, 146, 320n2, 321n19; advocacy model in, 111; antichoice tactics against, 325n96; in Colorado, 323n50; extralegal, 94; feminist, 93, 105, 125, 317n114; and free speech zones, 143; and health education, 222; professional model in, 111